# Psychology and Pathophysiological Outcomes of Eating

*Edited by Akikazu Takada and Hubertus Himmerich*

Published in London, United Kingdom

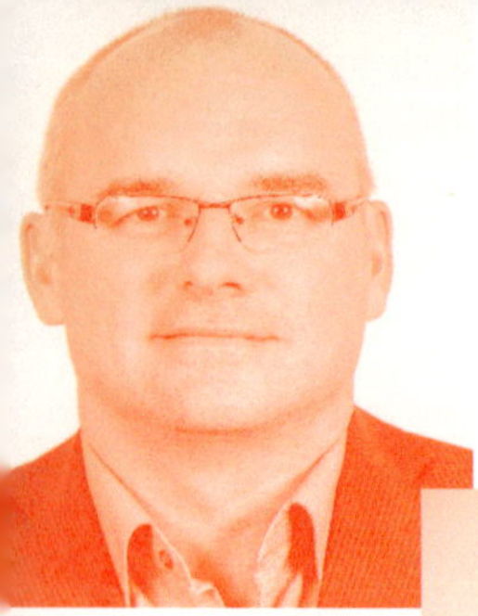
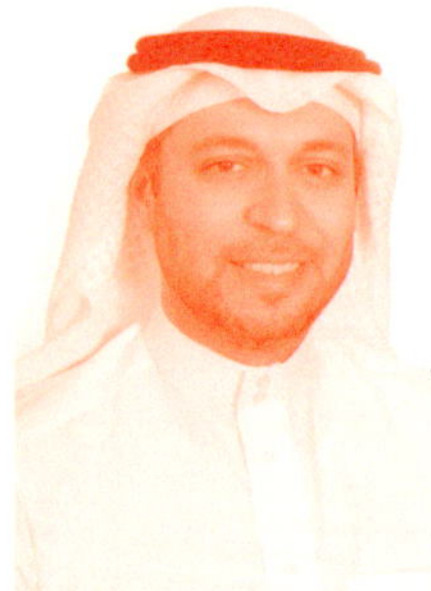
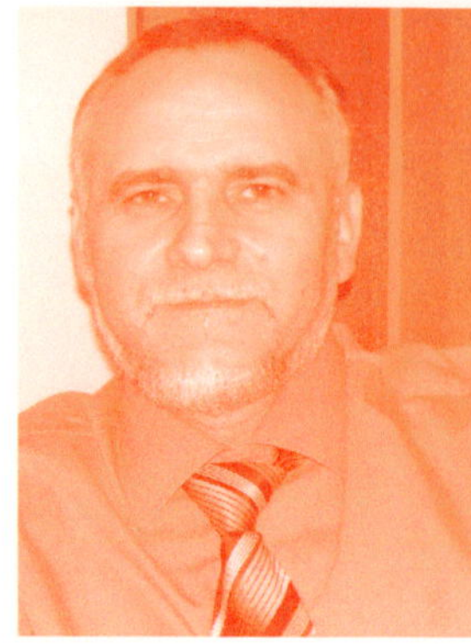
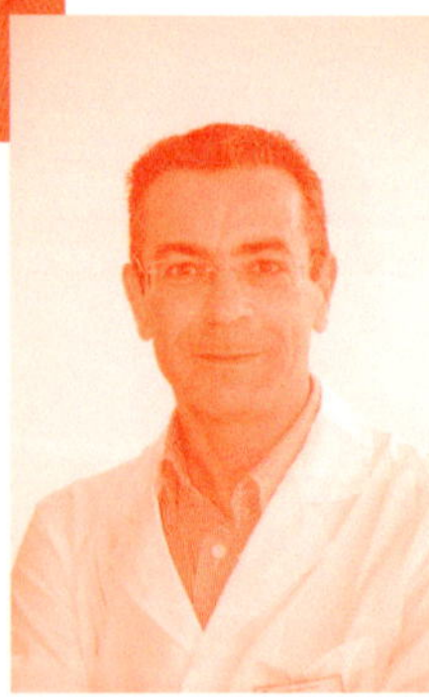
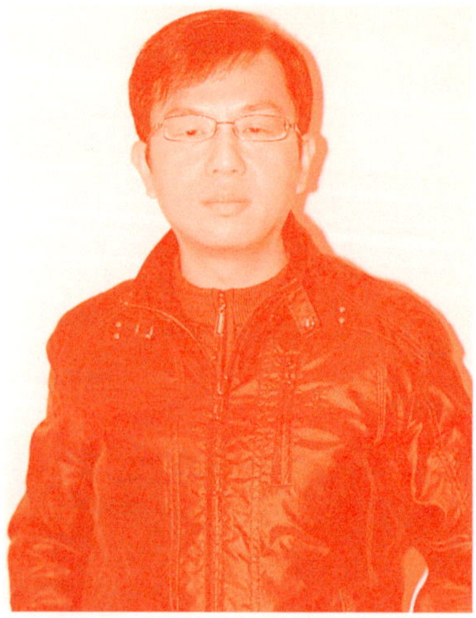
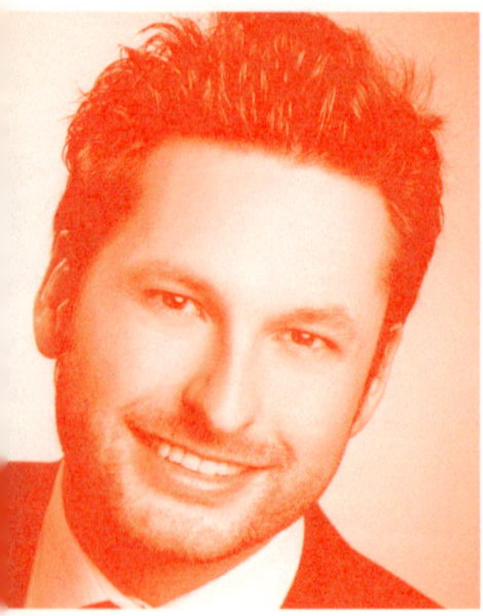
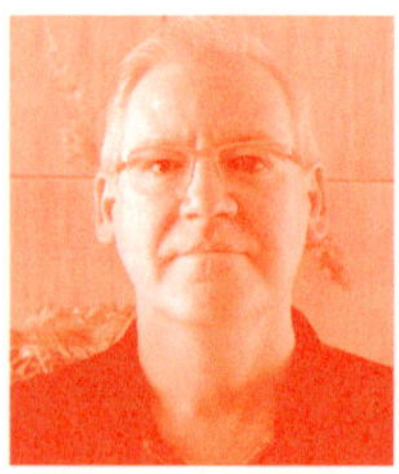

IntechOpen

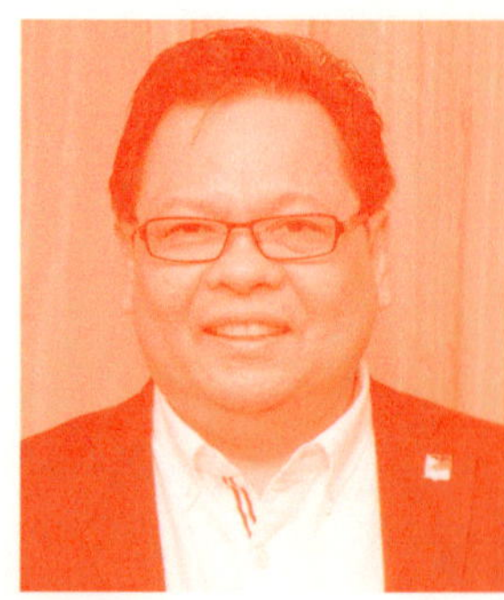
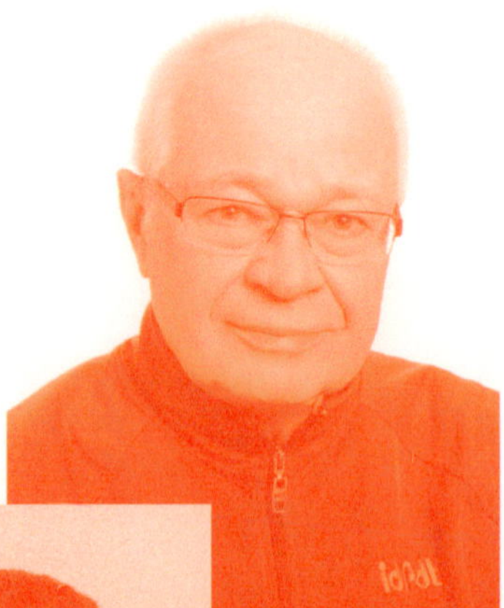
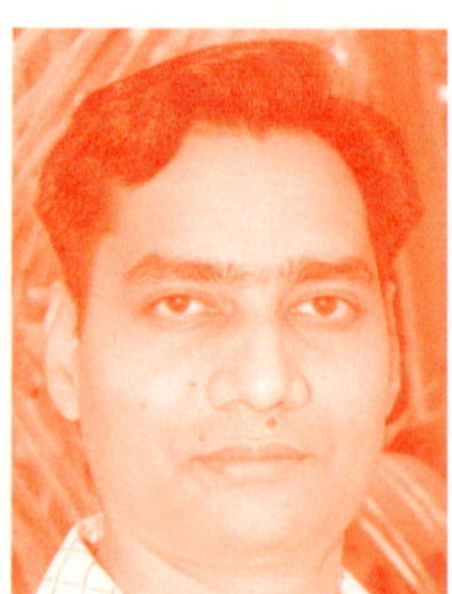
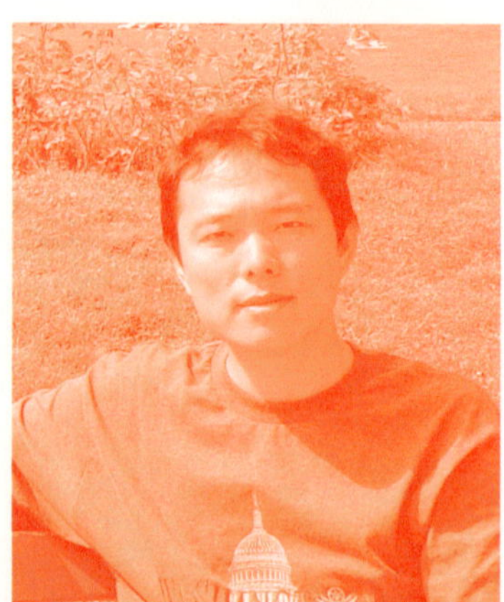
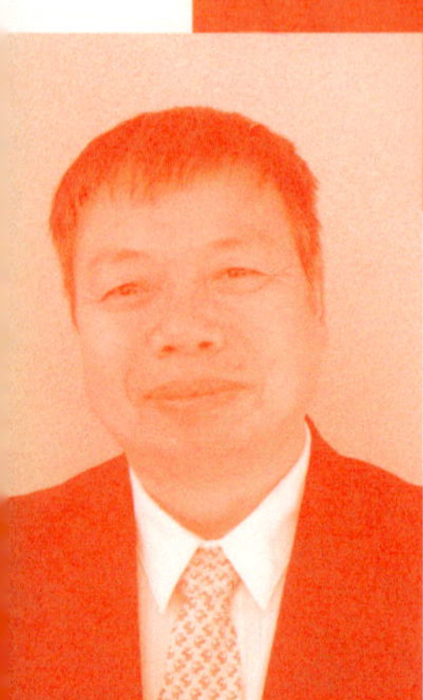
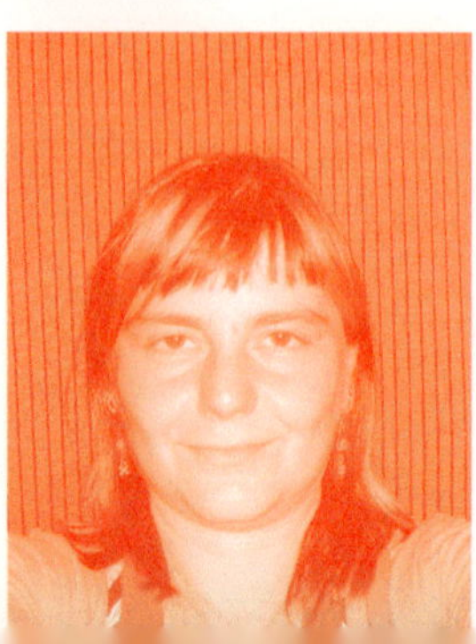

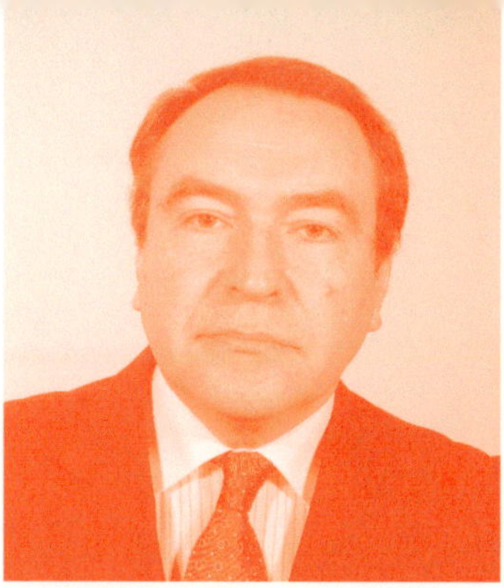

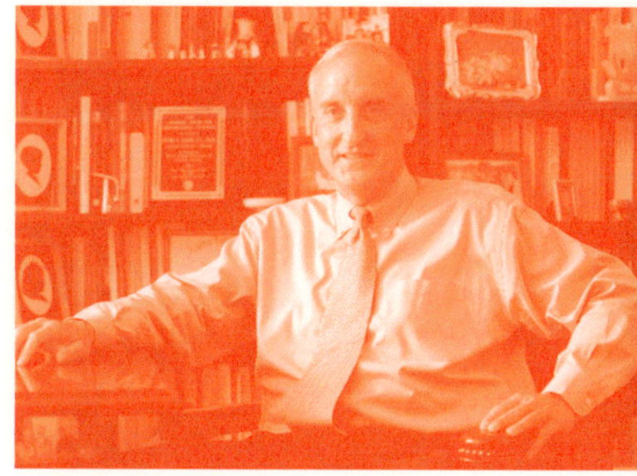

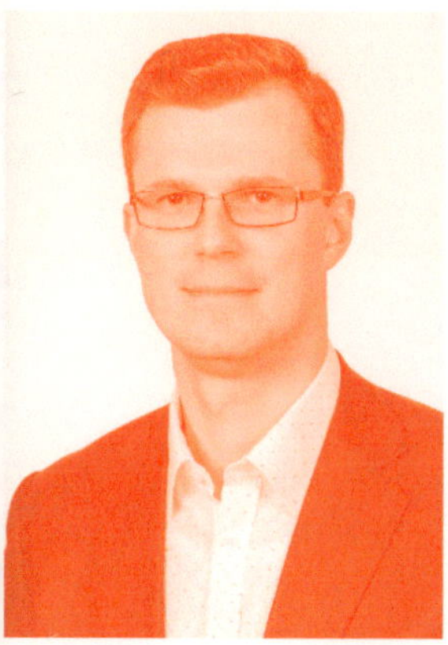

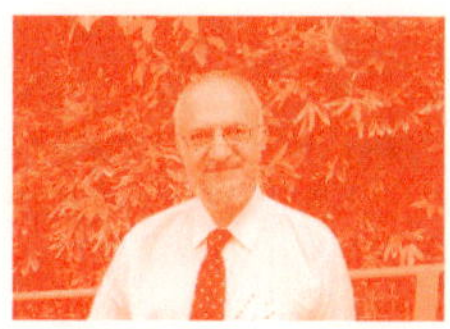

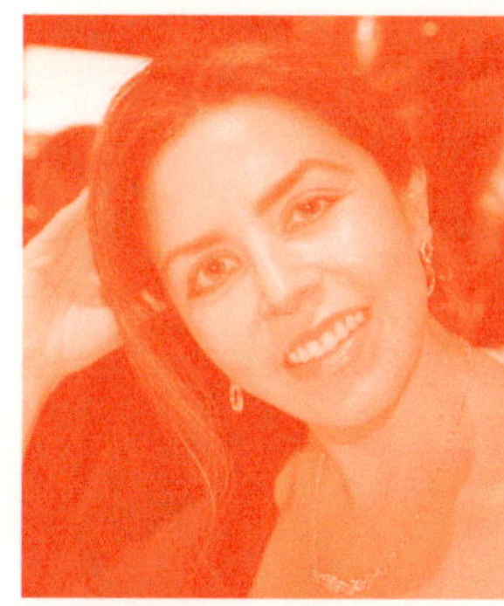

*Supporting open minds since 2005*

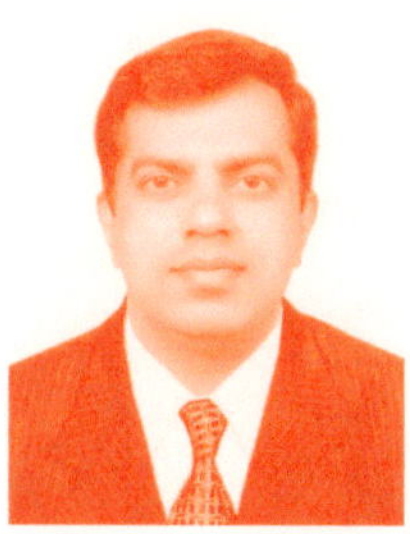

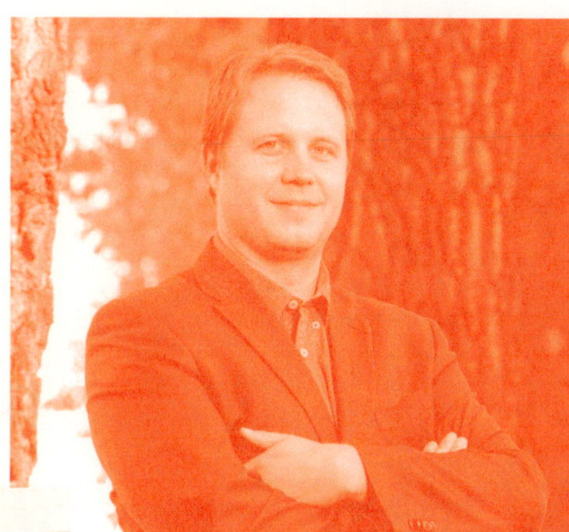

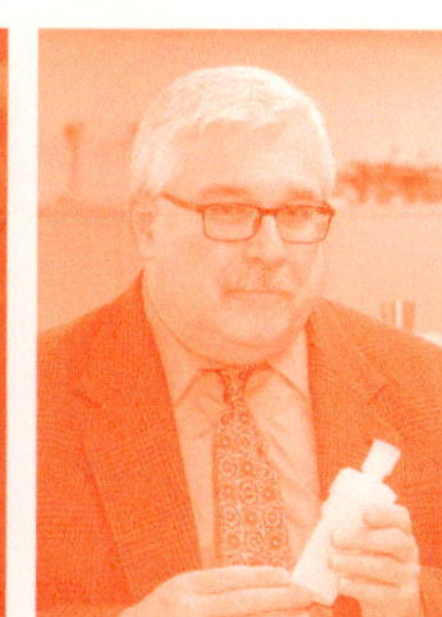

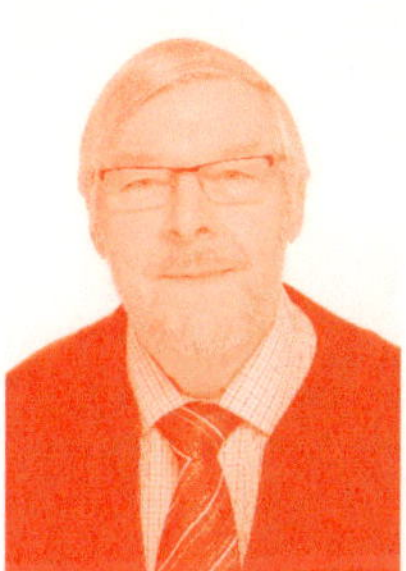

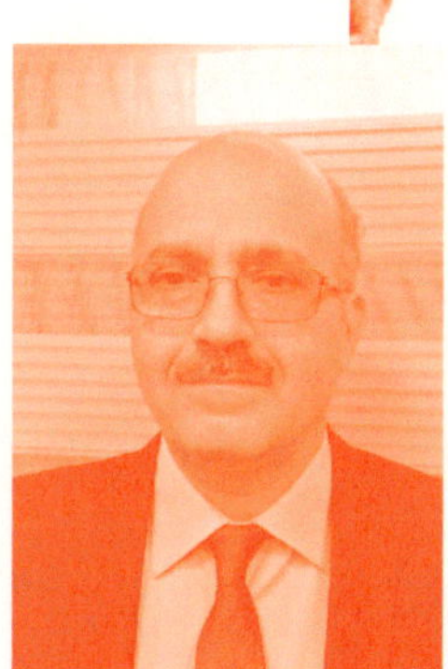

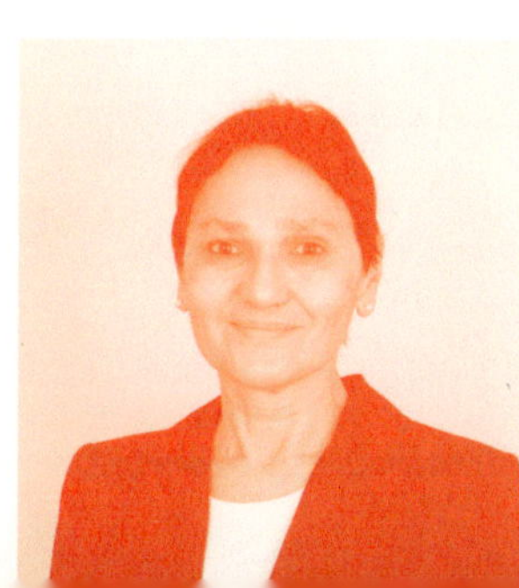

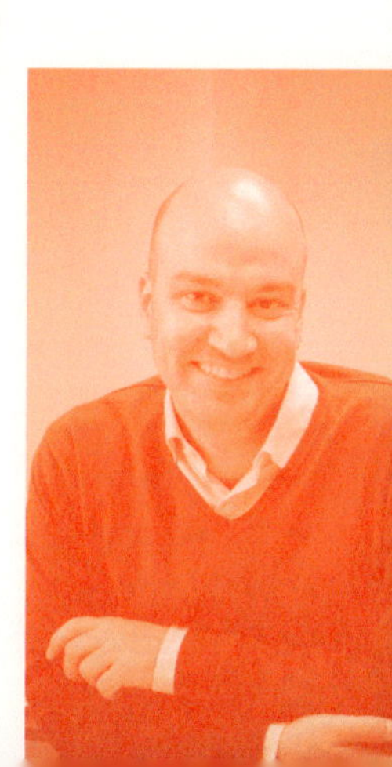

Psychology and Pathophysiological Outcomes of Eating
http://dx.doi.org/10.5772/intechopen.92917
Edited by Akikazu Takada and Hubertus Himmerich

Contributors
Akikazu Takada, Mariko Makino, Masahiro Hashizume, Mitsuo Yasushi, Yoshihiko Kanno, Mizuo Mifune, Takashi Yamamoto, Kayoko Ueji, Tadashi Inui, Haruno Mizuta, Shinichi Takahashi, Olariike Oyindasola Kayode, Junichiro Irie, Yuji Naito, Fatma Ibrahim Abdel-Latif Megahed, Salwa Abbas Ali Hassan, Hassan Ali Abdelwahid, Hanaa Kassem Farg, Shradha Mistri, Tatsuro Egawa, Kohei Kido, Takumi Yokokawa, Mami Fujibayashi, Katsumasa Goto, Tatsuya Hayashi, Keisha C. Gobin, Jennifer S. Mills, Joel D. Katz, Takeshi Inagaki, Tomohiro Suzuki, Tetsuro Komatsu, Hiroshi Shibata, Takayoshi Sasako, Kohjiro Ueki, Fumiko Shimizu, Yukie Ishii, M. Ogawa, Tetsuya Takao, Tomohisa Takagi, Ryo Inoue



First published in London, United Kingdom, 2021 by IntechOpen
IntechOpen is the global imprint of INTECHOPEN LIMITED, registered in England and Wales, registration number: 11086078, 5 Princes Gate Court, London, SW7 2QJ, United Kingdom
Printed in Croatia

British Library Cataloguing-in-Publication Data
A catalogue record for this book is available from the British Library

Additional hard and PDF copies can be obtained from orders@intechopen.com

Psychology and Pathophysiological Outcomes of Eating
Edited by Akikazu Takada and Hubertus Himmerich
p. cm.
Print ISBN 978-1-83968-776-1
Online ISBN 978-1-83968-777-8
eBook (PDF) ISBN 978-1-83968-778-5

For EU product safety concerns:
IN TECH d.o.o., Prolaz Marije Krucifikse Kozulić 3, 51000 Rijeka, Croatia, info@intechopen.com or visit our website at intechopen.com.

# Meet the editors

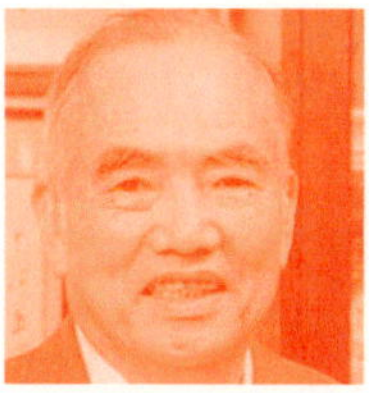

Akikazu Takada was born in Japan, 1935. After graduation from Keio University School of Medicine and finishing his post-graduate studies, he worked at Roswell Park Memorial Institute NY, USA. He then took a professorship at Hamamatsu University School of Medicine. In thrombosis studies, he found the SK potentiator that enhances plasminogen activation by streptokinase. He is very much interested in simultaneous measurements of fatty acids, amino acids, and tryptophan degradation products. By using fatty acid analyses, he indicated that plasma levels of trans-fatty acids of old men were far higher in the US than Japanese men. . He also showed that eicosapentaenoic acid (EPA) and docosahexaenoic acid (DHA) levels are higher, and arachidonic acid levels are lower in Japanese than US people. By using simultaneous LC/MS analyses of plasma levels of tryptophan metabolites, he recently found that plasma levels of serotonin, kynurenine, or 5-HIAA were higher in patients of mono- and bipolar depression, which are significantly different from observations reported before. In view of recent reports that plasma tryptophan metabolites are mainly produced by microbiota. He is now working on the relationships between microbiota and depression or autism.

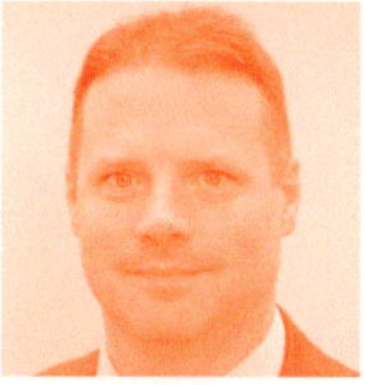

Dr. Hubertus Himmerich is a clinical senior lecturer for eating disorders at King's College London and a consultant psychiatrist on an inpatient ward for patients with eating disorders at Bethlem Royal Hospital, London, UK. Following medical school, Dr. Himmerich received his scientific and clinical training at the Max Planck Institute of Psychiatry, Germany, and the Universities of Mainz and Marburg, Germany. Afterwards, he worked as a consultant psychiatrist at the RWTH Aachen University Hospital and Professor of Neurobiology of Affective Disorders at the University of Leipzig, Germany. He has led and performed national and international scientific projects with researchers from Europe, Australia, and North America, and he has published more than 160 articles in peer-reviewed scientific journals, books, and book chapters.

# Contents

# Preface

An increased prevalence of obesity and disordered eating behavior has been reported in both developed and developing countries. In affected people, obesity and its physical and mental health consequences evolve slowly over time. In combination with an increasingly aging population, obesity particularly threatens the health and functional independence of older adults.

Many lifestyle interventions, psychological treatments, and diets have been proposed to fight this growing epidemic. However, an overarching and generally accepted scientific concept of disorders associated with disturbed food intake is still lacking.

This book provides up-to-date scientific insight into the psychology and the pathophysiological outcomes of eating. It covers the influence of lifestyle, circadian rhythm, sleep, and fragrant odors on appetite and weight regulation; the impact of glucose, sucrose, lactate, and ketone bodies on the brain; the consequences of glycation stress on the skeletal muscle; clinically relevant facets of electrolyte balance, bile acid, and glucose metabolism; pathophysiological and therapeutic aspects of diabetes, hypertension, and steatohepatitis; and the consequences and outcomes of energy-depleted conditions and eating disorders.

We are very proud of the high scientific level of the contributions in this book. We believe this volume provides noteworthy information about food, eating behavior, and metabolic diseases.

**Akikazu Takada**
Hamamatsu University School of Medicine,
Japan

**Hubertus Himmerich**
King's College London,
UK

Section 1

# Foods Intakes and the Central Nervous System

Chapter 1

# Attenuation of Food Intake by Fragrant Odors: Comparison between *Osmanthus fragrans* and Grapefruit Odors

*Takashi Yamamoto, Kayoko Ueji, Tadashi Inui and Haruno Mizuta*

## Abstract

Odors affect various physiological and mental activities. Previous studies in rats have shown that the odors of grapefruit and *Osmanthus fragrans* (OSM, fragrant tea olive) attenuate food intake, leading to a reduction in body weight gain, but it is not yet clear whether the causative mechanisms underlying these effects are the same for both odors. The first part of the present study revealed that grapefruit odor had no effect on the expression of feeding-related neuropeptides, in contrast to the previous finding that OSM odor suppresses orexigenic and activates anorexigenic neuropeptides in the hypothalamus of the rat. The second part revealed that OSM odor activated the parasympathetic nerve, in contrast to the previous finding demonstrating that grapefruit odor activates sympathetic nerve activity. The third part was performed to confirm the previous findings about the effects of OSM odor on appetitive reactions in humans. In human subjects, we found that continuous exposure to OSM odor attenuated appetite and consumption of snacks (cookies) and improved mood, when evaluated using the POMS (Profile of Mood States) data from university students. In conclusion, OSM odor attenuated appetite and decreased food intake in humans, and the underlying causative mechanisms differed from those mediating the effects of grapefruit odor, specifically in terms of the expression of hypothalamic feeding-related neuropeptides and autonomic nerve activity.

**Keywords:** odor, *Osmanthus fragrans*, grapefruit, feeding behavior, feeding-related neuropeptides, autonomic nerve, total mood disturbance

## 1. Introduction

Overeating leads to obesity, which heightens the risk of several chronic illnesses including hypertension, diabetes, high blood triglycerides, heart disease, stroke, kidney problems and cancer. One of the causes of overeating is palatability of foods, especially those containing sweet and fatty substances, which often promote ingestion over homeostatic repletion [1–3]. It is suggested that the palatability-induced ingestion is based on a sequential release of brain substances such as β-endorphin, dopamine and orexigenic neuropeptides, corresponding to palatability (liking), motivation (wanting), and actual intake (eating), respectively [3–7]. Any attempts to suppress actions of one or more of these brain substances could be an effective approach to prevent from overeating.

Odors produce various physiological, psychoemotional, and behavioral reactions depending on their qualities and hedonic tones [8–15]. Concerning food intake behavior, it is our common experience that odors associated with pleasant foods enhance appetite, but repellent odors reduce appetite. Interestingly, some fragrant odors attenuate ingestive behavior and body weight gain. Studies using rats have demonstrated that grapefruit odor inhibits food intake, leading to a reduction in body weight gain. It is plausible that this effect is mainly caused by activation of sympathetic nerve activity, which enhances energy consumption and suppresses appetite [16, 17]. Another example is the odor of *Osmanthus fragrans* (OSM, fragrant tea olive), which also attenuates food intake in rats [18]. This effect, however, is suggested to be due to the reduced expression of feeding-related neuropeptides in the hypothalamus. More precisely, Yamamoto *et al.* [18]. demonstrated that OSM odor decreased the messenger ribonucleic acid (mRNA) expression of orexigenic neuropeptides, such as agouti-related protein (AgRP), melanin-concentrating hormone (MCH), neuropeptide Y (NPY), and orexin, and increased the expression of anorexigenic neuropeptides, such as cocaine and amphetamine regulated transcript (CART) and proopiomelanocortin (POMC). It is also suggested that, in rats, OSM odor decreased the motivation to eat, food intake, and body weight, as well as caused sluggish masticatory movements [19].

OSM is an evergreen shrub that has been grown in Eastern Asia, especially in China, for more than 2500 years [20]. It produces small clusters of flowers in the late summer and autumn. The flowers are small, pale yellow, yellow, or orange-yellow and have a strong fragrant scent of ripe peaches or apricots. Because of its favorable fragrance, tea, wine, and jam with OSM flowers are traditionally very popular and are enjoyed on a daily basis in far-east Asia, especially in Taiwan and China. Since it has been traditionally believed to exert good effects on physical and mental health, the OSM plant has also been utilized as a Chinese herbal medicine. Among the volatile compounds of the scent of OSM, the essential ones are $\gamma$-decalactone, $\beta$-ionone, dihydro-$\beta$-ionone, linalool oxides [18, 21].

Although both grapefruit and OSM odors suppress appetite, food intake and body weight gain, the underlying causative mechanisms appear to differ to those described above. However, there are a lack of comparative data on the possible effects of grapefruit odor on feeding-related neuropeptides and effects of OSM odor on autonomic nerve activity. The present study, therefore, was designed to examine possible effects of grapefruit odor on the expression of orexigenic and anorexigenic neuropeptides in rats. We also examined effects of OSM odor, together with odors of lavender, jasmine, and milk on the autonomic nervous activity in humans. Finally, we examined how OSM odor affects appetitive reactions in humans.

## 2. Methods

### 2.1 Measurement of mRNAs for feeding-related neuropeptides

A total of 18 Wistar male rats were used. They were randomly divided into experimental and control groups (n = 9 each). Rats were individually housed in plastic cages, with freely available food and water, in a temperature- and humidity-controlled room (23°C, 60%). All animals were handled in accordance with the procedures outlined in the Guide for the Care and Use of Laboratory Animals (National

Institute of Health Guide), and this study was approved by the institutional committee on animal research (Animal Research Committee of Kio University).

The experimental rats received grapefruit essential oil as an olfactory stimulus with the same method as described in our previous paper [18]. Briefly, a drop (100 μl) of the oil was put on a filter paper, which was inserted between two metal mesh plates, and placed on the floor of the cage. The control rats were exposed to a filter paper containing a drop of water instead of the olfactory stimulus. The brains were removed 60 min after the onset of stimulation and the hypothalamus was removed, and preserved at −80 degrees. To examine the changes in the expression of mRNAs for prepro-orexin, MCH, AgRP, NPY, CART, and POMC, we used the same quantitative real time (RT)-PCR technique as that in the previous study [18].

### 2.2 Effects of odors on autonomic nerve activity

We used the essential oils of lavender, jasmine, milk (these three are products of Takasago International Corp. Japan), and *Osmanthus fragrans* (product of Argeville, France) as olfactory stimuli, and distilled water as an odorless control stimulus. To examine the effects of odors on autonomic nerve activity, a total of 60 university students (20—21 years old, 54 females and six males) were used. They were all in good health, without symptoms of nasal congestion, and their olfactory sensitivity was within the normal range, as judged using a T & T olfactometer [22, 23]. They were randomly divided into four groups (n = 15 each). Subjects in each group sniffed either one of the four odors (diluted to 2.5% with triethyl citrate) soaked in filter papers fixed in front of each subject's nose; the control stimulus was prepared in the same way. The order of presentation of the odors and control stimuli was counterbalanced within the group. Heart rate variation (HRV) was measured with a pulse analyzer device (TAS9, YKC Co. Ltd., Tokyo, Japan). This device was designed to evaluate autonomic nervous activity using acceleration pulse waves obtained from the tip of the index finger of the left hand. HRV was recorded for five minutes for each stimulus under the relaxed condition in a seated position following rest for 15 minutes.

The technical procedures and physiological interpretation of the HRV analysis have been reported by a number of researchers [24–29] with a useful guideline for HRV measurement and physiological interpretation [30]. The heart rate data were transferred to a personal computer, and the frequency domain measurements of HRV were determined by spectral analysis using fast Fourier transformation. The power spectrum was decomposed into its frequency components and quantified in terms of the relative power of each component. We used three frequency domain variables as an index of HRV. These frequency domain variables included low-frequency (LF: 0.04—0.15 Hz), high-frequency (HF: 0.15—0.40 Hz) and the ratio of LF to HF (LF/HF). The LF component reflects both parasympathetic and sympathetic nervous activities, the HF component reflects parasympathetic nervous activity, and the LF/HF ratio is considered an index of sympathetic nervous activity.

### 2.3 Effects of odors on feeding behavior

We used two odor stimuli (lavender and OSM), which were the same as those described in the previous section, and an odorless control stimulus (distilled water). To examine the effects of odors on feeding behavior, another cohort of 66 university students (20—21 years old, 60 females and six males) who belonged to one class of a nutritional course from Kio University were used. Experiments were conducted every Wednesday in three consecutive weeks.

The time schedule of an experimental day is shown in **Figure 1**. The experiment started at 12:00. After checking the physical condition, the subjects were randomly

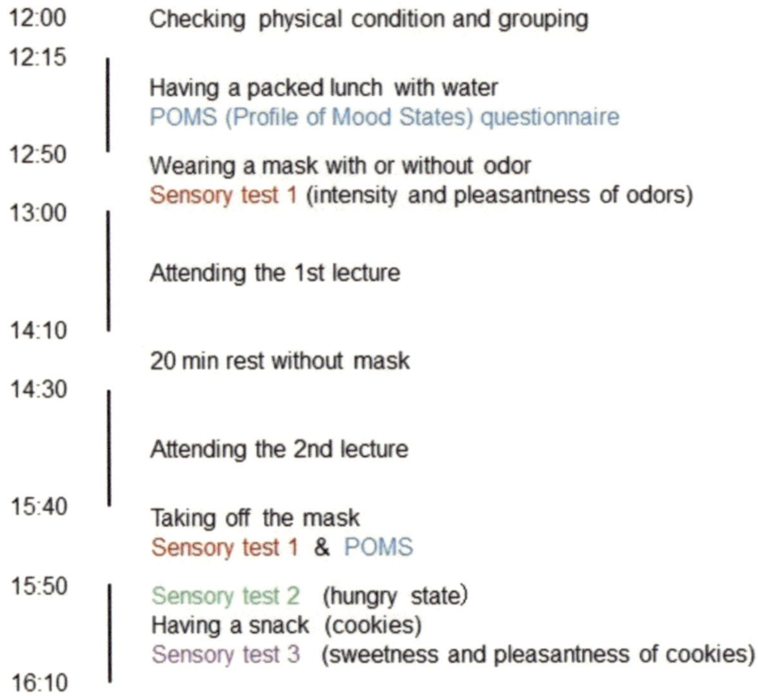


**Figure 1.**
*Time schedule of the conducted experiments on Wednesday. Subjects participated in the experiment with different odor stimuli on another two Wednesdays for three consecutive weeks.*

divided into three groups of 22 subjects. Each subject was served with a box lunch and a bottle of water and ate the lunch between 12:15 and 12:50 (**Figure 2**). Then, each subject wore a mask with a small pocked inside in which a filter paper (one cm x five cm) was inserted (**Figure 3**). The filter papers were infiltrated with a few drops of 2.5% OSM, 2.5% lavender oil, or non-odor distilled water. Each group received either OSM odor, lavender odor, or no odor-containing filter papers during a lecture on the first experimental day. Similarly, on the second and third experimental days, each group received a different stimulus (of the three stimuli). Thus, every subject received all three stimuli throughout the three experimental days. Subjects attended two lectures with a 20-minute intermission from 13:00-to-15:40.

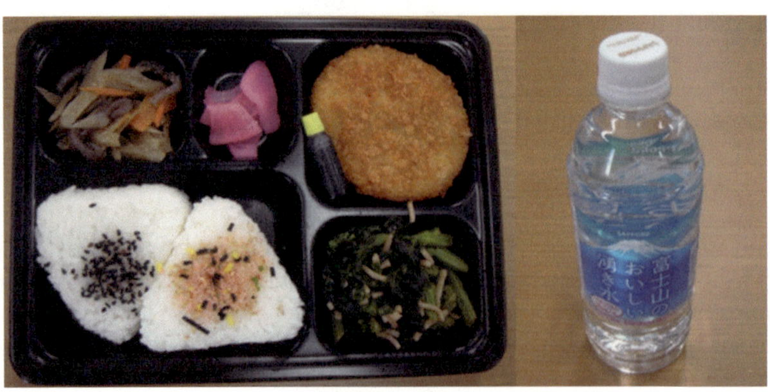

**Figure 2.**
*A box of lunch and a bottle of water served on the first experimental day. A different box of lunch was served on the second and third experimental days.*

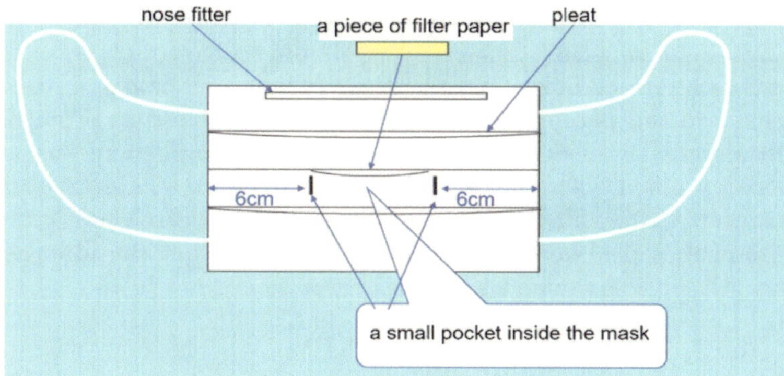


**Figure 3.**
*A mask with a filter paper in an inside pocket. The filter paper was soaked with 2.5%* Osmanthus fragrans *(OSM) for the OSM group, 2.5% lavender for the lavender group or odorless distilled water for the control group.*

They took off their masks during the intermission and wore the masks again with new filter papers just before the second lecture. After stimulation, each subject was given a package of snacks, containing 16 pieces of small cookies (Bourbon Petit with French Butter flavor, Bourbon Co. Niigata, Japan), and they were allowed to eat them freely, as much as they desired (**Figure 4**). The numbers of leftover cookies were counted and compared among the three odor groups.

The following sensory tests were assessed in each subject. To evaluate intensity and pleasantness of odors (sensory test 1 in **Figure 1**), the subjects were asked to select the score from one of five values ranging from 1 (very weak), 2 (weak), 3 (neutral), 4 (strong) to 5 (very strong) soon after putting masks and soon after taking off masks. To evaluate the level of hunger (sensory test 2), the subjects selected the score from one of five values from 1 (not hungry), 2 (slightly hungry), 3 (medium), 4 (moderately hungry) to 5 (very hungry). To evaluate the sweetness and pleasantness of the cookies (sensory test 3), the subjects selected scores from one of five values, ranging from 1 (very weak) to 5 (very strong), soon after eating the cookies.

To examine mood changes before and after odor stimulation, we administered the Profile of Mood States (POMS), a short-form questionnaire translated into Japanese (Kaneko Shobo Co. Ltd. Tokyo, Japan), after finishing lunch (or before odor stimulation) and after taking off the mask (or after odor stimulation). The POMS test consisted of 35 questions about the current mood state. The 35 questions were classified into six subscales: T—A (tension and anxiety), D (depression and dejection), A—H (anger and hostility), V (vigor), F (fatigue), and C (confusion). The subjects selected

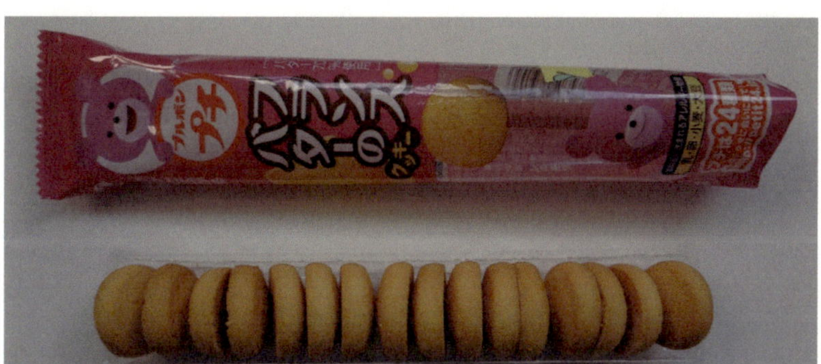

**Figure 4.**
*A commercially available package of 16 small cookies served as snack after taking off mask.*

the score from one of five values from 0 (not at all) to 4 (extremely). Total mood disturbance (TMD) was calculated by subtracting V from the sum of the other five subscale scores in each subject. Lower TMD scores were indicative of an improved mood.

For the experiments in humans (as described above), the study protocol was approved in advance by the Ethics Committee of Kio University and was performed in accordance with the Declaration of Helsinki of the World Medical Association. All subjects received an explanation of the nature of the research and agreed with the study protocol. We did not tell subjects about the names of the odors used in the experiments. All subjects signed written informed consent.

### 2.4 Data analysis

A two-way analysis of variance (ANOVA) was used to compare the expression of the feeding-related neuropeptides between grapefruit odor and non-odor conditions. To examine the effects of the four odors on the autonomic nerve activity in humans, a two-tailed paired $t$-test was used to compare each odor with the non-odor condition. With regards to the effects of odors on feeding behavior in humans, intensity and pleasantness scores of odors, and sweetness and palatability scores of cookies between OSM and lavender odors were analyzed using the Mann–Whitney $U$ test, and comparisons of hunger scores and cookie intake among OSM, lavender, and control groups were performed using the Friedman test and *post hoc* Wilcoxon signed rank test. Values of $P < 0.05$ were considered statistically significant. Statistical analyses were performed using a software program (IBM SPSS Statistics, ver. 25).

## 3. Results

### 3.1 Effects of grapefruit odor on the feeding-related neuropeptides in rats

The expression of mRNAs for the hypothalamic orexigenic neuropeptides, such as AgRP, MCH, NPY and orexin, and anorexigenic neuropeptides, such as CART and POMC, was measured using a real-time polymerase chain reaction (RT-PCR) on the rat hypothalamic specimens taken 60 minutes after the onset of grapefruit odor stimulation. The results were compared to those of similar samples taken from non-odor control rats. **Figure 5** shows the expression of mRNAs for four orexigenic and two anorexigenic neuropeptides in the control and experimental groups. A two-way analysis of variance (ANOVA) with peptide (gene expression of six peptides) and odor (water and grapefruit) revealed a statistically significant main effect of peptide [$F(5;96) = 8.76$, $P < 0.001$]. However, there were no main effects of odor and no peptide-odor interaction.

### 3.2 Effects of OSM odor on the autonomic nerve activity in humans

The effects of four kinds of odors (lavender, jasmine, OSM, and milk) on autonomic nerve activity, in terms of frequency analysis, are graphically summarized in **Figure 6**. The mean high frequency (HF) component of R-R variation (variability of the time interval between R waves), an indicator of the parasympathetic activity, was statistically significantly ($P < 0.05$, paired $t$-test) higher for lavender and OSM, and highly significantly ($P < 0.01$) lower for milk compared with the comparative value for the non-odor control. The mean low frequency/high frequency (LF/HF) score, an indicator of sympathetic activity, was significantly ($P < 0.05$) lower for lavender and OSM than for controls.

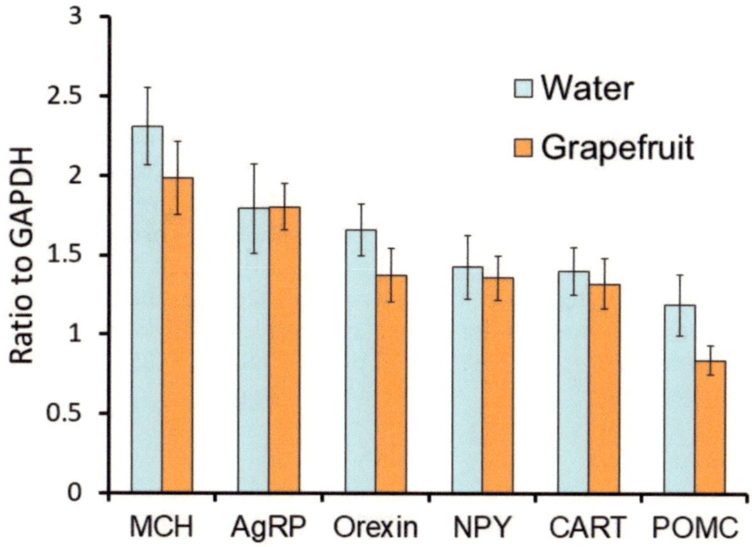


**Figure 5.**
*Effects of grapefruit odor on the expression of mRNAs for feeding-related neuropeptides in the hypothalamus of rats. Values are means ± SE. No difference was detected between the grapefruit odor group and the non-odor control group (two-way ANOVA, P > 0.05).*

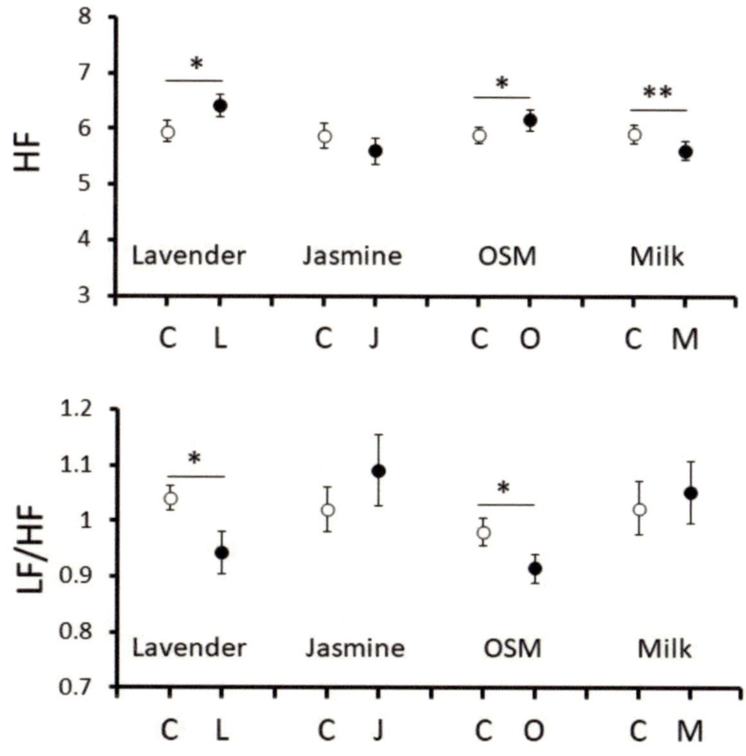


**Figure 6.**
*Effects of odors on autonomic nerve activity. Odors are lavender (L), jasmine (J), OSM (O) and milk (M). C, non-odor control; HF, high-frequency component; LF, low-frequency component. Values are means ± SE. Asterisks denote that the autonomic activity in the presence of the odor is significantly different from that in non-odor condition (two-tailed paired t-test). * P < 0.05, ** P < 0.01. OSM,* Osmanthus fragrans.

### 3.3 Effects of OSM odor on feeding behavior in humans

#### *3.3.1 Intensity and pleasantness scores of odors*

Five minutes after wearing masks with OSM odor, lavender odor or non-odor distilled water, the intensity score for the odors was 3.8 ± 0.9 (mean ± standard deviation [SD], n = 66) and 4.3 ± 0.7 (n = 66) for OSM and lavender groups, respectively. Soon after taking off the masks, the intensity score was significantly (Mann–Whitney *U* test, $P < 0.05$) lowered to 2.6 ± 1.0 and 2.8 ± 1.0, respectively. Five minutes after wearing masks, the pleasantness score for the odors was 2.2 ± 0.8 and 2.6 ± 1.0 for OSM and lavender groups, respectively, and soon after taking off masks, the pleasantness score was elevated to 2.5 ± 0.8 ($P < 0.05$) and 2.7 ± 0.9 ($P > 0.05$), respectively.

#### *3.3.2 Hunger score*

Before and after eating cookies, we asked subjects how they evaluated their hunger status. The number of subjects was counted at each level, ranging from no-hunger (1), slightly hungry (2), medium hunger (3), moderately hungry (4), and very hungry (5). Since the numbers of subjects belonging to the no-hunger and very hungry groups were so small, we categorized the subjects into three groups: not hungry (1 + 2), medium hunger (3) and hungry (4 + 5), and the results for OSM, lavender, and control groups are shown in **Figure 7–A**. The proportion among the three levels was significantly ($P < 0.05$, Friedman test and *post hoc* Wilcoxon signed rank test) different between OSM and control groups before eating cookies, indicating that OSM odor reduces hunger in the subjects. After eating, no difference was detected among the three groups (**Figure 7–B**).

#### *3.3.3 Cookie intake*

After offering a snack package to each subject, which contained 16 pieces of small cookies that could be consumed at will, we counted the remaining cookies. The number of leftover cookies varied greatly among the subjects. To examine any difference of odor effects on cookie eating, the subjects were divided into three

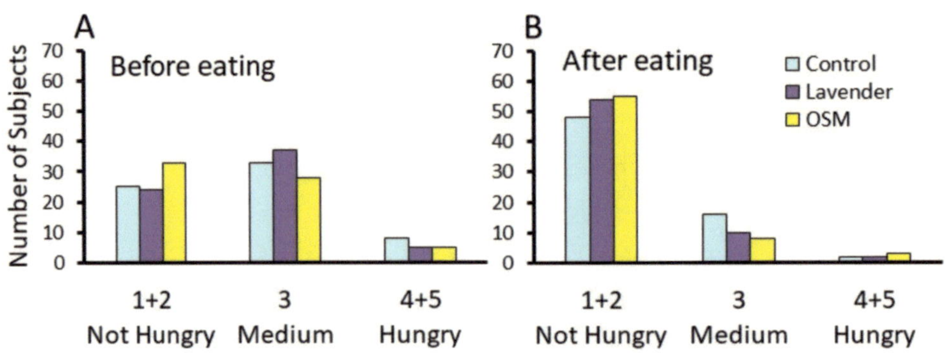


**Figure 7.**
*Proportion of hunger status. The numbers of subjects in the OSM, lavender, and non-odor control groups are expressed in three categories of hunger status (1, no-hunger; 2, slightly hungry; 3, medium hunger; 4, moderately hungry; 5, very hungry) before and after eating snacks. The hunger status before snack eating was different between OSM and control groups (Friedman test, post hoc Wilcoxon signed rank test, P < 0.01). OSM,* Osmanthus fragrans.

subgroups: a high-eating group (with leftovers ranging from zero-to-four cookies), a moderate-eating group (leftovers ranging from five-to-nine cookies), and a low-eating group (leftovers ranging from 10-to-16 cookies). The number of subjects belonging to each subgroup is shown for the three odor conditions in **Figure 8**. The graphical representation suggests that the subjects in OSM group ate less than those in control group, and this difference was statistically significant (Friedman test and *post hoc* Wilcoxon signed rank test, $P < 0.05$). No statistically significant difference was detected between either the OSM and lavender groups or between the lavender and control groups.

#### *3.3.4 Sweetness and palatability scores*

The palatability score for the cookies was 4.1 ± 0.7 (n = 66), 4.1 ± 0.6 (n = 66), and 4.2 ± 0.6 (n = 66) (mean ± SD) for OSM, lavender, and non-odor control groups, respectively. The sweetness score for the cookies was 3.5 ± 0.8, 3.6 ± 0.7 and 3.6 ± 0.7, respectively. No statistically significant difference in sweetness or palatability was observed among the three groups.

#### *3.3.5 Total mood disturbance score*

Total mood disturbance (TMD) scores of the Profile of Mood States (POMS) test are shown in **Figure 9**. The basal mood after lunch (or before putting on the odor mask) varied among the three groups: in the two odor (OSM and lavender) groups and the non-odor control group, the mean TMD scores were standardized to one. The rates of change in mood soon after taking off the mask (or before eating the cookie snack) were compared among the three groups. Statistically significantly (two-tailed paired *t*-test, $P < 0.01$) low TMD scores were detected after exposure to OSM odor, indicating a state of improved mood, while no significant difference was detected between pre- and post-mask-wearing in both the lavender and control groups.

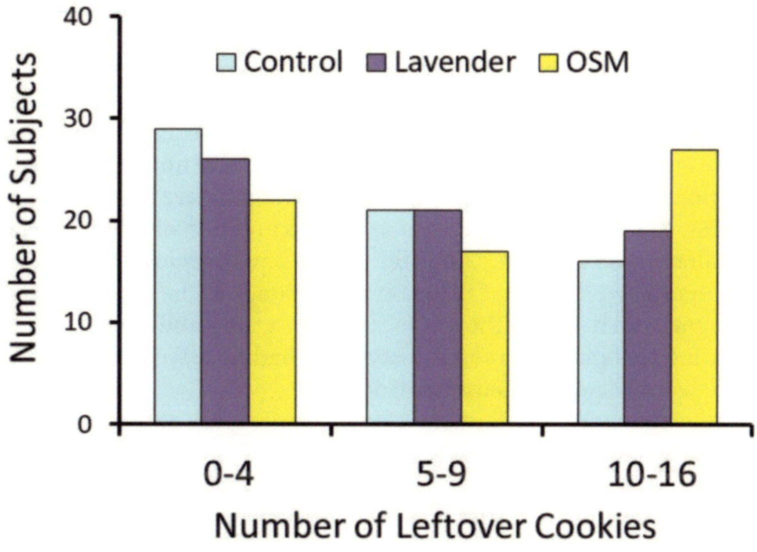


**Figure 8.**
*The numbers of leftover cookies in the three groups. The numbers of subjects who left a small number (zero-to-four) of cookies, a moderate (five-to-nine) number of cookies, and many (10–16) cookies are shown for the OSM, lavender, and non-odor control groups. The OSM group ate fewer cookies compared with the control group (Friedman test, post hoc Wilcoxon signed rank test, P = 0.05). OSM,* Osmanthus fragrans.

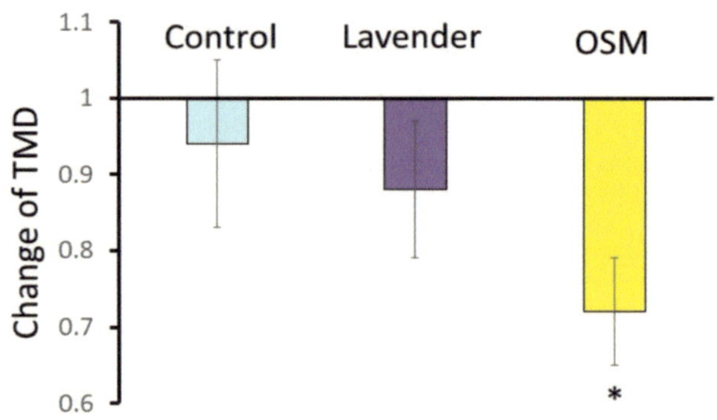


**Figure 9.**
*Total mood disturbance (TMD) scores before and after odor stimulation. The relative TMD score is shown after odor stimulation when the score before odor stimulation was set at unity. A statistically significant difference was apparent for OSM odor between the pre- and post-odor stimulation scores (two-tailed paired t-test). * $P < 0.05$. OSM,* Osmanthus fragrans.

## 4. Discussion

Previous studies in our laboratory have demonstrated that the odor of OSM attenuates food intake in rodents [18]. The present study was designed to confirm this effect in humans and also to compare the underlying causative mechanisms, in terms of autonomic nerve activity and expression of mRNA for feeding-related neuropeptides, between the OSM odor and grapefruit odor, which also attenuates food intake and body weight gain [16, 17, 31].

### 4.1 Feeding-related neuropeptides

It is well established that feeding-related neuropeptides in the hypothalamus play important roles in the elicitation, maintenance, and cessation of appetite and food intake [3, 32, 33]. Previously, our research group revealed that the neural information of OSM odor decreased mRNA expression of orexigenic neuropeptides (AgRP, NPY, MCH, and orexin) and increased expression of anorexigenic neuropeptides (CART and POMC) [18]. These findings are suggested to be, at least in part, the causative mechanisms underlying the effects of OSM odor on the decreased motivation to eat, sluggish masticatory movements, and the resulting reduction in body weight [18, 19]. Since comparative data are not available for the grapefruit odor, the present study examined the expression of feeding-related neuropeptides following exactly the same method we have previously used for the OSM odor. Consequently, we could not detect any difference in the expression of feeding-related neuropeptides between the grapefruit odor group and non-odor control group, indicating that grapefruit odor essentially had no effect on the expression of hypothalamic feeding-related neuropeptides.

### 4.2 Autonomic nerve activity

Fragrant odors are known to affect the autonomic nerve activity. For example, the odors of rose flowers [13, 15], lavender [34–36], and yuzu [37] activate parasympathetic neurons, whereas those of lemon [38], jasmine [39] and grapefruit [13, 17, 38, 40] activate sympathetic nerve activity. To our knowledge, there is only one previously published study that suggests that the OSM odor stimulates parasympathetic activity in humans [41]; therefore, more research is required to confirm these findings.

To examine how the OSM odor affects autonomic nerve activity in humans, we used the fingertip photoplethysmogram (PPG) to monitor autonomic nervous activation. Analysis of fingertip PPG signals is an important tool for assessing pulse wave components and their relation to vascular health. Several studies have demonstrated that the PPG waveform can provide clinical information on the dynamics of the autonomic nervous system, as well as the activity of the left ventricle, vascular aging, and arterial stiffness [42–44]. Although PPG is easy to set up, convenient, simple, and inexpensive, with only a single fingertip sensor, it has been proven that electrocardiogram and PPG signal recordings can be interchanged for heart rate variation (HRV) analysis including the time and frequency domains [45]. The PPG technique is also utilized for the assessment of arterial wall stiffening during aging [46] and for the assessment of the index of the periodontal condition [47].

The present HRV analysis on the basis of PPG has revealed that lavender odor significantly stimulates parasympathetic nerve activity, which is in agreement with previous results [34–36]. Jasmine odor tended to be a sympathetic activator, but the effect was not significant, which may have reflected an inter-individual difference in the preference for this odor, as suggested by Inoue *et al.* [48] and Kuroda *et al.* [49]. The important finding is that OSM odor significantly stimulated the parasympathetic nerve activity, which is opposite in action to grapefruit odor, which is a well-established sympathetic activator in animals [38] and humans [13, 40]. The milk odor, which was used as a control (or counter-part) odor for the OSM odor [18], tended to stimulate the sympathetic nerve activity.

The differences in the physiological actions between the OSM and grapefruit odors (as mentioned above) should be derived from the difference in volatile compounds in these odors. There are more than 10 active compounds detected in OSM odor, including major volatiles (such as ocimene, ionone, linalool, capraldehyde, and decalactone) [21, 50]. The major active volatile compound in grapefruit odor is limonene; additional compounds include myrcene, pinene, and linalool [51, 52]. It is noted that not only the major volatiles but some volatiles with low content also contribute to aroma [50]. Further study is required to elucidate the specific role of each compound.

### 4.3 Effects of odors on cookie intake

To confirm our previous findings in rodents that the OSM odor attenuates appetite and food intake, we elaborated on an experimental design in which the effect of OSM odor on snack eating behavior was examined in university students. Since OSM odor activates parasympathetic nerve activity (as described above), we selected lavender odor which also stimulates parasympathetic nerve activity for a comparable stimulus. Although sweetness and palatability of cookies were not different after exposure to OSM or lavender odors and in non-odor control group, we found that the hunger level, TMD score, and the numbers of cookies eaten significantly changed in the OSM group, compared with lavender and control groups. After exposure to the odors, subjects in the OSM group felt less hungry than those exposed to lavender or subjects in the control group, suggesting that appetite is reduced after exposure to OSM odor. Consequently, the consumption of cookies after OSM odor was less than that after lavender or non-odor conditions. Such effects in feeding behavior are not due to disagreeable feelings to OSM odor because pleasantness of OSM odor after exposure was not statistically significantly different from that of lavender odor. Moreover, mood states were significantly improved after exposure to OSM odor compared with lavender odor or non-odor conditions, as shown by the POMS data. Thus, the previous finding that the odor of OSM decreases food intake in rodents was modestly confirmed in humans through the present experimental paradigm.

## 4.4 Application

How could the findings of this present study be utilized in our daily life? As it is expected that appetite and meal size could be reduced under the presence of OSM odor, you will be more satisfied (satiated) with a smaller meal size that otherwise would not fulfill your appetite (**Figure 10**). Repeating this procedure at every meal, you could adjust yourself to eating smaller meals, which could possibly lead to a reduction in body weight. To examine this possibility, we performed a pilot study [53] where five females were exposed to OSM odor daily from the hour of rising to bedtime for 12 days. For delivery of the odor, each subject hung a small case containing a filter paper soaked in OSM essential oils around their neck. At the end of the experiment, the subjects showed a reduction in total body fat and body weight, compared with five females in the non-odor control group. For a practical use, it is necessary to elucidate the most effective and convenient method of odor exposure, or exposure duration. A proper use of the OSM odor as well as grapefruit odor could be an attractive and promising tool to promote ecological eating and to improve and promote good health.

A limitation of our study pertains to the selection of subjects and the duration of odor stimulation. The number of subjects was not enough to analyze the results in terms of sex differences because the number of male subjects was too small to be compared with female subjects. Subjects wore masks with odor continuously for 70 minutes and another 70 minutes, separated by a 20-minute-intermission without masks. Adaptation to odors is a well-known phenomenon: repeated or prolonged exposure to an odorant leads to decreases in olfactory sensitivity to that odorant [54–56]. According to Inoue *et al.* [48], five-minutes continuous exposure to the odor of jasmine tea affected autonomic nerve responses for more than 60 minutes, suggesting that our prolonged odor presentation may have not been necessary. Proper duration of exposure and concentration of the odor should be determined more precisely in future studies.

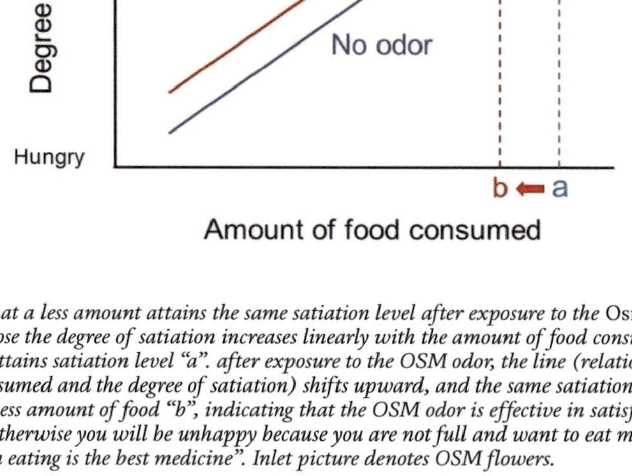


**Figure 10.**
*A model showing that a less amount attains the same satiation level after exposure to the* Osmanthus fragrans *(OSM) odor. Suppose the degree of satiation increases linearly with the amount of food consumed, the amount of food intake "a" attains satiation level "a". after exposure to the OSM odor, the line (relationship between the amount of food consumed and the degree of satiation) shifts upward, and the same satiation level "a" can be attained by taking less amount of food "b", indicating that the OSM odor is effective in satisfying appetite with a smaller volume, otherwise you will be unhappy because you are not full and want to eat more. A proverb says that "moderation in eating is the best medicine". Inlet picture denotes OSM flowers.*

## 5. Conclusion

The present human experiments have shown that OSM odor is agreeable and elicits sedative effects, improves mood, attenuates hunger, and reduces food intake. Grapefruit odor, which has also been shown to attenuate food intake, activates sympathetic nerve activity and had no effects on expression of feeding-related neuropeptides in rats, which is contrary to the results obtained for OSM odor, indicating the difference of causative neural mechanisms between the two odors. Exposure to OSM odor before eating and that to grapefruit odor after eating may be recommended as the effective practical use for preventing from overeating and obesity.

## Acknowledgements

The essential oils of odors were supplied by Ryouichi Komaki of the Seisyo Aroma Institute, Kanagawa, Japan. We are grateful to Ryouichi Komaki, Masao Kubota, Satomi Kunieda, and Yuji Minematsu for their contributions (preparing, executing, and analysis the data) to the human feeding behavior experiment. This work was supported by JSPS KAKENHI (Grant Number 17 k00835 to T.Y.) and a grant for Project Research from Kio University.

## Author contributions

TY and KU designed the study, KU and TI performed the experiments on humans and animals, respectively, HM performed the data analyses, TY wrote the manuscript, and all authors reviewed and approved the paper.

## Competing interests

The authors declare no competing interests.

## Author details

Takashi Yamamoto[1*], Kayoko Ueji[1], Tadashi Inui[2] and Haruno Mizuta[1]

1 Department of Nutrition, Faculty of Health Science, Kio University, Nara, Japan

2 Department of Oral Physiology, Graduate School of Dental Medicine, Hokkaido University, Kita-ku, Sapporo, Hokkaido 060-8586, Japan

*Address all correspondence to: ta.yamamoto@kio.ac.jp

## References

[1] Lucas F, Sclafani A. Hyperphagia in rats produced by a mixture of fat and sugar. Physiology&Behavior. 1990;47:51-55. DOI: 10.1016/0031-9384(90)90041-2

[2] Saper CB, Chou TC, Elmquist JK. The need to feed: homeostatic and hedonic control of eating. Neuron. 2002;36:199-211. DOI: 10.1016/s0896-6273(02)00969-8

[3] Furudono Y, Ando C, Yamamoto C, Kobashi M, Yamamoto T. Involvement of specific orexigenic neuropeptides in sweetener-induced overconsumption in rats. Behavioral Brain Research. 2006;175:241-248. DOI: 10.1016/j.bbr.2006.08.031

[4] Berridge KC. Food reward: brain substrates of wanting and liking. Neuroscience and Biobehavioral Reviews. 1996;20:1-25.

[5] Yamamoto T, Sako N, Maeda S. Effects of taste stimulation on β-endorphin levels in rat cerebrospinal fluid and plasma. Physiology&Behavior. 2000;69:345-350. DOI: 10.1016/s0031-9384(99)00252-8

[6] Tsuji T, Yamamoto T, Tanaka S, Bakhshishayan S, Kogo M. Analyses of the facilitatory effect of orexin on eating and masticatory muscle activity in rats. Journal of Neurophysiology. 2011;106:3129-3135. DOI: 10.1152/jn.01108.2010

[7] Yamamoto T. Central mechanisms of taste: Cognition, emotion and taste-elicited behaviors. Japanese Dental Science Review. 2008;44:91-99. DOI: 10.1016/j.jdsr.2008.07.003

[8] Nagai M, Wada M, Usui N, Tanaka A, Hasebe Y. Pleasant odors attenuate the blood pressure increase during rhythmic handgrip in humans. Neuroscience Letters. 2000;289:227-229. DOI: 10.1016/s0304-3940(00)01278-7

[9] Buchbauer G, Jirovetz L, Jager W, Plank C, Dietrich H. Fragrance compounds and essential oils with sedative effects upon inhalation. Journal of Pharmaceutical Scienses. 1993;82:660-664. DOI: 10.1002/jps.2600820623

[10] Manley CH. Psychophysiological effect of odor. Critical Reviews in Food Science and Nutrition. 1993;33, 57-62. DOI: 10.1080/10408399309527612

[11] Komori T, Fujiwara R, Tanida M, Nomura J, Yokoyama MM. Effects of citrus fragrance on immune function and depressive states. Neuroimmunomodulation. 1995;2:174-180. DOI: 10.1159/000096889

[12] Alaoui-Ismaili O, Vernet-Maury E, Dittmar A, Delhomme G, Chanel J. Odor hedonics: connection with emotional response estimated by autonomic parameters. Chemical Senses. 1997;22: 237-248. DOI: 10.1093/chemse/22.3.237

[13] Haze S, Sakai K, Gozu Y. Effects of fragrance inhalation on sympathetic activity in normal adults. Japanese Jaurnal of Pharmacology. 2002;90:247-253. DOI: 10.1254/jjp.90.247

[14] Shepherd GM. Smell images and the flavour system in the human brain. Nature. 2006;444: 316-321. DOI: 10.1038/nature05405

[15] Igarashi M, Song C, Ikei H, Ohira T, Miyazaki Y. Effect of olfactory stimulation by fresh rose flowers on autonomic nervous activity. Journal of Alternative and Complementary Medicine. 2014;20:727-731. DOI: 10.1089/acm.2014.0029

[16] Nagai K, Niijima A, Horii Y, Shen J, Tanida M. Olfactory stimulatory with grapefruit and lavender oils change autonomic nerve activity and

physiological function. Autonomic Neuroscience. 2014;185:29-35. DOI: 10.1016/j.autneu.2014.06.005

[17] Shen J, Niijima A, Tanida M *et al.* Olfactory stimulation with scent of grapefruit oil affects autonomic nerves, lipolysis and appetite in rats. Neuroscience Letters. 2005;380:289-294. DOI: 10.1016/j.neulet.2005.01.058

[18] Yamamoto T, Inui T, Tsuji T. The odor of *Osmanthus fragrans* attenuates food intake. Scientific Reports. 2013;3:1518. DOI: 10.1038/srep01518

[19] Tsuji T, Inui T, Kida K *et al.* The odor of *Osmanthus fragrans* affects masticatory muscle activities due to changes of feeding-related neuropeptides. Chemical Senses. 2014;39:670. DOI: 10.1038/srep01518

[20] Kewscience, Plants of the World, *Osmanthus fragrans* Lour. http://powo.science.kew.org/taxon/urn:lsid:ipni.org:names:610878-1

[21] Deng C, Song G, Hu Y. Application of HS-SPME and GC-MS to characterization of volatile compounds emitted from Osmanthus flowers. Annali di Chimica. 2004;94:921-927. DOI: 10.1002/adic.200490114

[22] Takagi SF. A standardized olfactometer in Japan. A review over ten years. Annals of the New York Academy of Sciences. 1987;510:113-118. DOI: 10.1111/j.1749-6632.1987.tb43476.x

[23] Hong SM, Park IH, Kim KM, Shin JM, Lee HM. Relationship between the Korean version of the sniffin' stick test and the T & T olfactometer in the Korean population. Clinical and Experimental Otorhinolaryngology. 2011;4:184-187. DOI: 10.3342/ceo.2011.4.4.184

[24] Tanaka M, Mizuno K, Tajima S, Sasabe T, Watanabe Y. Central nervous system fatigue alters autonomic nerve activity. Life Sciences. 2009;84: 235-239. DOI: 10.1016/j.lfs.2008.12.004

[25] Mizuno K. Mental fatigue caused by prolonged cognitive load associated with sympathetic hyperactivity. Behavioral and Brain Functions. 2009;84:235-239. DOI: 10.1186/1744-9081-7-17

[26] Park CK, Lee S, Park HJ, Baik YS, Park YB, Park YJ. Autonomic function, voice, and mood states. Clinical Autonomic Research. 2010;2:103-110. DOI: 10.1007/s10286-010-0095-1

[27] Leti T, Bricout VA. Interest of analyses of heart rate variability in the prevention of fatigue states in senior runners. Autonomic Neuroscience. 2012;173: 14-21. DOI: 10.1016/j.autneu.2012.10.007

[28] Vigo C, Gatzemeier W, Sala R *et al.* Evidence of altered autonomic cardiac regulation in breast cancer survivors. Journal of Cancer Survivorship. 2015;9:699-706. DOI: 10.1007/s11764-015-0445-z

[29] Kume S, Nishimura Y, Mizuno K *et al.* Music improves subjective feelings leading to cardiac autonomic nervous modulation: A Pilot Study. Frontiers in Neuroscience. 2017;10;11:108.DOI: 10.3389/fnins.2017.00108.

[30] Task Force of the European Society of Cardiology and the North American Society of Pacing and Electrophysiology, Heart rate variability. Standards of measurement, physiological interpretation, and clinical use, American Heart Association, Inc. 1996;17:354-381.

[31] Tanida M, Niijima A, Shen J, Nakamura T, Nagai K. Olfactory stimulation with scent of essential oil of grapefruit affects autonomic neurotransmission and blood pressure. Brain Research. 2005;1058:44-55. DOI: 10.1016/j.brainres.2005.07.048

[32] Arora SA. Role of neuropeptides in appetite regulation and obesity--a review. Neuropeptides 2006;40:375-401 DOI: 10.1016/j.npep.2006.07.001

[33] Boughton CK, Murphy KG. Can neuropeptides treat obesity? A review of neuropeptides and their potential role in the treatment of obesity. British Journal of Pharmacology. 2013;170:1333-1348. DOI: 10.1111/bph.12037

[34] Shen J,Niijima A, Tanida M *et al.* Olfactory stimulation with scent of lavender oil affects autonomic nerves, lipolysis and appetite in rats. Neuroscience Letter. 2005;383:188-193. DOI: 10.1016/j.neulet.2005.04.010

[35] Duan X, Tashiro M, Wu D *et al.* Autonomic nervous function and localization of cerebral activity during lavender aromatic immersion. Technol and Health Care. 2007;15:69-78. DOI: 10.3233/THC-2007-15201

[36] Matsumoto T, Asakura H, Hayashi T. Does lavender aromatherapy alleviate premenstrual emotional symptoms?: a randomized crossover trial. Journal of Alternative and Complementary Medicine. 2013;7:12. DOI:10.1751-0759-7-12. DOI: 10.1186/1751-0759-7-12

[37] Matsumoto T, Kimura T, Hayashi T. Aromatic effects of a Japanese citrus fruit-yuzu (*Citrus junos* Sieb. Ex Tanaka)-on psycoemotional states and autonomic nervous system activity during the menstrual cycle: a single-blind randomized controlled crossover study. Biopsychosocial Medicine. 2013;10:11. DOI: 10.1186/s13030-016-0063-7

[38] Niijima A, Nagai K. Effect of olfactory stimulation with flavor of grapefruit oil and lemon oil on the activity of sympathetic branch in the white adipose tissue of the epididymis. Experimental Biology and Medicine. 2003;228:1190-1192. DOI: 10.1177/153537020322801014

[39] Hongratanaworakit T. Stimulating effect of aromatherapy massage with jasmine oil. Natural Product Communication. 2010;5:157-162 DOI: 10.1177/1934578X1000500136

[40] Herz RS. Aromatherapy facts and fictions: a scientific analysis of olfactory effects on mood, physiology and behavior. International Journal of Neuroscience. 2009;119:263-290. DOI: 10.1080/00207450802333953

[41] Hozumi H, Hasegawa S, Tsunenari T *et al.* Aromatherapies using *Osmanthus fragrans* oil and grapefruit oil are effective complementary treatments for anxious patients undergoing colonoscopy: A randomized controlled study. Complementary Therapies of Medicine. 2017;34:165-169. DOI: 10.1016/j.ctim.2017.08.012

[42] Nitzan M, Babchenko A, Khanokh B, Landau D. The variability of the photoplethysmographic signal: a potential method for the evaluation of the autonomic nervous system. Physiological Measurement. 1998;19:93-102. DOI: 10.1088/0967-3334/19/1/008

[43] Huotari M, Vehkaoja A, Maatta K, Kostamovaara J. Photoplethysmography and its detailed pulse waveform analysis for arterial stiffness. Journal of Structural Mechanics. 2011;44:345-362.

[44] Elgendi M. On the analysis of fingertip photoplethysmogram signals. Current Cardiology Reviews. 2012;8:14-25. DOI: 10.2174/157340312801215782

[45] Ahn JM. Heart rate variability (HRV) analysis using simultaneous handgrip electrocardiogram and fingertip photoplethysmogram. Journal of the Association for Information System. 2013;5:164-170.

[46] Hong KS, Park KT, Ahn JM. Aging index using photoplethysmography for a healthcare device: comparison with brachial-ankle pulse wave velocity. Healthcare Informatics Research. 2015;21:30-34. DOI: 10.4258/hir.2015.21.1.30

[47] Furuta M, Tomofuji T, Ekuni D *et al.* Relationship between periodontal

condition and arterial properties in an adult population in Japan. Oral Disease. 2010;16:781-787. DOI: 10.1111/j.1601-0825.2010.01688.x

[48] Inoue N, Kuroda K, Sugimoto A *et al*. Autonomic nervous responses according to preference for the odor of jasmine tea. Bioscience, Biotechnology, Biochemistry. 2003;67:1206-1214. DOI: 10.1271/bbb.67.1206

[49] Kuroda K, Inoue N, Ito Y *et al*. Sedative effects of the jasmine tea odor and R-linalool, one of its major odor components, on autonomic nerve activity and mood states. European Journal of Applied Physiology. 2005;95:107-114. DOI: 10.1007/s00421-005-1402-8

[50] Cai X, Mai RZ, Zau JJ *et al*. Analysis of aroma-active compounds in three sweet osmanthus (*Osmanthus fragrans*) cultivars by GC-olfactometry and GC-MS. Journal of Zhejiang University. Science B. 2014;15:638-48. DOI: 10.1631/jzus.B1400058

[51] Ren JN, Tai YN, Dong M *et al*. Characterisation of free and bound volatile compounds from six different varieties of citrus fruits. Food Chemistry. 2015;185:25-32. DOI: 10.1016/j.foodchem.2015.03.142

[52] González-Mas MC, Rambla JL, López-Gresa MP, Blázquez MA, Granell A. Volatile compounds in *citrus* essential oils: a comprehensive review. Fronties in Plant Science. 2019;10:12. DOI: 10.3389/fpls.2019.00012

[53] Kunieda S, Komaki R, Ishikawa N *et al*. The odor of *Osmanthus fragrans* helps to suppress appetite. Chemical Senses. 2014;39:651-652.

[54] Dalton P. Psychophysical and behavioral characteristics of olfactory adaptation. Chemical Senses. 2000;25:487-492. DOI: 10.1093/chemse/25.4.487

[55] Pellegrino R, Sinding C, de Wijk RA, Hummel T. Habituation and adaptation to odors in humans. Physiolgy & Behavior. 2017;177:13-19.

[56] Pierce AM, Simons CT. Olfactory adaptation is dependent on route of delivery. Chemical Senses. 2018;43: 197-203. DOI: 10.1093/chemse/bjy007

Chapter 2

# Lactate and Ketone Bodies Act as Energy Substrates as Well as Signal Molecules in the Brain

*Shinichi Takahashi*

## Abstract

Astroglia or astrocytes, the most abundant cells in the brain, are interposed between neuronal synapses and the microvasculature in the brain's gray matter. This unique anatomical location allows astroglia to play pivotal roles in brain metabolism as well as in the regulation of cerebral blood flow. In particular, astroglial cellular metabolic compartmentation exerts supportive roles in dedicating neurons to the generation of action potentials and protects neurons against the oxidative stress associated with their high energy consumption. Key products of astroglia include lactate and ketone bodies (beta-hydroxybutyrate and acetoacetate), which can also be produced avidly by muscle and liver, respectively. Therefore, brain cells, skeletal muscles, and hepatocytes constitute a metabolic compartmentation in the whole body. In this chapter, I will focus on brain cells, especially astroglia, since the impairment of normal astroglial function can lead to numerous neurological disorders including stroke, neurodegenerative diseases, and neuro-immunological diseases. I will also discuss the metabolic responses of brain cells in terms of food consumption and exercise. A better understanding of the astroglial metabolic response is expected to lead to the development of novel therapeutic strategies for diverse neurological diseases.

**Keywords:** astrocyte, astroglia, brain-derived neurotrophic factor, beta-hydroxybutyrate, fatty acids, glucose

## 1. Introduction

"Eating", especially glucose ingestion is essential for brain function. When we get tired either physically or mentally, we may want "sweet stuff". Some people prefer "fatty food". These unconscious impulses imply fundamental roles of glucose and fatty acid in the brain. The human brain is a complex, organized organ consisting of numerous cell types including neurons and glial cells [1, 2]. In addition, the microvasculature, which supplies oxygen and glucose, is also an essential component [3]. The human adult brain weighs 1.4 kg, or approximately 2% of the body weight, and consumes 20% of the total oxygen consumption and 25% of the glucose consumption in the body (**Figure 1**) [4, 5]. Brain function mainly consists of intellectual information processing, which is based on the generation of action potentials resulting from ionic flux across the cellular membrane. The ratio of the cerebral metabolic rate of oxygen ($CMR_{oxy}$) to glucose ($CMR_{glc}$) consumption

**Measured**

Brain (1.4 kg) = 70 kg (2% of total body weight)

Averaged $CMR_{glc}$ = 31 μmol/100 g/min (25% of total body glucose consumption)

Averaged $CMR_{oxy}$ = 156 μmol/100 g/min (20% of total body oxygen consumption)

**$CMR_{oxy}/CMR_{glc}$ = 156/31 = 5.0**

**Theoretical**

$C_6H_{12}O_6 + 6O_2 = 6CO_2 + 6H_2O + 38ATP$

**$CMR_{oxy}/CMR_{glc}$ = 6 / 1 = 6.0**

**Figure 1.**
*Cerebral metabolic rate of glucose ($CMR_{glc}$) and oxygen ($CMR_{oxy}$) in human adults (adapted from [4]).*

is approximately 6, implying the complete oxidation of one molecule of glucose (6 carbon molecules) for every 6 molecules of oxygen, producing $CO_2$ and $H_2O$ (**Figure 1**) [4, 5]. The first step in glucose metabolism is glycolysis, which generates 2 ATPs; pyruvate/lactate is the end-product of glycolysis, and this product then enters the tricarboxylic acid (TCA) cycle, where ATP is produced more efficiently (resulting in 36 ATPs). Continuous ATP production is essential to generate action potentials, maintaining consciousness as well as intellectual function. Surprisingly, however, ATP production in the brain is solely dependent on glucose and oxygen as energy substrates [4, 5]. Moreover, these essential energy substrates must be supplied from outside of the brain through the microvasculature, since there is virtually no storage of glucose or oxygen in the brain. As a result, even a short period of cessation in cerebral blood flow (CBF) induces an immediate impairment of brain function [6]. Longer periods of ischemia cause irreversible damage to brain cells, making the restoration of function in stroke patients difficult even after vigorous rehabilitation [6, 7].

Regarding the maintenance and restoration of brain function, the topic of synaptic plasticity is essential. The theoretical basis of the beneficial effects of physical exercise on brain function relies on the facilitation of synaptic transmission and plasticity. Brain-derived neurotrophic factor (BDNF) plays a pivotal role in maintaining the neural network, improving its function, and restoring the network after damage [8, 9]. BDNF is a neurotrophic factor that was identified in the pig brain for the first time in 1982 [9]. BDNF, which is produced in both neurons and glial cells, improves a wide variety of neuronal functions including both motor functions and memory [8, 9]. Physical exercise does, indeed, improve not only motor function, but also mental function [10–12]. Unfortunately, however, the exact mechanism by which physical exercise induces BDNF production in the brain has not yet been elucidated. Recently, two nutrient molecules that are closely related to brain energy metabolism have become points of focus: lactate [13, 14] and beta-hydroxybutyrate (BHB) [15, 16]. The former is an end-product of glycolysis, and the latter is a type of ketone body, which are metabolites of fatty acid produced through beta-oxidation. Importantly, the concentrations of both lactate and BHB have been widely recognized as being elevated after exercise as a result of increases in their production by skeletal muscle and in the liver, respectively. Furthermore, both lactate and BHB are transported into the brain via monocarboxylate transporters (MCTs) (**Figure 2**) [17]. Therefore, lactate and BHB are also cable of acting as signal molecules resulting in BDNF production in the brain.

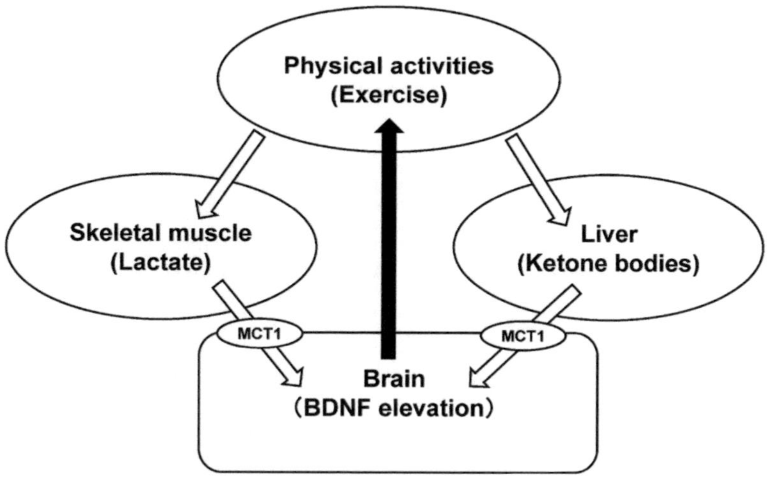


**Figure 2.**
*Physical activity, brain, muscle, liver, and BDNF: hypothetical model 1. BDNF, brain-derived neurotrophic factor; MCT1, monocarboxylate transporter 1 (expressed on brain microvessels).*

As described above, brain energy metabolism is solely dependent on exogenous glucose and oxygen supplied from outside the brain under normal physiological conditions [4, 5]. Importantly, however, it has also long been known that exogenous lactate and BHB can fuel the brain as alternative energy substrates under non-physiological conditions such as starvation, insulin-resistance and so on [4, 5]. Lactate enters the TCA cycle of the neurons after the conversion of acetyl-CoA by the pyruvate dehydrogenase complex (PDHC), while BHB can enter the TCA cycle directly without the action of PDHC (**Figure 3**) [4, 5]. These mechanisms imply that the exercise-induced production of lactate and BHB provides (1) energy substrates for the short-term maintenance of brain function, and (2) signal molecules capable of inducing BDNF production in the brain for the long-term maintenance of brain plasticity.

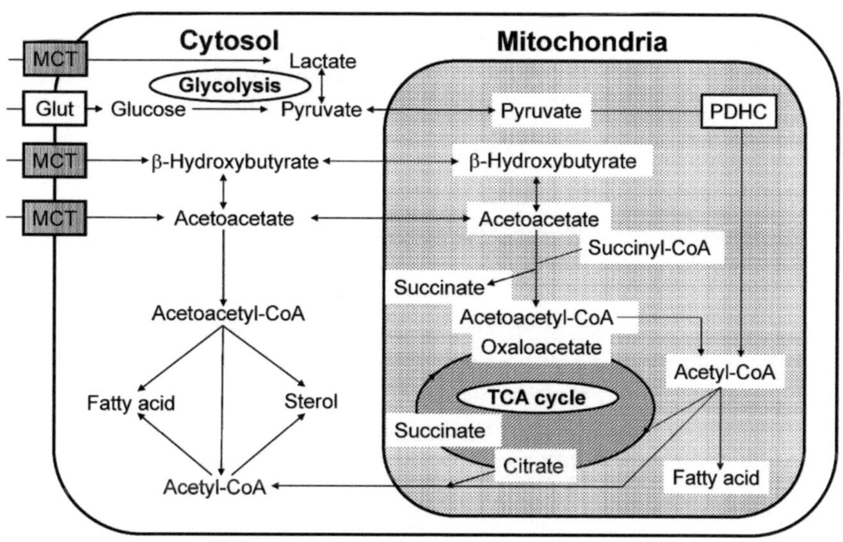


**Figure 3.**
*Transportation and metabolic pathway of lactate and ketone bodies (β-hydroxybutyrate and acetoacetate) into neural cells. MCT, monocarboxylate transporter; Glut, glucose transporter; TCA, tricarboxylic acid; PDHC, pyruvate dehydrogenase complex.*

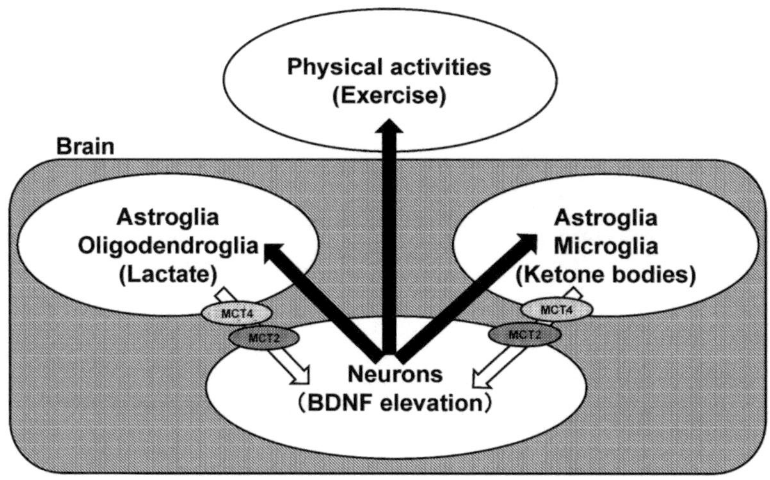


**Figure 4.**
*Physical activity, brain (neurons and glial cells), muscle, liver, and BDNF: hypothetical model 2. BDNF, brain-derived neurotrophic factor; MCT2, monocarboxylate transporter 2 (expressed on neurons), MCT4, monocarboxylate transporter 4 (expressed on astroglia).*

The brain, muscle, and liver therefore compose a metabolic network that is linked through physical exercise. Of note, physical exercise (voluntary movement) is initiated by neuronal excitation (**Figure 2**) [4, 5]. Generally, the functional activation of the brain increases both local $CMR_{glc}$ and local $CMR_{oxy}$ to produce more ATPs. Under normal resting conditions, neither lactate nor BHB is present in the blood in sufficient quantities to be transported into the brain because of the slow transportation kinetics of MCTs [4, 5]. As a result, their roles as energy substrates for the brain seem to be limited. Importantly, however, the brain itself, or more exactly its astroglia, can produce both lactate and BHB upon neuronal excitation (**Figure 4**) [3–5]. Our research has focused on the metabolic compartmentalization between neurons and glial cells [18–27], revealing that astrocytes produce both lactate and BHB, both of which can fuel neurons as energy substrates, via processes that are coupled with neuronal excitation [3]. Accumulating evidence supporting the actions of exogenous lactate and BHB as signal molecules that induce BDNF converge in this intracerebral metabolic compartment between neurons and astrocytes, where astrocyte-derived lactate and BHB support neuronal function in terms of both energy metabolism and synaptic plasticity [3].

## 2. Sources and roles of exercise-induced lactate and ketone bodies in the brain

Physical activity is known to elevate lactate levels in the blood [13, 14]. Since physical activities are beneficial for the maintenance of both mental and physical health, an exploration of the mechanisms by which physical exercise improves neuronal function is an important target. Energetically, human brain function is solely dependent on the oxidative metabolism of glucose [4, 5]. Glucose is continuously supplied by the blood stream, since virtually no glucose storage exists in the brain. Besides the brain, only the testis is known to rely on glucose as an energy substrate [4, 5].

Glucose in the blood is taken up by glucose transporter 1 (Glut1) in the endothelium of brain microvessels [3–5, 17]. In addition to this glucose transporter, MCTs expressed in the brain microvessels allow lactate and ketone bodies (especially BHB) to cross the blood–brain barrier (BBB) [3–5, 17]. Neural cells (neurons and glia) are thus able to take up glucose, lactate, and BHB via glucose transporters or MCTs (**Figure 2**) [17]. Once lactate or BHB is transported into the brain cells, they enter the TCA cycle to act as energy substrates, similar to glucose (**Figure 3**). Although neither lactate nor BHB is an efficient energy substrate because of the slow transportation kinetics of MCTs, elevations in their blood concentrations allow them to act as energy sources supplied externally from the brain [3–5]. The concentrations of both lactate and BHB do, indeed, increase after physical exercise [28, 29]. The sources of the elevated lactate and BHB levels in the blood after physical activity are the skeletal muscles and liver, respectively [3–5]. Under starvation and insulin-resistance in diabetic patients, glucose availability in the peripheral tissue is limited, and BHB can fuel brain function in the place of glucose.

In addition to their roles as energy substrates, both lactate and BHB can improve brain function through synaptic plasticity. Ample evidence supports BDNF being a key molecule in the induction of neuronal plasticity [8, 9]. BDNF is a member of the neurotrophin family and is produced in neurons as well as glial cells [8, 9]. BDNF promotes neurite outgrowth, facilitates synaptic transmission, and regenerates the neuronal network. Recent evidence suggests that both lactate and BHB, which are produced outside the brain during physical exercise, act as signal molecules in the brain after crossing the BBB [13–16]. Lactate induces BDNF expression, and this action of lactate is dependent on the activation of Sirtuin1 deacetylase. Silent information regulator 1 (SIRT1) increases the levels of the transcriptional coactivator peroxisome proliferator-activated receptor gamma coactivator 1-alpha (PGC-1$\alpha$) and the secreted molecule fibronectin type III domain-containing protein 5 (FNDC5), which are known to mediate BDNF expression [13, 14]. In contrast, BHB induces BDNF expression by acting as a direct Class I histone deacetylase (HDAC) inhibitor. By inhibiting HDAC2 and HDAC3 and by preventing their recruitment to BDNF promoter I, BHB induces BDNF expression [15, 16].

## 3. Lactate production and consumption in the brain

In addition to skeletal muscles, numerous cells in the body generate lactate. Especially under a hypoxic/anoxic state, virtually all cell types generate lactate through glycolysis, since the further oxidation of lactate in the mitochondrial TCA cycle is inhibited because of oxygen unavailability [3–5]. Importantly, even under a sufficient supply of oxygen, lactate production can occur (aerobic glycolysis). Although brain function is dependent on the complete oxidation of glucose, cellular differences in the cell types should be noted. In fact, astroglia seem to be more glycolysis-dependent, compared with neurons (**Figure 5**) [3, 23]. Astroglia exhibit normal mitochondrial function and are capable of oxidizing glucose as well as lactate/pyruvate in mitochondria (**Figures 6–8**), albeit lactate/pyruvate does not seem to be an ideal substrate [3, 23].

Astroglial endfeet envelope brain microvessels as well as synapses (**Figure 9**) [30–32]. This anatomical location of astroglia seems to be suitable for the direct uptake of glucose from the microvessels [3]. Glucose is metabolized glycolytically in the astroglial cytosol, generating lactate/pyruvate (**Figure 9**). In contrast to neurons, however, ATP consumption by astroglia is much smaller than that by neurons, since astroglia do not generate action potentials. In fact, approximately one half of the total neuronal ATP consumption reflects $Na^+$,$K^+$-ATPase activity, which restores and maintains the ionic gradient across the cell membrane to maintain the generation of action potentials [4, 5]. Astroglial $Na^+$,$K^+$-ATPase also plays

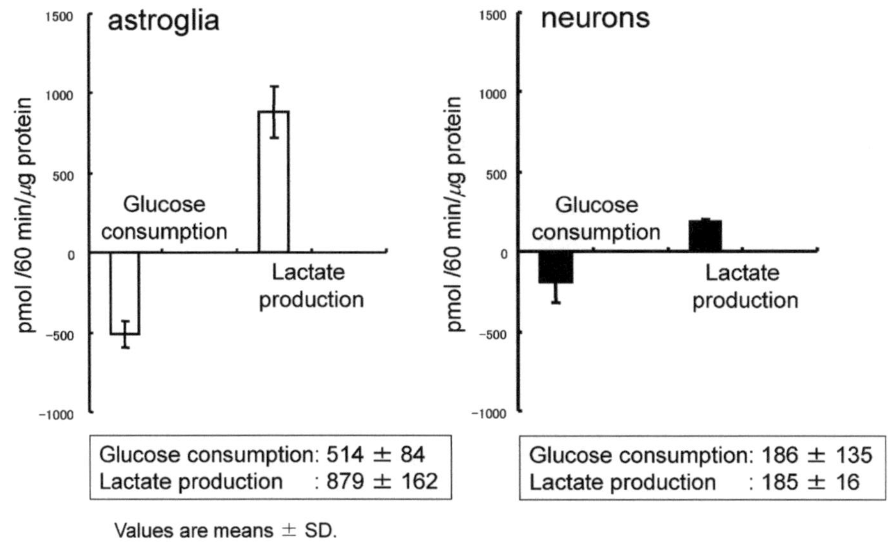


**Figure 5.**
*Glucose consumption and lactate production measured directly in culture medium for rat astroglia and neurons (adapted from [23]).*

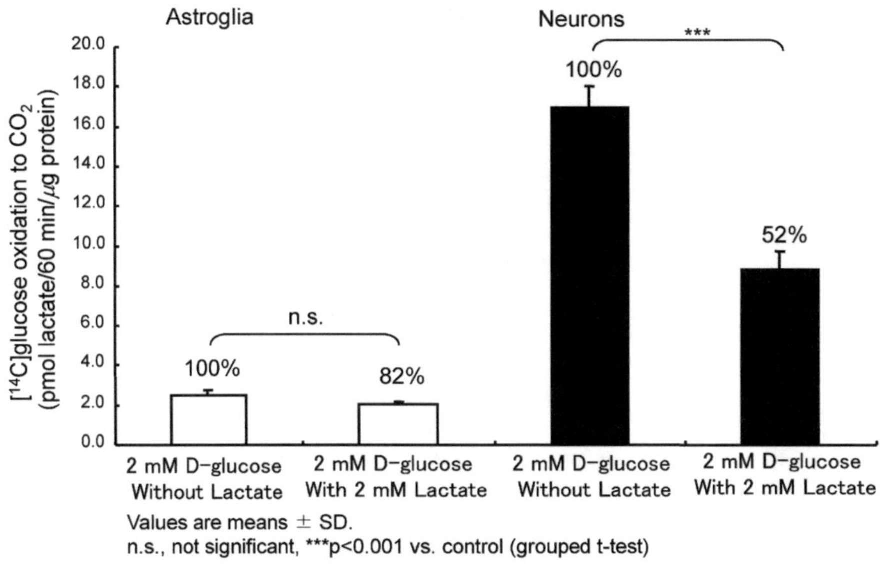


**Figure 6.**
*Competition assay 1: [$^{14}$C]glucose oxidation is inhibited by lactate by approximately half in neurons but not in astroglia (adapted from [23]).*

a role in maintaining the ionic gradient, and this helps astroglia to take up glutamate released into the synaptic cleft (**Figure 9**) [3, 18, 33]. Glutamate is the most widely distributed excitatory transmitter, and primary motor neurons in the motor cortex release glutamate, which in turn activates secondary motor neurons in the spinal cord to induce muscle contraction. Whether glutamate re-uptake stimulates astroglial $CMR_{glc}$ and $CMR_{oxy}$ remains controversial [3, 18, 33–53]. In an in vitro culture model, at least, the application of glutamate increased glucose consumption (**Figure 10**) as well as lactate production (**Figure 11**), suggesting the activation of glycolysis in an $CMR_{oxy}$-independent manner [3, 18, 33].

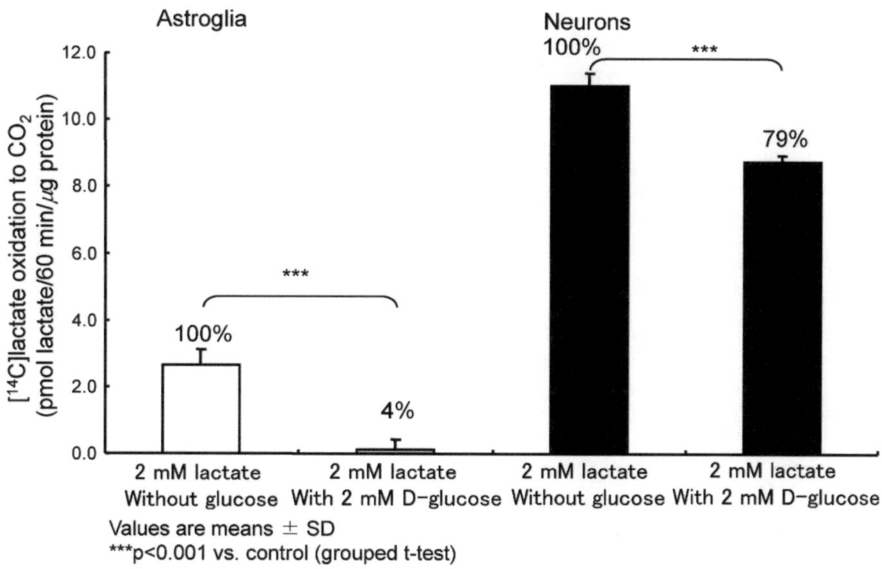


**Figure 7.**
*Competition assay 2: [$^{14}$C]lactate oxidation is somewhat inhibited by glucose in neurons but is markedly inhibited in astroglia (adapted from [23]).*

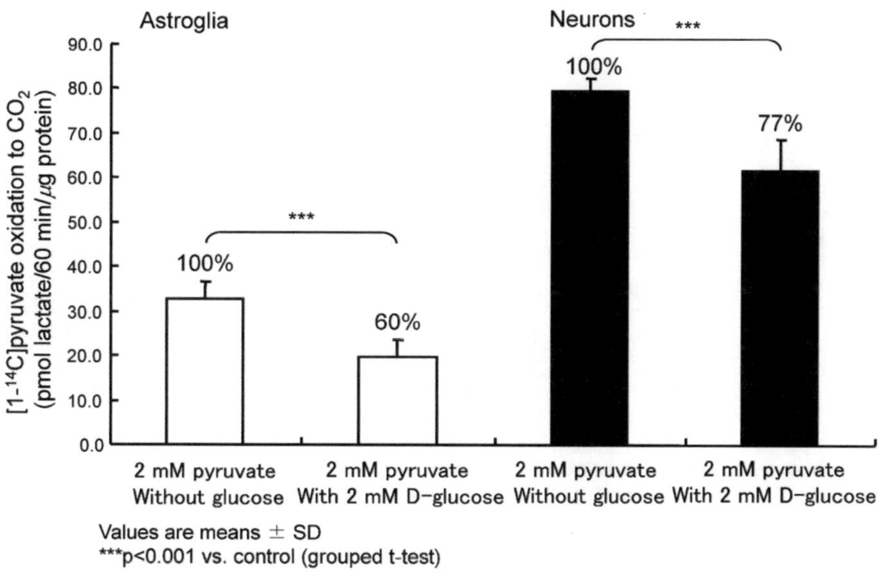


**Figure 8.**
*Competition assay 3: [1-$^{14}$C]pyruvate oxidation is somewhat inhibited by glucose in neurons.*

## 4. Primary astroglia from rodent brain and human iPS cell-derived astroglia

Classically, cultured astroglia prepared from rats or mice have been used to assess the metabolic properties of astroglia in vitro [3]. Basal glucose consumption by cultured rodent astroglia seems to be comparable to that by cultured rodent neurons. Interestingly, however, the amount of lactate that is released into the culture media is much higher in astroglial cultures than in neuronal cultures (**Figure 5**) [3, 23],

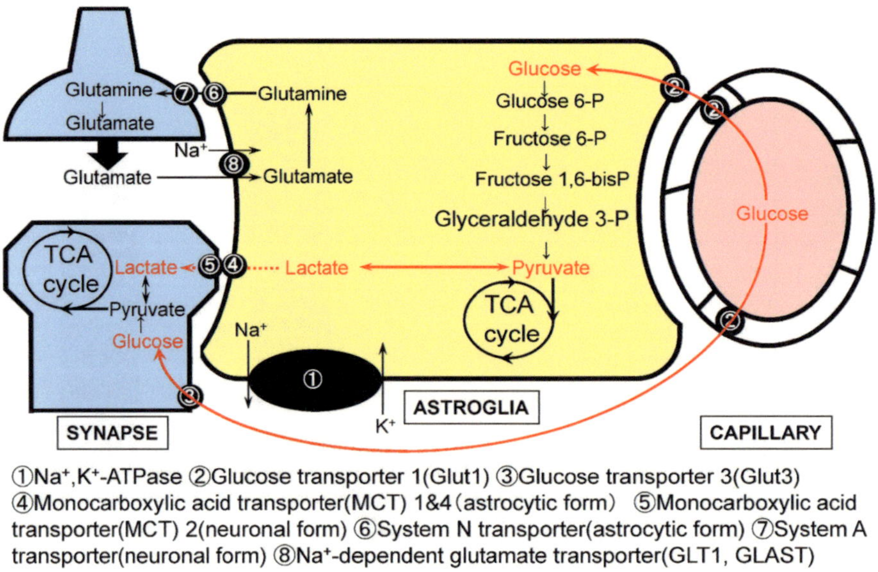


**Figure 9.**
*Astrocyte-neuron lactate shuttle hypothesis (ANLSH) (adapted from [3]).*

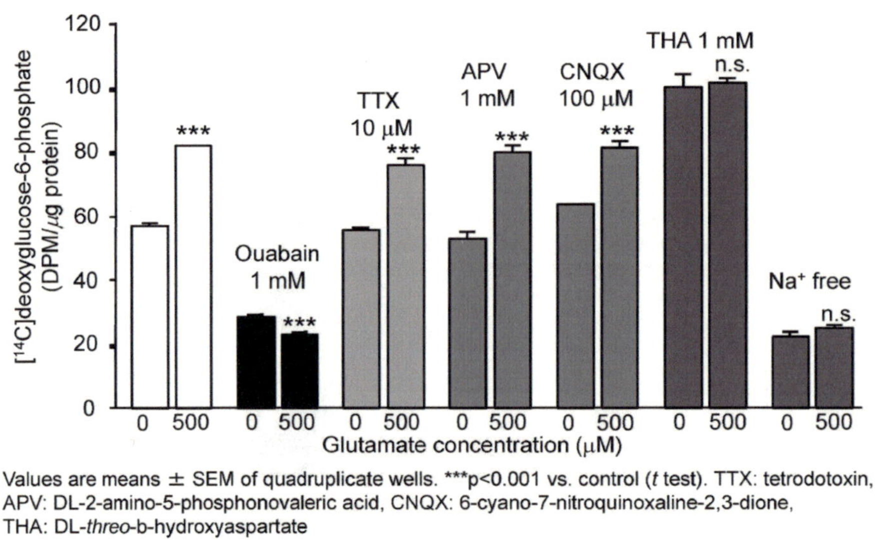


**Figure 10.**
*Glutamate stimulates [$^{14}$C]deoxyglucose phosphorylation through a $Na^+$-dependent glutamate transporter in rat cultured astroglia (adapted from [18]).*

suggesting the occurrence of active aerobic glycolysis in astroglia. Although the glucose consumption of astroglia seems to be comparable to that of neurons, the in vivo location of astroglia in the brain may make glucose uptake more suitable [30–32]. In contrast, neurons are not in direct contact with microvessels. Therefore, avid glucose uptake by cultured neurons may not reflect glucose metabolism in vivo. Of course, glucose supplied from the microvessels diffuses into the extracellular space and can be taken up by neurons via their glucose transporters (Glut 3) (**Figure 9**) [3, 17]. In addition to glucose, lactate generated by astroglia and released into the extracellular space can also be taken up by neurons via neuronal MCT2 (**Figure 9**) [3, 17]. When both glucose and lactate are available, cultured neurons metabolize lactate preferentially (**Figures 6** and 7) [3, 23].

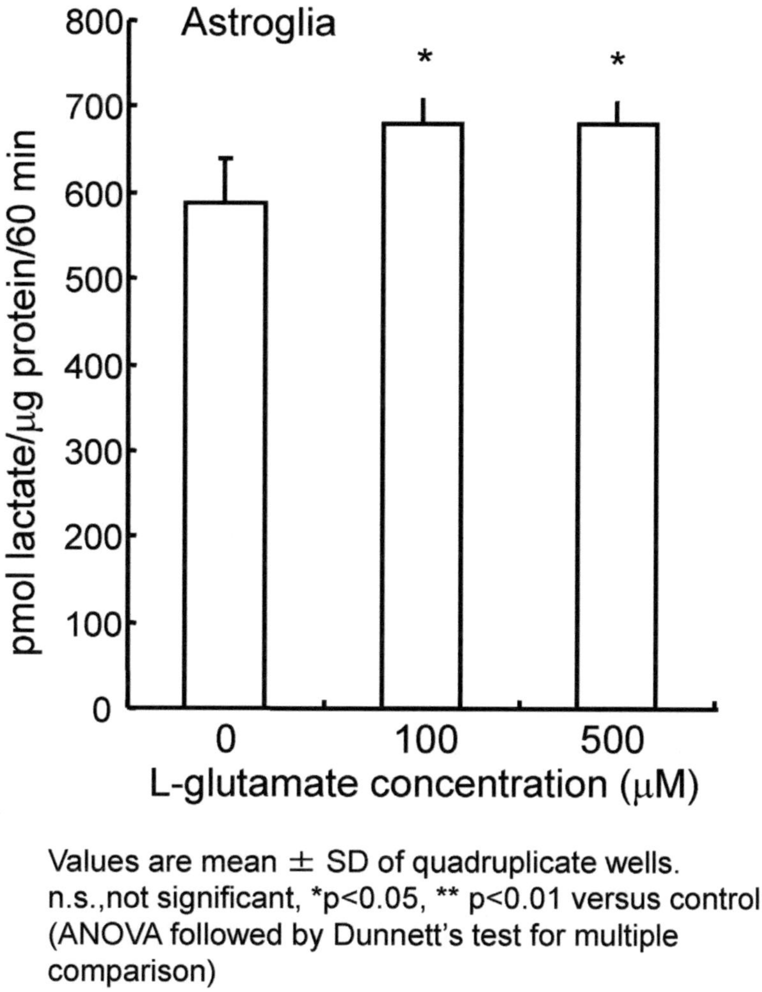


**Figure 11.**
*Effects of L-glutamate on lactate release measured directly in culture medium for rat astroglia (adapted from [23]).*

Neuronal activation causes glutamate release in the synaptic cleft. The maximal concentration of glutamate can reach 1 mM, which is toxic to neurons. To prevent glutamate toxicity, the end-feet of astroglia, which envelope the synapse (tripartite synapse) [32], remove glutamate via glutamate transporters together with the co-transportation of $Na^+$ based on an inwardly lower $Na^+$-gradient across the membrane [3, 16, 33]. This inwardly lower ionic concentration gradient is maintained by $Na^+$,$K^+$-ATPase; thus, ATP production requires glucose as an energy substrate. So far, cultured astroglia typically show high glucose utilization and lactate production, and these profiles are exaggerated by the addition of glutamate. Recently, we evaluated astroglia that had differentiated from human induced-pluripotent stem (iPS) cells and observed the conservation of similar metabolic profiles [54]. These results suggest that glutamate uptake enhances the consumption of glycolysis-derived ATP. Of note, glutamate in astroglia is converted into glutamine and recycled back to neurons (glutamate-glutamine cycle) (**Figure 5**) [3]. In addition, some of this glutamate is converted to alfa-ketoglutarate and utilized as a TCA cycle substrate (**Figure 12**) [3–5]. The capacity for glutamate oxidation is greater in astroglia than in neurons (**Figure 13**) [unpublished data]. Moreover, recent findings

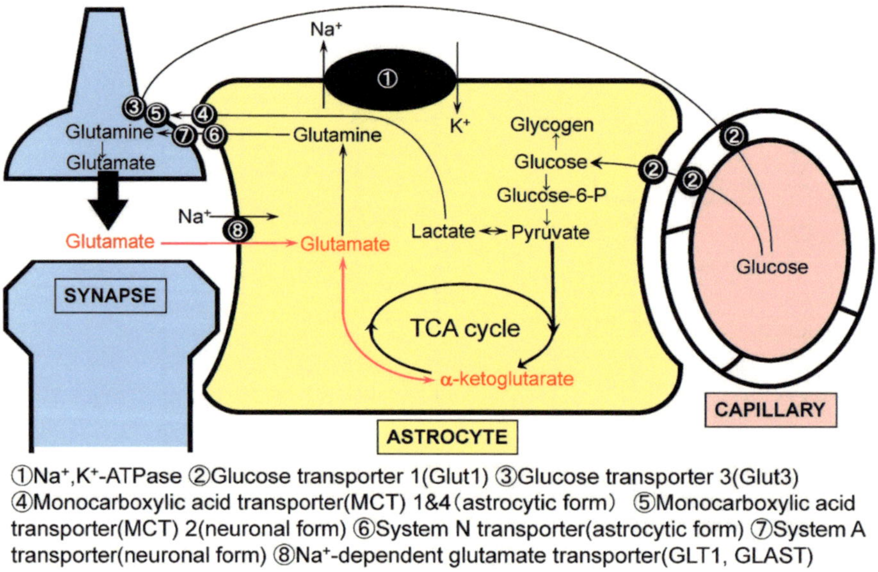


**Figure 12.**
*Glutamate taken up by $Na^+$-dependent glutamate transporters enhances astroglial energy metabolism (both glycolytic and/or oxidative) (adapted from [3]).*

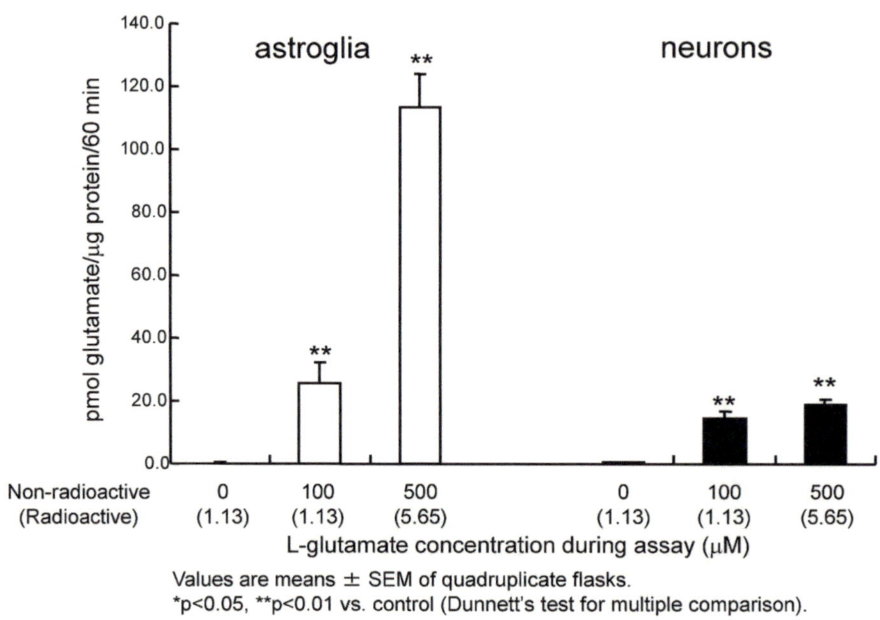


**Figure 13.**
*[1-$^{14}$C]glutamate oxidation ($CO_2$ production from glutamate) in astroglia and neurons.*

suggest that malate, an intermediate TCA metabolite, contributes to lactate production through its conversion into lactate via malic enzyme (**Figure 14**) [3].

## 5. Fates of lactate produced by astroglia

Whether lactate produced and released from astroglia can be used as an energy substrate by neurons has long been debated [36–53]. Theoretically, MCT4 in astroglia

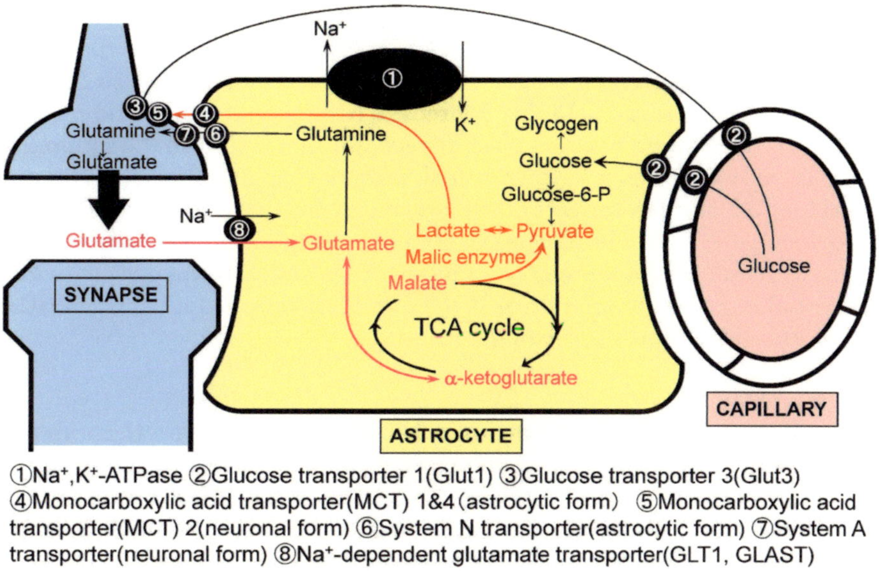


**Figure 14.**
*Glutamate taken up by $Na^+$-dependent glutamate transporters enhances lactate production through a glycolytic pathway as well as through malic enzyme activation in astroglia (adapted from [3]).*

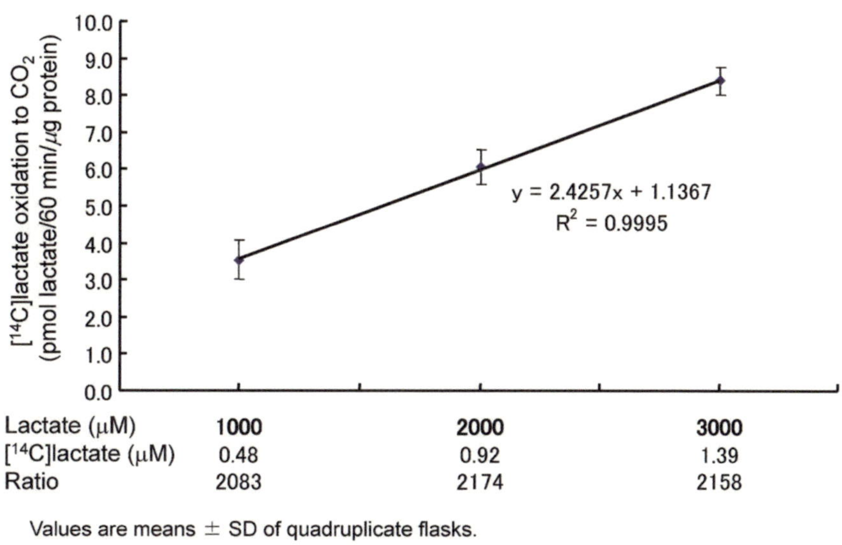


**Figure 15.**
*Increasing lactate concentrations (1–3 mM) enhance [$^{14}$C]lactate oxidation in cultured neurons (adapted from [23]).*

export lactate outside such cells, and MCT2 in neurons take up lactate [3, 17]. Once lactate enters a neuron, it could become a preferential energy substrate, compared with glucose; this pathway is known as the astrocyte-neuron lactate shuttle model (**Figure 5**) [3, 33]. In our in vitro culture model, increasing the concentrations of lactate enhanced the neuronal oxidation of lactate (**Figure 15**) [23]. The argument against this model is based on the high affinity of MCT2, which results in the rapid saturation of lactate transportation into neurons [52, 53]. Thus, astroglial lactate production does not favor neuronal lactate utilization. The validity of this model should be elucidated in vivo.

Lactate plays a role as a signal molecule. BDNF expression can also be induced by lactate through the activation of Sirtuin1 deacetylase. SIRT1 increases the levels of the transcriptional coactivator PGC-1α and the secreted molecule FNDC5, known to mediate BDNF expression [13, 14]. Moreover, hydroxycarboxylic acid receptor 1 (HCAR1) has been found to act as a lactate receptor that results in the suppression of neuronal activity [55–57]. Lauritzen et al. showed that HCAR1 at the BBB was essential for mediating the effects of exercise on angiogenesis in a mouse model [56]. Furthermore, lactate binding to HCAR1 on neurons inhibits adenylate cyclase and thus decreases cAMP, thereby reducing neuronal activity and gene regulation. The potential negative modulation of BDNF production by lactate through HCAR1 should be examined more closely in the future.

## 6. Astroglia produce ketone bodies, which serve as neuronal energy substrates

In addition to BHB, acetoacetate and acetone are listed as ketone bodies. During starvation, ketone body production by hepatocytes in the liver is enhanced [3–5]. Astroglia in the brain function similar to hepatocytes and generate more ketone bodies than neurons (**Figure 16**) [3, 25]. The production of BHB is regulated by the AMP/ATP level, or the cellular energy state. AMP-activated protein kinase (AMPK) can sense a decrease in ATP and the resultant increase in AMP, which induces the activation of AMPK. Decreased malonyl-CoA stimulates the beta-oxidation of long-chain fatty acids, enhancing the production of acetoacetate and BHB. 5-Amino-1-b-D-ribofuranosyl-imidazole-4-carboxamide (AICAR), an activator of AMPK, stimulates these two ketone bodies in astroglia (**Figure 17**) [3, 25]. Similar to lactate, BHB is exported via MCT4 and is then imported into neurons through MCT2 and used as an alternative energy substrate [3, 17]. Unlike glucose-derived lactate, which needs to be converted to acetyl-CoA by PDHC to enter the TCA cycle, BHB enters the TCA cycle in an PDHC-independent manner. PDHC is susceptible to cellular stressors like reactive oxygen species (ROSs). Enhanced lactate production under brain ischemia triggers the accumulation of lactate. Unfortunately, however, re-perfusion therapy might not be helpful when PDHC is

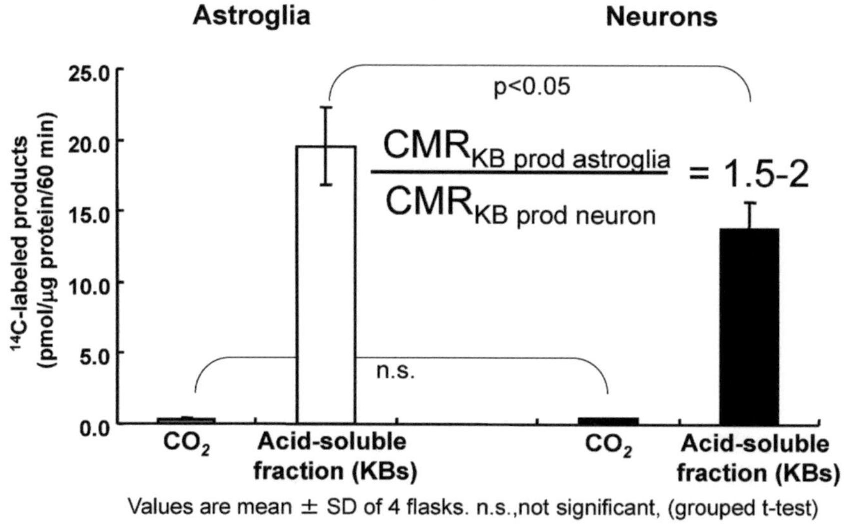


**Figure 16.**
*[1-$^{14}$C]palmitic acid (PA) derived-$CO_2$ and acid-soluble fractions (ketone bodies: KBs) in rat neurons and astroglia (adapted from [25]).*

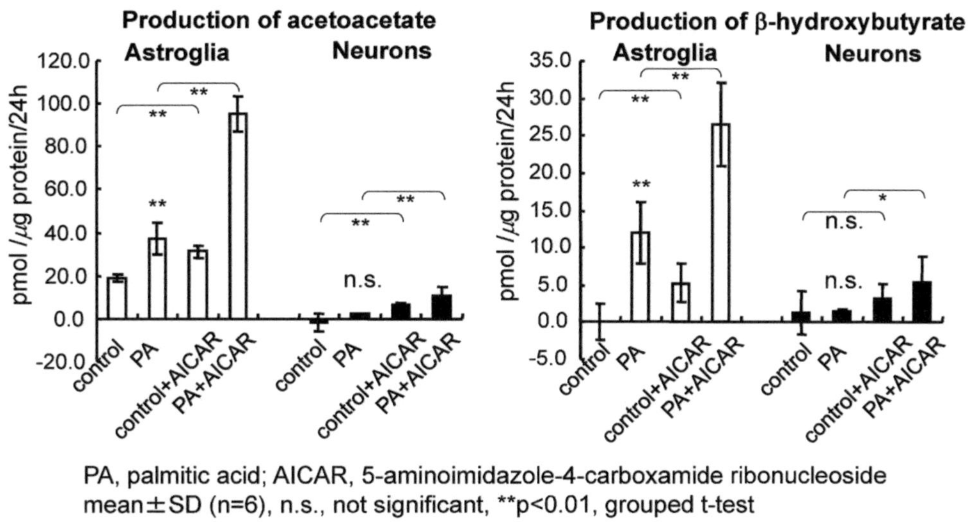


**Figure 17.**
*Ketogenesis by astroglia and neurons by 5-aminoimidazole-4-carboxamide ribonucleoside (AICAR), a cell-permeable activator of AMPK (500 μM) (adapted from [25]).*

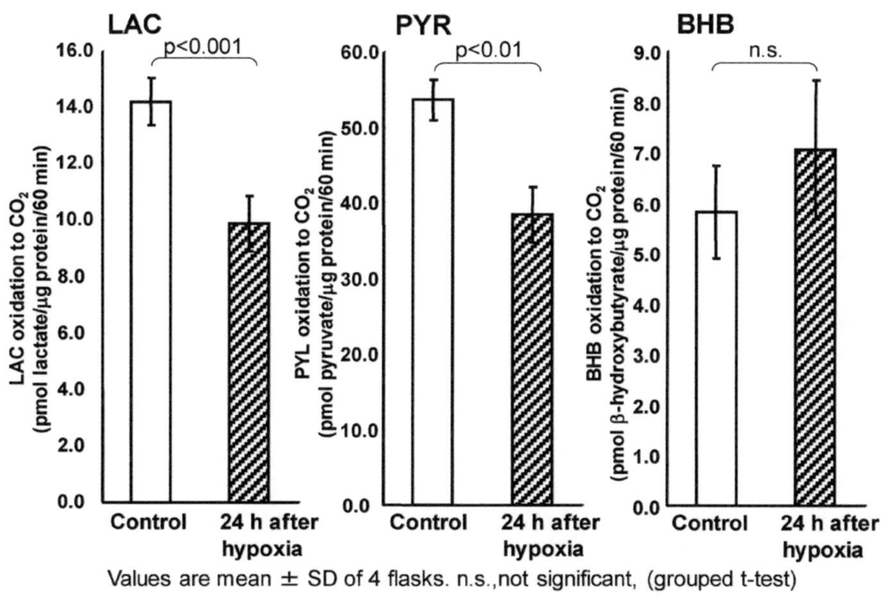


**Figure 18.**
*Effects of 1% hypoxia (24 h) on oxidative metabolism of lactate (LAC), pyruvate (PYR), or β-hydroxybutyrate (BHB) in neurons (adapted from [25]). Neuronal utilization (oxidative metabolism) of LAC and PYR was significantly reduced after hypoxia, while BHB oxidation was preserved.*

damaged, since lactate is incapable of being utilized even in the presence of re-supplied oxygen (**Figure 18**). In contrast, neurons can utilize BHB instead of lactate, and ATP production can be restored after re-oxygenation (**Figure 18**) [3, 25].

## 7. BHB acts as an HDAC inhibitor and as a ligand of HCAR2

Vigorous physical exercise induces BHB production by the liver, but astroglial BHB production under similar conditions has not been confirmed.

Liver-derived BHB acts as a direct Class I HDAC inhibitor. By inhibiting HDAC2 and HDAC3 and preventing their recruitment to the BDNF promoter I, BHB induces BDNF expression [15, 16]. As described above, ischemic insults do, indeed, activate astroglial BHB production. Therefore, BHB-induced BDNF may help neuronal regeneration after ischemic damage. Further study is warranted. BHB released from astroglia also acts as a ligand of hydroxycarboxylic acid receptor 2 (HCAR2) and exerts neuroprotective effects by activating HCAR2, which in turn promotes the downstream activation of silent information regulator 1 (SIRT1) and inhibits nuclear factor-kappa B (NFκB) to protect against oxidative stress [58–61].

## 8. BHB can play a role in remyelination in the white matter of the brain

In terms of functional recovery, both the neuronal structure and myelination are essential [3, 7]. As for the energy supply, the white matter axons of neurons are myelinated by oligodendrocytes. The astroglial end-feet are in direct contact with neurons only at Ranvier nodes, implying that neither glucose nor lactate can reach neurons easily. In fact, axonal metabolic demand is fulfilled by lactate supplied by oligodendrocytes. How lactate is generated by oligodendrocytes remains to be elucidated. Since astroglial end-feet are suitable for the uptake of glucose from microvessels, lactate generated in astroglia could be transported to oligodendrocytes; alternatively, a pathway involving the direct uptake of glucose by oligodendrocytes could be involved. Importantly, myelin damage (demyelination) can occur in various neurological disorders, while the remyelinating capacity can potentially restore damaged myelin (remyelination). Myelin cholesterol synthesis is essential for such a process, and BHB could be a possible substrate [62–65]. Moreover, BDNF reportedly facilitates myelination [66].

## 9. Summary

Brain function is dependent on glucose, which is supplied from outside the brain as food. The unavailability of glucose forces the brain to utilize ketone bodies, especially BHB. In addition to glucose and BHB, lactate is another possible energy source for the brain. Physical exercise enhances the production of both lactate and BHB. The former is generated in skeletal muscles, while the latter is generated in liver hepatocytes. Interestingly, astroglia can generate both lactate and BHB inside the brain upon neuronal excitation. Astroglia-derived lactate and BHB can serve as alternative energy substrates, since physical activities are initiated by neuronal excitation, which cause astroglia to generate lactate and BHB inside the brain. Irrespective of the origins of lactate and BHB, both can be transported into neurons and simulate BDNF production, facilitating neurotransmission and synaptic plasticity. Thus, physical activity helps the human brain to function in a healthy manner through a metabolic compartment composed of glial cells, skeletal muscles, and liver.

## Acknowledgements

The author thanks the Departments of Neurology and Physiology, Keio University School of Medicine, for their support. This work was supported in part by JSPS KAKENHI Grant Number 19 K08002 and 17 K09762.

## Disclosure

The author declares no conflicts of interest.

## Abbreviations

| | |
|---|---|
| AICAR | 5-amino-1-b-D-ribofuranosyl-imidazole-4-carboxamide |
| AMPK | AMP-activated protein kinase |
| BHB | beta-hydroxybutyrate |
| BBB | blood–brain barrier |
| BDNF | brain-derived neurotrophic factor |
| CBF | cerebral blood flow |
| $CMR_{glc}$ | cerebral metabolic rate of glucose |
| $CMR_{oxy}$ | cerebral metabolic rate of oxygen |
| FNDC5 | fibronectin type III domain-containing protein 5 |
| Glut1 | glucose transporter 1 |
| Glut3 | glucose transporter 3 |
| HDAC | histone deacetylase |
| HCAR1 | ydroxycarboxylic acid receptor 1 |
| HCAR2 | hydroxycarboxylic acid receptor 2 |
| iPS cell | induced-pluripotent stem cell |
| MCTs | monocarboxylate transporters |
| NFκB | nuclear factor-kappa B |
| PGC-1α | peroxisome proliferator-activated receptor gamma coactivator 1-alpha |
| PDHC | pyruvate dehydrogenase complex |
| ROSs | reactive oxygen species |
| SIRT1 | silent information regulator 1 |
| TCA | tricarboxylic acid |

## Author details

Shinichi Takahashi[1,2]

1 Department of Neurology and Stroke, Saitama Medical University International Medical Center, Hidaka-shi, Saitama-ken, Japan

2 Department of Physiology, Keio University School of Medicine, Tokyo, Japan

*Address all correspondence to: takashin@tka.att.ne.jp

## References

[1] Somjen GG. Nervenkitt: notes on the history of the concept of neuroglia. Glia. 1988;1:2-9.

[2] Allen NJ, Barres BA. Neuroscience: Glia - more than just brain glue. Nature. 2009;457(7230):675-677.

[3] Takahashi S. Metabolic compartmentalization between astroglia and neurons in physiological and pathophysiological conditions of the neurovascular unit. Neuropathology. 2020 Apr;40(2):121-137.

[4] Clarke DD, Sokoloff L. Circulation and energy metabolism of the brain. In: Basic Neurochemistry: Molecular, Cellular, and Medical Aspects (Siegel G, Agranoff B, Albers RW, Fisher S, eds), 6th edn, Lippincott-Raven, Philadelphia, 1999, p.637-669.

[5] Dienel GA. Energy metabolism in the brain. In: From Molecules to Networks: an Introduction to Cellular and Molecular Neuroscience (Byrne JH, Roberts JL, eds), 2nd edn, Academic Press, London, 2009, p.49-110.

[6] Dirnagl U, Iadecola C, Moskowitz MA. Pathobiology of ischaemic stroke: an integrated view. Trends Neurosci. 1999;22:391-397.

[7] Janowski M, Wagner DC, Boltze J. Stem Cell-Based Tissue Replacement After Stroke: Factual Necessity or Notorious Fiction? Stroke. 2015;46:2354-2363.

[8] Binder DK, Scharfman HE. Brain-derived neurotrophic factor. Growth Factors. 2004;22:123-131

[9] Barde YA, Edgar D, Thoenen H. Purification of a new neurotrophic factor from mammalian brain. EMBO J. 1982;1:549-553.

[10] Cotman CW, Berchtold NC. Exercise: a behavioral intervention to enhance brain health and plasticity. Trends Neurosci. 2002;25:295-301

[11] Cotman CW, Berchtold NC, Christie LA. Exercise builds brain health: key roles of growth factor cascades and inflammation. Trends Neurosci. 2007;30:464-472.

[12] Wrann CD, White JP, Salogiannnis J, Laznik-Bogoslavski D, Wu J, Ma D, Lin JD, Greenberg ME, Spiegelman BM. Exercise induces hippocampal BDNF through a PGC-1alpha/FNDC5 pathway. Cell Metab. 2013;18:649-659.

[13] El Hayek L, Khalifeh M, Zibara V, Abi Assaad R, Emmanuel N, Karnib N, El-Ghandour R, Nasrallah P, Bilen M, Ibrahim P, Younes J, Abou Haidar E, Barmo N, Jabre V, Stephan JS, Sleiman SF. Lactate Mediates the Effects of Exercise on Learning and Memory through SIRT1-Dependent Activation of Hippocampal Brain-Derived Neurotrophic Factor (BDNF). J Neurosci. 2019;39:2369-2382.

[14] Müller P, Duderstadt Y, Lessmann V, Müller NG. Lactate and BDNF: Key Mediators of Exercise Induced Neuroplasticity? J Clin Med. 2020 Apr 15;9(4):1136.

[15] Sleiman SF, Henry J, Al-Haddad R, El Hayek L, Abou Haidar E, Stringer T, Ulja D, Karuppagounder SS, Holson EB, Ratan RR, Ninan I, Chao MV. Exercise promotes the expression of brain derived neurotrophic factor (BDNF) through the action of the ketone body beta-hydroxybutyrate. Elife. 2016 Jun 2;5:e15092.

[16] Norwitz NG, Hu MT, Clarke K. The Mechanisms by Which the Ketone Body D-beta-Hydroxybutyrate May Improve the Multiple Cellular Pathologies of Parkinson's Disease. Front Nutr. 2019 May 14;6:63.

[17] Simpson IA, Carruthers A, Vannucci SJ. Supply and demand in cerebral energy metabolism: the role of nutrient transporters. J Cereb Blood Flow Metab. 2007;27:1766-1791.

[18] Takahashi S, Driscoll BF, Law MJ, Sokoloff L. Role of sodium and potassium ions in regulation of glucose metabolism in cultured astroglia. Proc Natl Acad Sci U S A. 1995;92:4616-4620.

[19] Sokoloff L, Takahashi S, Gotoh J, Driscoll BF, Law MJ. Contribution of astroglia to functionally activated energy metabolism. Dev Neurosci. 1996;18:344-352.

[20] Takahashi S, Abe T, Gotoh J, Fukuuchi Y. Substrate-dependence of reduction of MTT: a tetrazolium dye differs in cultured astroglia and neurons. Neurochem Int. 2002;40:441-448.

[21] Abe T, Takahashi S, Fukuuchi Y. Reduction of Alamar Blue, a novel redox indicator, is dependent on both the glycolytic and oxidative metabolism of glucose in rat cultured neurons. Neurosci Lett. 2002;326:179-182.

[22] Abe T, Takahashi S, Suzuki N. Oxidative metabolism in cultured rat astroglia: effects of reducing the glucose concentration in the culture medium and of D-aspartate or potassium stimulation. J Cereb Blood Flow Metab. 2006;26:153-160.

[23] Takahashi S. Energy metabolism of neurons and astroglia. Cerebral Blood Flow and Metabolism (in Japanese). 2010;21:18-27.

[24] Takahashi S, Izawa Y, Suzuki N. Astroglial pentose phosphate pathway rates in response to high-glucose environments. ASN Neuro. 2012 Mar 22;4(2):e00078.

[25] Takahashi S, Iizumi T, Mashima K, Abe T, Suzuki N. Roles and regulation of ketogenesis in cultured astroglia and neurons under hypoxia and hypoglycemia. ASN Neuro. 2014 Sep 11;6(5):1759091414550997.

[26] Iizumi T, Takahashi S, Mashima K, Minami K, Izawa Y, Abe T, Hishiki T, Suematsu M, Kajimura M, Suzuki N. A possible role of microglia-derived nitric oxide by lipopolysaccharide in activation of astroglial pentose-phosphate pathway via the Keap1/Nrf2 system. J Neuroinflammation. 2016 May 4;13(1):99.

[27] Mashima K, Takahashi S, Minami K, Izawa Y, Abe T, Tsukada N, Hishiki T, Suematsu M, Kajimura M, Suzuki N. Neuroprotective Role of Astroglia in Parkinson Disease by Reducing Oxidative Stress Through Dopamine-Induced Activation of Pentose-Phosphate Pathway. ASN Neuro. 2018 Jan-Dec;10:1759091418775562.

[28] van Hall G. Lactate kinetics in human tissues at rest and during exercise. Acta Physiol (Oxf). 2010;199:499-508.

[29] Evans M, Cogan KE, Egan B. Metabolism of ketone bodies during exercise and training: physiological basis for exogenous supplementation. J Physiol. 2017;595:2857-2871

[30] García-Marín V, García-López P, Freire M. Cajal's contributions to glia research. Trends Neurosci. 2007;30:479-487.

[31] Mathiisen TM, Lehre KP, Danbolt NC et al. The perivascular astroglial sheath provides a complete covering of the brain microvessels: an electron microscopic 3D reconstruction. Glia. 2010;58:1094-1103.

[32] Araque A, Parpura V, Sanzgiri RP et al. Tripartite synapses: glia, the unacknowledged partner. Trends Neurosci. 1999;22:208-215.

[33] Pellerin L, Magistretti PJ. Glutamate uptake into astrocytes stimulates

aerobic glycolysis: a mechanism coupling neuronal activity to glucose utilization. Proc Natl Acad Sci USA. 1994;91:10625-10629.

[34] Souza DG, Almeida RF, Souza DO, Zimmer ER. The astrocyte biochemistry. Semin Cell Dev Biol. 2019 Apr 22. pii: S1084-9521(18)30071-5.

[35] Bordone MP, Salman MM, Titus HE, Amini E, Andersen JV, Chakraborti B, Diuba AV, Dubouskaya TG, Ehrke E, Espindola de Freitas A, Braga de Freitas G, Gonçalves RA, Gupta D, Gupta R, Ha SR, Hemming IA, Jaggar M, Jakobsen E, Kumari P, Lakkappa N, Marsh APL, Mitlöhner J, Ogawa Y, Paidi RK, Ribeiro FC, Salamian A, Saleem S, Sharma S, Silva JM, Singh S, Sulakhiya K, Tefera TW, Vafadari B, Yadav A, Yamazaki R, Seidenbecher CI. The energetic brain - A review from students to students. J Neurochem. 2019 Oct;151(2):139-165.

[36] Aubert A, Costalat R, Magistretti PJ, Pellerin L. Brain lactate kinetics: Modeling evidence for neuronal lactate uptake upon activation. Proc Natl Acad Sci U S A. 2005;102:16448-16453.

[37] Laughton JD, Bittar P, Charnay Y, Pellerin L, Kovari E, Magistretti PJ, Bouras C. Metabolic compartmentalization in the human cortex and hippocampus: evidence for a cell- and region-specific localization of lactate dehydrogenase 5 and pyruvate dehydrogenase. BMC Neurosci. 2007 May 23;8:35.

[38] Pellerin L, Bouzier-Sore AK, Aubert A, Serres S, Merle M, Costalat R, Magistretti PJ. Activity-dependent regulation of energy metabolism by astrocytes: an update. Glia. 2007;55:1251-1262

[39] Jolivet R, Allaman I, Pellerin L, Magistretti PJ, Weber B. Comment on recent modeling studies of astrocyte-neuron metabolic interactions. J Cereb Blood Flow Metab. 2010;30:1982-1986.

[40] Pellerin L, Magistretti PJ. Sweet sixteen for ANLS. J Cereb Blood Flow Metab. 2012;32:1152-1166

[41] Mazuel L, Blanc J, Repond C, Bouchaud V, Raffard G, Déglon N, Bonvento G, Pellerin L, Bouzier-Sore AK. A neuronal MCT2 knockdown in the rat somatosensory cortex reduces both the NMR lactate signal and the BOLD response during whisker stimulation. PLoS One. 2017 Apr 7;12(4):e0174990.

[42] Pellerin L. Neuroenergetics: Astrocytes Have a Sweet Spot for Glucose. Curr Biol. 2018;28:R1258-R1260.

[43] Dienel GA, Hertz L. Glucose and lactate metabolism during brain activation. J Neurosci Res. 2001;66:824-38

[44] Hertz L, Dienel GA. Lactate transport and transporters: general principles and functional roles in brain cells. J Neurosci Res. 2005;79:11-18.

[45] Hertz L, Peng L, Dienel GA. Energy metabolism in astrocytes: high rate of oxidative metabolism and spatiotemporal dependence on glycolysis/glycogenolysis. J Cereb Blood Flow Metab. 2007;27:219-249.

[46] Dienel GA, Ball KK, Cruz NF. A glycogen phosphorylase inhibitor selectively enhances local rates of glucose utilization in brain during sensory stimulation of conscious rats: implications for glycogen turnover. J Neurochem. 2007;102:466-478.

[47] Dienel GA. Astrocytes are 'good scouts': being prepared also helps neighboring neurons. J Cereb Blood Flow Metab. 2010;30:1893-1894.

[48] Dienel GA. Brain lactate metabolism: the discoveries and the

controversies. J Cereb Blood Flow Metab. 2012;32:1107-1138.

[49] Mergenthaler P, Lindauer U, Dienel GA et al. Sugar for the brain: the role of glucose in physiological and pathological brain function. Trends Neurosci. 2013;36:587-597

[50] Dienel GA, Cruz NF. Contributions of glycogen to astrocytic energetics during brain activation. Metab Brain Dis. 2015;30:281-298.

[51] Dienel GA. The metabolic trinity, glucose-glycogen-lactate, links astrocytes and neurons in brain energetics, signaling, memory, and gene expression. Neurosci Lett. 2017;637:18-25.

[52] Dienel GA. Lack of appropriate stoichiometry: Strong evidence against an energetically important astrocyte-neuron lactate shuttle in brain. J Neurosci Res. 2017;95:2103-2125.

[53] Dienel GA. Brain Glucose Metabolism: Integration of Energetics with Function. Physiol Rev. 2019;99:949-1045.

[54] Leventoux N, Morimoto S, Imaizumi K, Sato Y, Takahashi S, Mashima K, Ishikawa M, Sonn I, Kondo T, Watanabe H, Okano H. Human Astrocytes Model Derived from Induced Pluripotent Stem Cells. Cells. 2020 Dec 13;9(12):2680.

[55] Morland C, Lauritzen KH, Puchades M, Holm-Hansen S, Andersson K, Gjedde A, Attramadal H, Storm-Mathisen J, Bergersen LH. The lactate receptor, G-protein-coupled receptor 81/hydroxycarboxylic acid receptor 1: Expression and action in brain. J Neurosci Res. 2015;93:1045-1055.

[56] LauritzenKH,MorlandC,PuchadesM, Holm-HansenS,HagelinEM,LauritzenF, AttramadalH,Storm-MathisenJ,GjeddeA, Bergersen LH. Lactate receptor sites link neurotransmission, neurovascular coupling, and brain energy metabolism. Cereb Cortex. 2014 Oct;24(10):2784-2795.

[57] de Castro Abrantes H, Briquet M, Schmuziger C, Restivo L, Puyal J, Rosenberg N, Rocher AB, Offermanns S, Chatton JY. The Lactate Receptor HCAR1 Modulates Neuronal Network Activity through the Activation of Gα and Gβγ Subunits. J Neurosci. 2019;39:4422-4433.

[58] Graff EC, Fang H, Wanders D, Judd RL. Anti-inflammatory effects of the hydroxycarboxylic acid receptor 2. Metabolism. 2016;65:102-113.

[59] Rahman M, Muhammad S, Khan MA, Chen H, Ridder DA, Müller-Fielitz H, Pokorná B, Vollbrandt T, Stölting I, Nadrowitz R, Okun JG, Offermanns S, Schwaninger M. The β-hydroxybutyrate receptor HCA2 activates a neuroprotective subset of macrophages. Nat Commun. 2014 May 21;5:3944.

[60] Offermanns S, Schwaninger M. Nutritional or pharmacological activation of HCA(2) ameliorates neuroinflammation. Trends Mol Med. 2015;21:245-255.

[61] Parodi B, Rossi S, Morando S, Cordano C, Bragoni A, Motta C, Usai C, Wipke BT, Scannevin RH, Mancardi GL, Centonze D, Kerlero de Rosbo N, Uccelli A. Fumarates modulate microglia activation through a novel HCAR2 signaling pathway and rescue synaptic dysregulation in inflamed CNS. Acta Neuropathol. 2015;130:279-95.

[62] Koper JW, Lopes-Cardozo M, Van Golde LM. Preferential utilization of ketone bodies for the synthesis of myelin cholesterol in vivo. Biochim Biophys Acta. 1981;666:411-417.

[63] Poduslo SE, Miller K. Ketone bodies as precursors for lipid synthesis in neurons, astrocytes,

and oligodendroglia (myelin) in hyperthyroidism, hyperketonemia and hypoketonemia. Neurochem Int. 1991;18:85-88.

[64] Kadish I, Thibault O, BlalockEM, ChenKC, GantJC, PorterNM, Landfield PW.Hippocampal and cognitive aging across the lifespan: a bioenergetic shift precedes and increased cholesterol trafficking parallels memory impairment. J Neurosci. 2009;29:1805-1816.

[65] Kıray H, Lindsay SL, Hosseinzadeh S, Barnett SC. The multifaceted role of astrocytes in regulating myelination. Exp Neurol. 2016;283:541-549.

[66] Fulmer CG, VonDran MW, Stillman AA, Huang Y, Hempstead BL, Dreyfus CF. Astrocyte-derived BDNF supports myelin protein synthesis after cuprizone-induced demyelination. J Neurosci. 2014;34:8186-8196.

Chapter 3

# Roles of Glucose and Sucrose Intakes on the Brain Functions Measured by the Working Ability and Morris Maze

*Akikazu Takada, Fumiko Shimizu, Yukie Ishii, M. Ogawa and Tetsuya Takao*

## Abstract

Sugars such as glucose or sucrose are considered hazardous foods because their intakes lead to obesity, further causing diabetes mellitus (DM), or cardiovascular diseases. However, glucose is needed for many brain functions such as memory and emotion among others. Glucose induces the secretion of insulin, which is needed for transportation of tryptophan from the blood to the brain. Serotonin, which is converted from tryptophan, is important for mood stability, control of emotion, and feeding is inhibited by serotonin in the hypothalamus. We discuss transportation of glucose from the blood to the glia cells. After glycolysis of glucose in the glia lactic acid is transported to cells such as glutaminergic neurons. After the release from neurons glutamic acid is taken up into glia cells and further to neurons again. Sucrose is degraded into glucose and fructose in the intestine thus intake of sucrose increases plasma levels of glucose. We show that intake of sucrose enhanced memory measured by Morris maze in rats and improved the working ability in humans. Roles of glucose and sucrose intakes are discussed together with the function of serotonin in feeding.

**Keywords:** sucrose, glucose, feeding, glucose transporter, glutaminergic neuron, Morris maze, working ability, glycolysis, astrocyte, serotonin, hypothalamus

## 1. Introduction

Obesity is now a global burden [1, 2]. Increase in the prevalence of obesity has lead the American Heart Association (AHA) to call for actions to prevent the consequences of this epidemic [3, 4]. Recently, the AHA reviewed many weight-loss approaches for the management and treatment of obesity [5].

Foods such as fats, carbohydrates or sugar are considered to be causes of such increase in global obesity pandemic. Intakes of carbohydrates result in increase in release of insulin which suppresses the release of fatty acids into circulation, thus storage of fat in fat cells. So carbohydrate is blamed for increase in obesity.

The German Nutrition Society published guidelines in which relationships between carbohydrate intake and prevention of nutrition-related diseases are indicated [6]. The guideline proposes that high carbohydrate intake at the expense of total fat and saturated fatty acids reduces the concentrations of total, LDL, and HDL



IntechOpen

cholesterol. A high carbohydrate consumption at the expense of polyunsaturated fatty acids such as EPA or DHA increases total and LDL cholesterol. But reduces HDL cholesterol. Further, intake of high carbohydrate increases triglyceride concentration. High consumption of sucrose increases obesity and type2 diabetes mellitus (T2DM).

On the other hand, as stated later, glucose is needed for many brain functions such as memory, emotion, decision, motivation etc. Sucrose is degraded in the intestine and gives rise to glucose. Some studies show that sucrose intakes improve memory.

In the present review, we discuss the transportation of glucose from the blood to the brain, influences of glucose or sucrose on memory and working ability, and feeding.

## 2. Importance of glucose in the brain functions

It is now well known that glucose is important for a variety of brain functions. Late 20th century, the development of positron emission tomography (PET) made it possible to visualize the amount of glucose in discrete regions of the brain. For example, light stimulation increased the metabolism of cerebral glucose in the primary visual cortex [7].

The learning of a complex visuospatial motor task was shown to increase the use of glucose by the brain [8].

Summarizing data published, PET studies showed that cognitive demand increased glucose metabolism in localized regions of the brain. In PET studies radioactively labeled glucose appears in brain areas that are metabolically active within a few minutes after the injection into blood. These observations indicate that the brain relies on glucose when neurons are activated.

### 2.1 Transportation of glucose from blood to brain

Tsacopoulos et al. [9] indicated that capillaries of the brain are surrounded by glia cells and glucose uptaken is phosphorylated exclusively in glia cells, not in neurons.

In mammalian there is evidence that glutamate is a coupling signal between neuronal activation and glucose uptake by astrocytes [10, 11].

Astrocytes surround capillaries, which indicate that astrocytes form the first cellular barrier that glucose encounters in the brain. This suggests that astrocytes are likely sites of primary glucose uptake (**Figure 1**).

Schematic figure of the cytological relationships among capillary, astrocyte, and neuron. Processes of astrocytes surround capillaries (end-feet) and ensheath synapses. Receptors and uptake sites for neurotransmitters are on astrocytes. Astrocytes are ideally suited to sense synapse activity and to couple it with glucose uptake and its metabolism.

There are glucose transporters (55kDA Glut1) in the inner sites and outer sites of endothelial cells, and between astrocytes and capillaries (45kDA Glut1). There are Glut 3 transporters on walls of neurons [12].

Glut 1 and Glut 3 glucose transporters are present in the walls of capillaries and neurons (**Figure 2**).

Glucose transporters, Glut1 are located in the luminal and abluminal membranes of brain endothelial cells. There are small amounts of Glut 1 located in the cytoplasm and the largest fractions of Glut1 are at the abluminal membranes. The lower content of Glut1 at the luminal membrane may be due to the comparably high glucose concentration in this membrane, which is close to the plasma concentration.

There appears to be a tight coupling between $Na^{+}$ dependent glutamate uptake by astrocytes and glucose utilization [13] (**Figure 3**).

*DOI: http://dx.doi.org/10.5772/intechopen.99203*

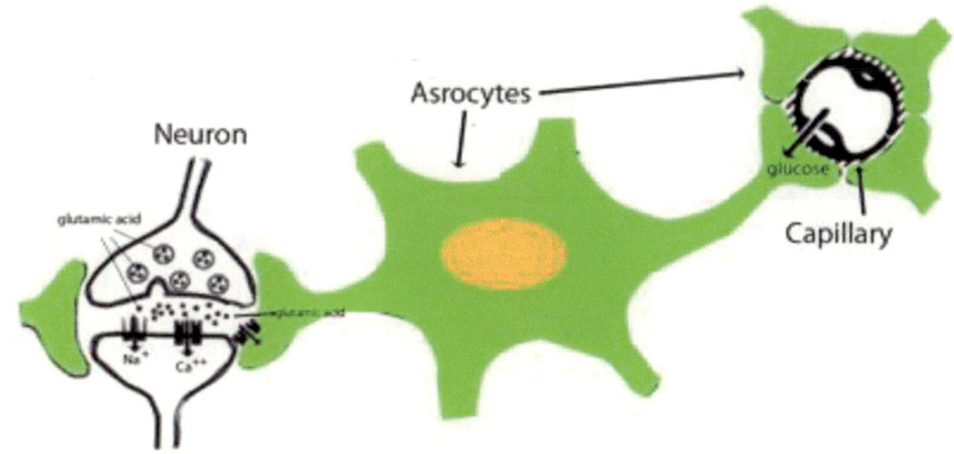


**Figure 1.**
*Capillary, astrocyte and neuron.*

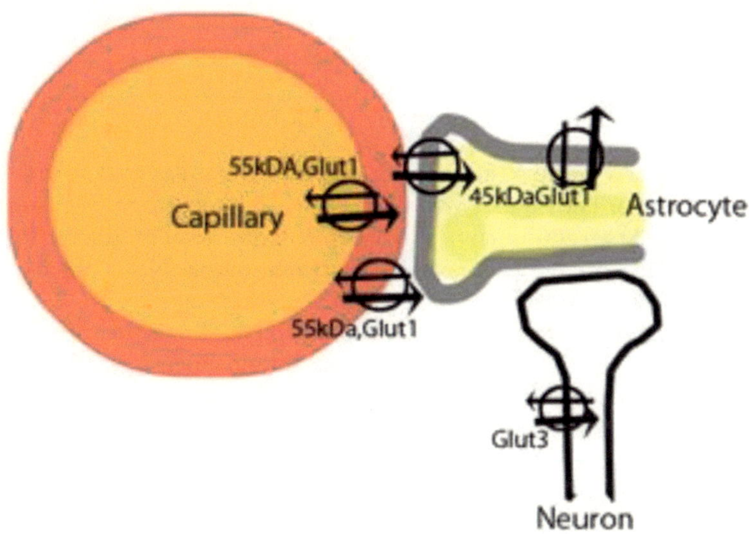


**Figure 2.**
*Glucose transporters in the walls of capillaries and the walls of neuron.*

Glutamate is cotransported with $Na^+$, causing increase in the concentration $Na^+$ in astrocytes, which activate the astrocyte $Na^+/K^+$-ATP ace. Activation of $Na^+/K^+$-ATPase stimulates glycolysis. Lactate released by astrocytes is taken up by neurons and become energy source of neurons.

When summarized, glucose is degraded by glycolysis in astrocytes which generates two molecules of ATP used for uptake of K+ and glutamate from the synaptic cleft. When neurons are active, glycolysis is more active, so that transportation of glucose from the blood to astrocytes increases.

### 2.2 Roles of glucose in memory

It has been known long time that glucose intake improves cognitive behaviors. In elderly humans, changes in blood glucose levels following ingestion of a glucose containing drink was shown to be significantly correlated with performances in the Wechsler memory scale [14].

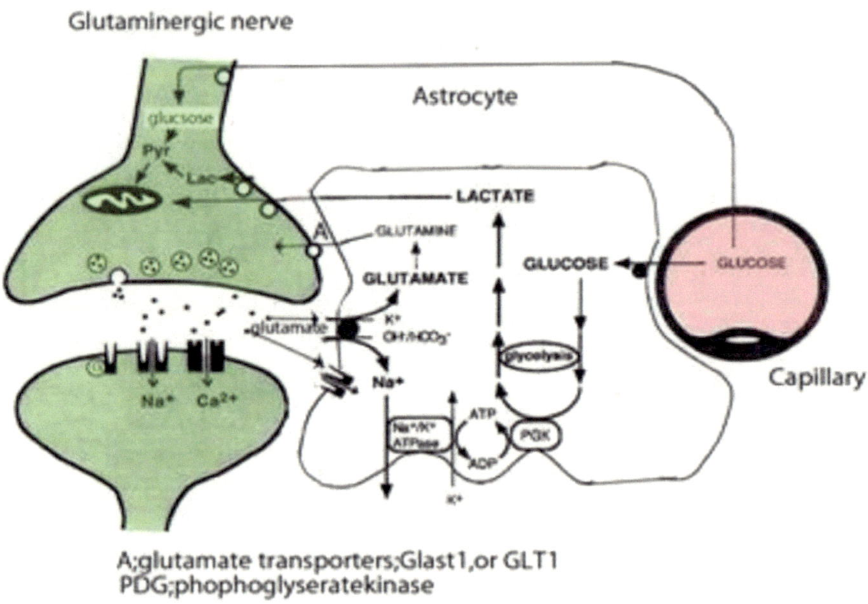


**Figure 3.**
*Transportation of glucose from the blood to neurons.*

Verbal fluency of a group of 80 females, aged 20, was measured after taking a glucose drink or placebo. The fluency was significantly higher after a glucose drink [15].

It was shown that an equilibrium starts between the level of glucose between blood and brain [16]. Such mechanism suggests that higher blood glucose levels promote better performance of brain functions.

The recall of a story was associated with blood glucose levels measured by Wechsler memory scale [17]. A positive correlation between blood glucose and forgetting was shown in young adults, thus those with higher initial blood glucose remember more.

There are various data indicating that glucose supply to the brain is necessary for maintaining good performances of brain functions.

In rats, systemic injections of glucose were shown to enhance learning and memory in many conditions. When microinjected into the specific sites of the brain, glucose levels increased and improved behavioral performances controlled by these sites [18].

Furthermore, glucose administration was shown to enhance memory in generally healthy aged rodents and humans. Glucose ingestion resulted in significant enhancement of performances on several tests including orientation, word recognition, and recall, narrative prose, and face recognition [19].

### 2.3 Glucose and memory measured by Morris maze experiments

As stated above, glucose intakes improve brain functions. Sucrose is degraded to glucose in the intestine and glucose is transported to the blood. A few systematic studies have been carried out as to the effects of sucrose on brain function [20, 21].

Morris used the delayed matching-to-place task which is an unusual variant of the water-maze protocols [22].

#### *2.3.1 Experimental procedures*

Wistar rats aged 11 weeks were trained in water to learn the location of the platform. Rats later learned to reach the platform in 15 min. After 6–12 trials. Rats were administered either glucose (2 g/8 ml/kg) or 8 ml/kg of water intraperitoneally. 24 hours later rats swam in Morris water maze and the ratio of stay at the platform (target) quarter to the rest of the area was measured. The distance to the target was also compared between glucose administered rats and the controls.

*2.3.2 Results*

**Figure 4** show that the ratio of stay in the target quarter in the test was larger after glucose was given, but data are not statistically significant.

Rats were given sucrose solution (10%) or sucralose solution (0.015%) or water as a control in a drinking bottle.

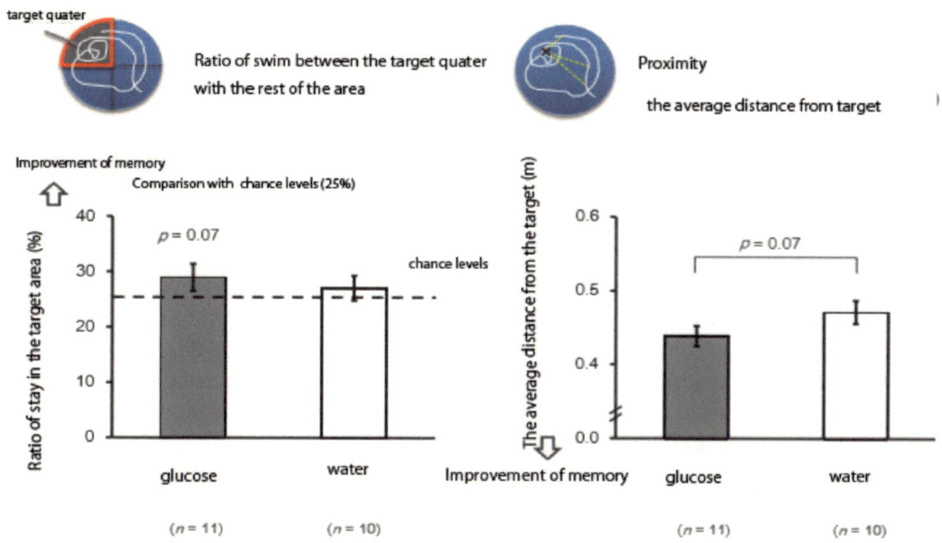


**Figure 4.**
*Effects of glucose administration on memory [23].*

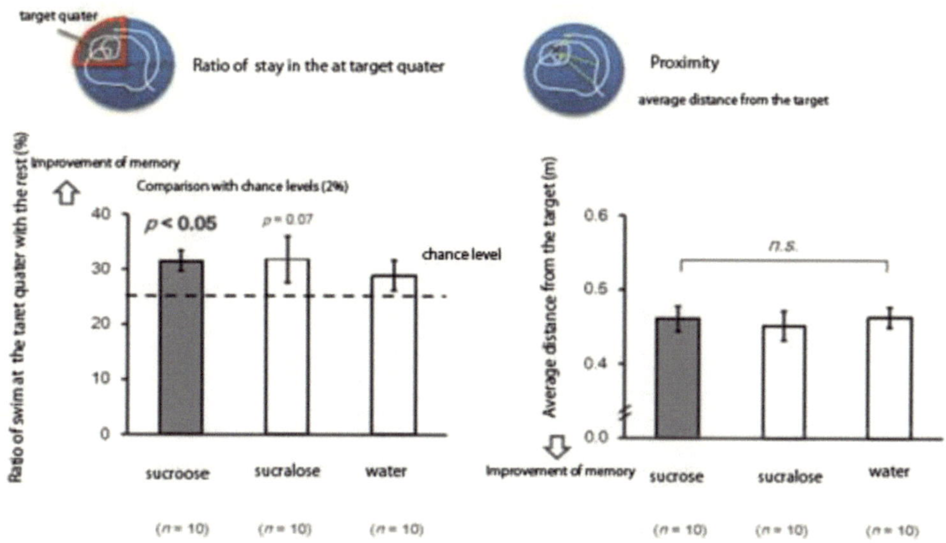


**Figure 5.**
*Effects of sucrose administration on the improvement of memory.*

**Figure 5** shows that rats given sucrose stayed at the target quarter significantly more compared with rats given sucralose. There was no significant decrease about the proximity measurements between rats given sucrose and sucralose.

These results clearly show that the administration of sucrose improved memory consolidation when compared with rats given sucralose in Morris maze experiments.

## 3. The working ability after administration of glucose, sucrose or fructose in young women

Female college students participated in the experiments. They took Uchida-Kraaepelin tests and drank solutions containing glucose, sucrose, fructose or water as controls.

### 3.1 Uchida-Kraepelin tests

There are numbers of a digit lined. Two numbers lined together are added [24, 25]. The number of the higher digit is described. This procedure is repeated for 1 min. Then the addition of numbers of the second line was performed, and repeated for 15 min. The total numbers added are calculated, and the numbers are compared before and after the experiment.

The working duty of 1 min. Was repeated 15 times then drinks were taken. After blood measurements at 30 min. Tests were repeated.

**Figure 6** shows that the working ability was significantly higher after the administration of sucrose, although there was a tendency for the working ability to increase after glucose or fructose administration, but not significantly.

We examined correlation coefficients between blood glucose levels and the working ability. Although there tends to be increase in the working ability with increase in blood glucose levels, but not significant.

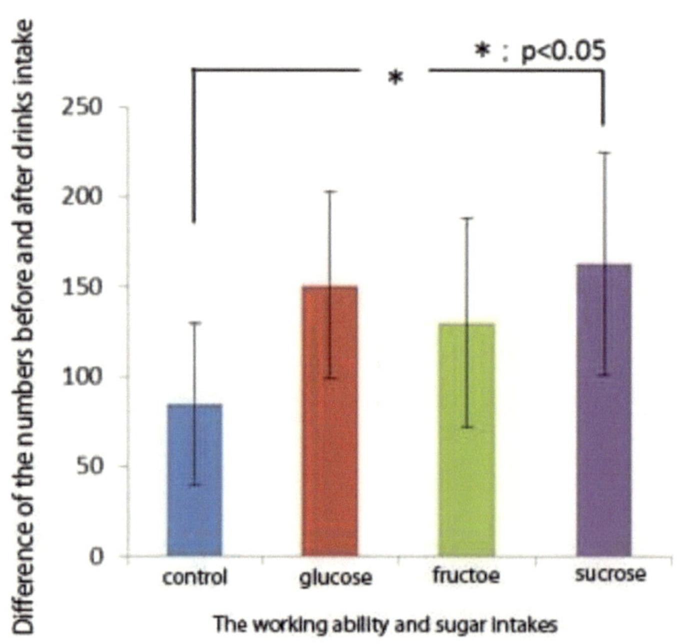


**Figure 6.**
*Relationship between sugar administration and the working ability.*

## 4. Transportation of tryptophan to the brain and conversion to serotonin

Central serotonergic neurons play important roles in a variety of functions in animals and humans (see Review [26]).

We wanted to know if serotonin affects feeding by using injection of MAO inhibitor such as tranylcypromine (TC) intra peritoneally or by microinjection of TC into the hypothalamus.

At first, we injected TC intraperitoneally into rats and measured changes in body weights and foods intake [27].

**Figure 7** shows that after the injection of TC in rats body weights decreased and amounts of food intakes decreased significantly.

**Figure 8** shows that micro infusion of TC solution into the paraventricular nucleus of hypothalamus resulted in dramatic decrease of food intakes and body weight. These data suggest that serotonin inhibited feeding.

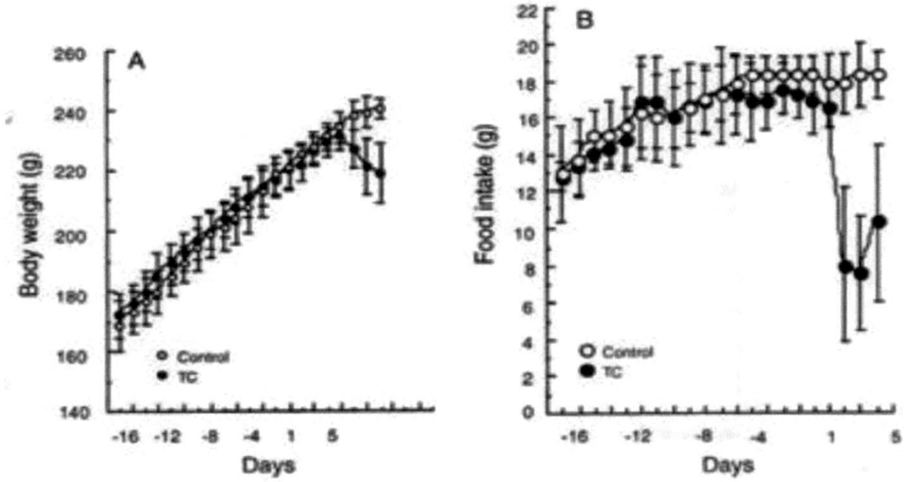


**Figure 7.**
*Growth curves of rats administered with TC or vehicle.*

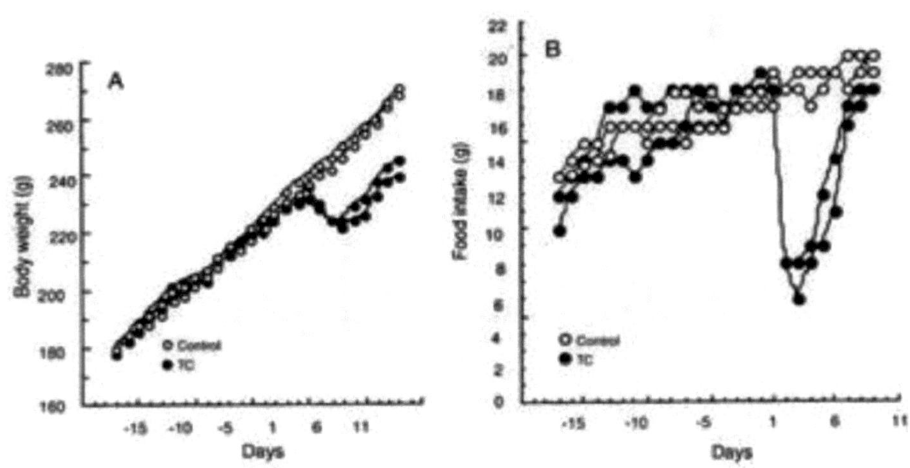


**Figure 8.**
*Changes in body weight and amounts of food intakes after the injection of TC into hypothalamus.*

## 5. Discussion

Obesity pandemic is a great concern for not only health professionals but lay people. Because of such concern, weight loss diets often recommended are the restriction of either carbohydrates or fats. Low fat diets were popular in late 20th century, but carbohydrate restriction became popular in recent years. The proponents of carbohydrate restriction claim that this diet decreased insulin secretion which causes elevated release of free fatty acids from adipose tissues and elevated fat oxidation and energy expenditure. The restriction of carbohydrates was reported to decrease body fat more than restriction of dietary fat [28–30].

On the other hand it is well known that glucose is needed for many brain functions. Although neurons can use lactic acid astrocytes need glucose, which is degraded by glycolysis. ATP produced during glycolysis is used for the uptake of glutamate released from activated neurons [13, 31–33].

Since the administration of glucose or sucrose improved memory functions stated above, we must pay attention to maintaining good brain function in choosing carbohydrate restricted diets.

Glucose ingestion increases blood glucose levels, further insulin levels. Burtman's group showed that insulin is needed for the transportation of tryptophan from blood to brain [34, 35].

Tryptophan is converted in the brain to serotonin, further melatonin [36].

**Figure 9** shows that tryptophan absorbed from the intestine is transported to the brain in the presence of insulin. 5HT; serotonin.

Serotonin is important for many brain functions such as emotion, feeding, sleep resilience or satiety. We showed that increase in serotonin by intraperitoneal injection or by infusion into the hypothalamus of tranylcypromine resulted in inhibition of feeding (**Figures** 7 and **8**).

Thus, glucose administration indirectly affects brain functions by increasing the concentration of serotonin in the brain.

Finally we should not forget the possibility of increased pleasure, thus increased motivation due to the stimulation of pleasure centers such as Nucl.Accumbens by sweet taste of sucrose as reviewed by Berridge and Kringelbach [37].

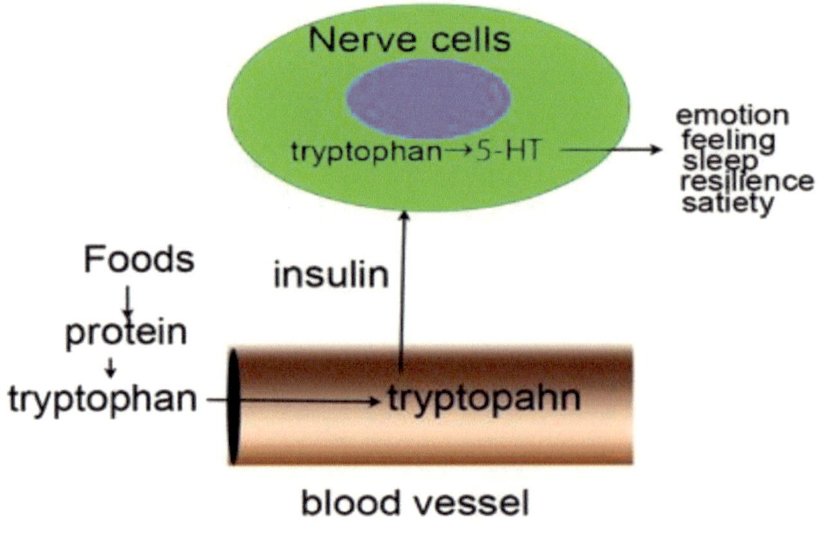


**Figure 9.**
*Tryptophan transport from blood to brain.*

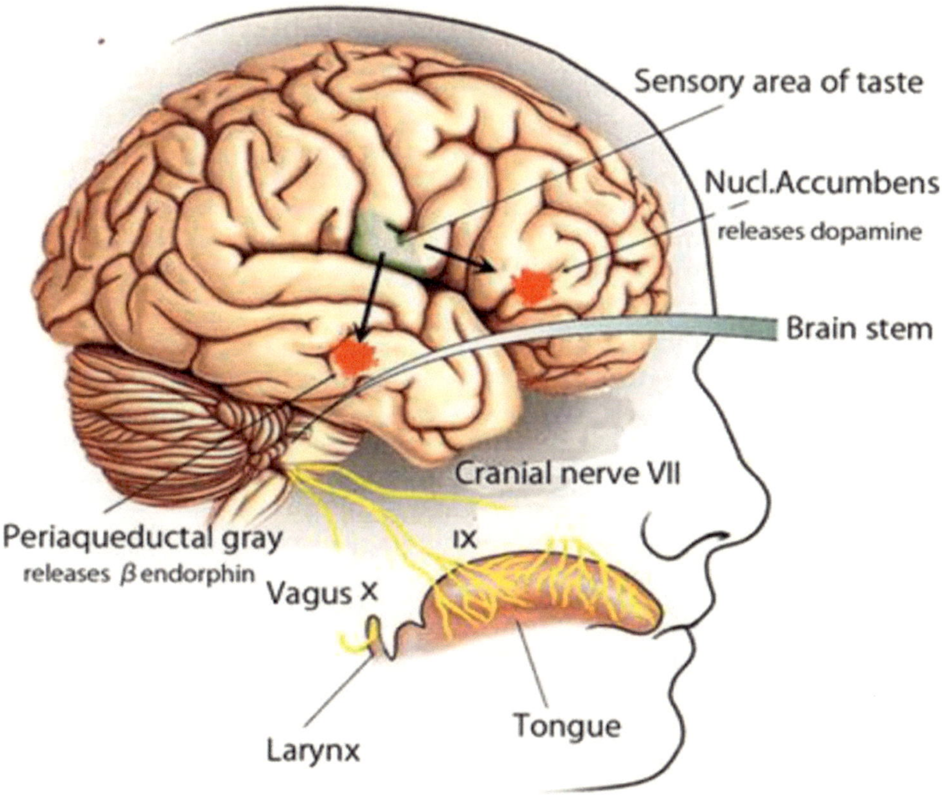


**Figure 10.**
*Brain areas related to the stimulations by taking palatable foods.*

**Figure 10** shows a schematic representation of brain areas stimulated by palatable foods such as sucrose.

Sucrose applied to the taste buds on the tongue stimulates afferent fibers of cranial nerves such as IX or VII, which send informations of the taste to sensory areas of the brain. The stimulations of the taste area further activate Nucl.Accumbens, releasing dopamine and the periaqueductal gray in the midbrain, releasing βendorphin. Such stimulation may enhance the motivation [38, 39].

## 6. Conclusion

Since brain needs glucose for variety of functions, attention must be paid to glucose when various diets related to glucose administration are discussed.

## Conflicts of interest

There is no conflict of interest for any author.

## Author details

Akikazu Takada[1*], Fumiko Shimizu[2], Yukie Ishii[2], M. Ogawa[2] and Tetsuya Takao[2]

1 Faculty of Life and Environmental Sciences, Showa Women's University, Tokyo, Japan

2 International Projects on Food and Health (NPO), Tokyo, Japan

*Address all correspondence to: takada-1a@kmd.biglobe.ne.jp

## References

[1] Eckel RH, York DA, Rossner S, Hubbard V, Caterson I, St Jeor ST, Hayman LL, Mullis RM, Blair SN; American Heart Association. Prevention conference VII: Obesity, a worldwide epidemic related to heart disease and stroke: Executive summary. Circulation. 2004;110: 2968-2975.

[2] World Health Organization. Obesity: Preventing and managing the global epidemic [WHO Technical report series #894]. 2000. Geneva. World Health Organization.

[3] Eckel RH. Obesity and heart disease: A statement for healthcare professionals from the nutrition committee, American Heart Association. Circulation. 1997;96:3248-3250.

[4] Eckel RH, Krauss RM. American Heart Association call to action: Obesity as a major risk factor for coronary heart disease. AHA Nutrition Committee. Circulation. 1998;97:2099-2100.

[5] Klein S, Burke LE, Bray GA, Blair S, Allison DB, Pi-Sunyer X, Hong Y, Eckel RH; American Heart Association Council on nutrition, physical activity, and metabolism. Clinical implications of obesity with specific focus on cardiovascular disease: A statement for professionals from the Am heart association council on nutrition, physical activity, and metabolism: Endorsed by the Am college of cardiology foundation. Circulation. 2004;110:2952-2967.

[6] Hauner H, Bechthold A, Boeing H, Brönstrup A, Buyken A, Leschik-Bonnet E, Linseisen J, Schulze M, Strohm D, Wolfram G Evidence-based guideline of the German nutrition society: Carbohydrate intake and prevention of nutrition-related diseases.; German Nutrition Society. Ann Nutr Metab. 2012;60 Suppl 1:1-58. doi: 10.1159/000335326.

[7] Reivich M, Alavi A. Positron emission tomographic studies of local cerebral glucose metabolism in humans in physiological and pathophysiological conditions. Adv Metab Disord. 1983;10:135-176. doi: 10.1016/b978-0-12-027310-2.50010-4.

[8] Haier RJ, Siegel Jr BV, MacLachlan A, Lottenberg ES, Buchsbaum MS. Regional glucose metabolic changes after learning a complex visuospatial/motor task: A positron emission tomographic study. Brain Res. 1992;570(1-2):134-143. doi: 10.1016/0006-8993(92)90573-r.

[9] Tsacopoulos M, Eviquoz-Mercicr V, Pcrrottct P. Buchncr E Honeybee retinal glial cells transform glucose and supply the neurons with metabolic substrates. Proc Natl Acad Sci USA.1988;85: X727-8731.

[10] Pcllcrin L, Magistretti PJ (1994) Glutamate uptake into astrocytcs stimulates aerobic glycolysis: A mechanism coupling neuronnl activity to glucose utilization. Proc Natl Acad Sci USA. 1994,91;10625-10629.

[11] Takahashi S, Driscoll BF, Law MJ, Sokoloff L. Role of sodium and potassium ions in regulation of glucose metabolism in cultured astroglia. Proc Nat1 Acad Sci USA. 1995, 92:4616-4620.

[12] Duelli R, Kuschinsky W. Brain glucose transpoters: Relationship to local energy demand. New Physiological Sciences. 2001; 16:71-76. doi: 10.1152/physiologyonline.2001.16.2.71.

[13] Takahashi S, Driscoll BF, Law MJ, Sokoloff L. Role of sodium and potassium ions in regulation of glucose metabolism in cultured astroglia. Proc Nat1 Acad Sci USA 1993; 92:4616-4620.

[14] Hall JLL Gonder-Frederick A, Chewning WW, Silveira J, Gold PE.

Glucose enhancement of performance on memory tests in young and aged humans. Neuropsychologia 1989;27:1129-1138.doi: 10.1016/0028-3932(89)90096-1.

[15] Benton D, Parker PY, Donohoe RT. The supply of glucose to the brain and cognitive functioning. Biosoc Sci. 1996;28::463-479. doi: 10.1017/s0021932000022537.

[16] Lund-Anderson H. Transort of glucose from blood to brain. Physiol. Rev. 1998; 59:305-352.

[17] Benton D, Owen D, Parker P. Blood glucose, memory and attention. 1995; Neurpsychologia 1994; 32:595-607.

[18] Gold PE. Role of glucose in regulating the brain and cognition. American Journal of Clinical Nutrition. 1995;61(4Suppl.): 0875-9858.

[19] Manning CA, Rogozzino ME, Gold PE. Glucose enhancement of memory in patients with probable senile dementia of the Alzheimer's type. Neurobiology of Aging. 1993;14:523-528.

[20] van der Zwaluw, N.L., van de Rest, O., Kessels, R.P., de Groot, L.C.,2014 Short-term effects of glucose and sucrose on cognitive performance and mood in elderly people. J Clin Exp Neuropsychol. 36, 517-527

[21] Zamora Navarro S, Pérez llamas F importance of sucrose in cognitive functions: Knowledge and behavior. 2013 Nutr Hosp. Suppl 4:106-111.

[22] Morris RG. Developments of a water-maze procedure for studying spatial learning in rats. 1984 J. Neurosci. Methods 11, 47-60.

[23] Takada A, Ogawa M. Sucrose and brain functions. Obesity: Open Access 2018; 4:1-5. doi.org/10.16966/2380-5528.135

[24] Ogawa, M., Shimizu. F., Ishii, Y., Takao, T., Takada, A. effects of glucose and sucrose administration on the working ability of young women. 2018 Integrative Food, Nutrition and Metabolism 5, 1-4.

[25] Sugimoto, K., Kanai, A., Shoji, N. 2009, The Effectiveness of the Uchida-Kraepelin Test for Psychological Stress: An Analysis of Plasma and Salivary Stress Substances. Biopsychosoc Med. 3, 3-5. doi: 10.1186/1751-0759-3-5

[26] Serotonin in the central nervous system and periphery. 1995.ed. Takada A, Curzon G. International Congress series No. 1088. ISBM 0-444-s1965-7.

[27] Takada Y, Nagai N, Tkahashi H, Urano T, Takada A. Increased serotonergic activities inhibit feedings and cause arousal responses in rats. Biogenic amine 1998; 14:67-77.

[28] Westman EC, Feinman RD, Mavropoulos JC, Vernon MC, Volek JS, Wortman JA, Yancy WS, Phinney SD. Low-carbohydrate nutrition and metabolism. Am J Clin Nutr. 2007; 86:276-284.

[29] Taubes, G. Why we Get Fat and What to Do about it. New York: Alfred A. Knopf; 2011.

[30] Ludwig DS, Friedman MI. Increasing adiposity: Consequence or cause of overeating? JAMA. 2014; 311:2167-2168.

[31] Parker JC, Hoffman JF The role of mcmhranc phosphoglyccratc kinasc in the control of glycolytic rate by active cation transport in human red blood cells. J Gen Physiol 1967; 60:893-916.

[32] Lipton P, Heimbach CJ. Mechanism of extracellular K' stimulation of protein synthesis in the in vitro hippocampus. J Nourochem 1978; 31: 1299-1308.

[33] Lynch RM, B&ban RS. Coupling of aerobic glycolysis and Na' K +-ATPaqc in renal cell line MDCK. Am J Physiol 1987; 253:C269-C276.

[34] Fernstrom JD, Wurtman RJ. Brain serotonin content: Increase following ingestion of carbohydrate diet. Science. 1971;174:1023-1025

[35] Fernstrom JD, Wurtman RJ. Brain serotonin content: Physiological regulation by plasma neutral amino acids. Science. 1972;178:414-416.

[36] Takada A, Shimizu F, Ishii Y, Ogawa M, Takao T. Glucose or sucrose intakes and plasma levels of essential and nonessential amino acids new insights into metabolic syndrome. Ed. Takada A. DOI: 10.5772/intechopen. 92257.

[37] Berridge KC. Measuring hedonic impact in animals and infants: Microstructure of affective taste reactivity patterns. Neurosci Biobehav Rev. 2000;24:173-198. doi: 10.1016/ s0149-7634(99)00072-x.

[38] Berridge KC, Kringelbach ML. Pleasure systems in the brain, Neuron. 2015; 86: 646-664. doi:10.1016/j. neuron.2015.02.018.

[39] Bartoshuk L. The measurement of pleasure and pain. Perspectives on Psychological Science. 2014; 9:91-93.

Chapter 4

# Circadian Clock, Sleep, and Diet

*Junichiro Irie*

## Abstract

Circadian rhythm is a fundamental process of sustaining metabolic homeostasis by predicting changes in the environment. This is driven by biological clocks, which operate within a 24-h period to orchestrate daily variation of metabolism and sleep. The central clock in the hypothalamus is the master keeper of the circadian rhythm and is primarily reset by light, while the feeding-fasting rhythm, that is, nutritional stimulus, entrains peripheral clocks in peripheral organs such as the intestine and liver. Nutritional stimuli are important modulators of peripheral circadian rhythms and may affect the central clock and sleep homeostasis through metabolic alterations. In this chapter, I will summarize the significance of circadian rhythm and sleep in metabolic regulation as well as discuss the impact that diet has on circadian rhythm and sleep.

**Keywords:** circadian rhythm, sleep, clock gene, intestinal microbiota, jet lag

## 1. Introduction

The term circadian rhythm refers to the natural and internal process that regulates the sleep-wake cycle in all mammals, and repeats about every 24 h, which is almost the same as the rotation of the earth. Circadian rhythm is not only an important mechanism for the sleep-wake cycle, but also for the homeostasis of endocrine and metabolic systems that rely on the body to predict and adapts to changing environments during daytime and nighttime. Since the circadian rhythm is maintained even in the absence of light stimulation, this rhythm is called the "circadian clock" and determines diurnal fluctuations such as blood pressure and body temperature [1]. In mammals, the suprachiasmatic nucleus (SCN) in the hypothalamus of the brain is the master keeper of circadian rhythms, and it also controls the circadian rhythms of other organs. Animals in which the SCN has been damaged are unable to perform circadian activities, and the transplantation of the SCN restores their circadian rhythm. SCN neurons form a network and transmit circadian rhythms by transcription factors CLOCK, BMAL1, and Period (Per) and Cryptochrome (CRY), which suppress their activities.

Although the circadian clock is best known for producing 24-h cycle rhythms in movements, metabolism, and hormones, a circadian rhythm also exists in peripheral organs, including the liver and digestive tract. These rhythms are called peripheral clocks. In addition to the rhythms of clock genes in peripheral organs, nutritional stimuli, such as diet, have also been shown to modulate circadian rhythms in peripheral organs. Furthermore, the circadian rhythms in peripheral organs likely affect the central clocks and *vice versa*.

In this chapter, we will focus on the role that circadian rhythms play in systemic metabolism as well as the role that nutritional stimuli play in circadian rhythm and sleep.

## 2. The circadian rhythms and metabolic regulation

Circadian rhythms can be found in humans, including a sleep-wake rhythm, an eating-hunger rhythm, and hormonal fluctuations that occur on a roughly 24-h cycle that is synchronized with the light-dark cycle [2]. This rhythm is mainly driven by the biological clock, which in mammals consists of a central clock located in the hypothalamus and a peripheral clock in other organs. Light is the main environmental synchronizer of the central clock, while eating and motion synchronize the peripheral clock. Optical signals are transmitted from the central clock to peripheral organs, such as the skin and muscles, and regulate the circadian rhythm of the cell cycle and insulin sensitivity [3].

In mammals, the circadian clock is mainly tuned by transcription factors called Circadian Locomotor Output Cycles Kaput (CLOCK) and brain and muscle ARNT-like protein-1 (BMAL1), which form a heterodimer and activate transcription of target genes in the light phase [4, 5]. They target genes that suppress biological clocks such as Per (Period) and Cry (Cryptochrome), which suppress the transcription of CLOCK-BMAL1 in the dark phase [5]. The clock gene circuit is also regulated by the nuclear receptors retinoic acid receptor-related orphan receptor (ROR) and REV-ERB, which regulate Bmal1 gene expression positively and negatively, respectively. In addition to the transcriptional feedback loop of clock genes, various oscillations of gene expression are modulated by the regulation of transcription factors other than clock genes [6].

Circadian rhythms in the expression of genes and proteins have also been observed in peripheral organs such as the liver and intestine. In fact, approximately 30% of gene expression in the intestinal tract shows a circadian rhythm, and this is also observed in the proliferation of intestinal epithelium and intestinal permeability. A circadian rhythm can also be observed in the blood concentration of triglyceride-rich lipoproteins synthesized in the intestinal tract [7, 8]. Furthermore, clock genes such as Clock and Bmal1 are expressed in the gastrointestinal tract, and their expression is particularly high in the lower gastrointestinal tract and large intestine, with the expression site found mainly in the epithelial layer rather than the mucosal layer [8].

These clock genes affect the functions of the intestine by altering the expression of target genes, such as sodium-glucose cotransporter (SGLT) 1, which is involved in glucose absorption and peptide transporter (PEPT) 1, which is involved in peptide absorption. In mice, the transporter involved in glucose uptake increases in the dark phase, while the peptide transporter increases during the light phase. Similarly, a diurnal variation was observed in lipid absorption, and the number of genes involved in lipid absorption increased in the dark phase. Additionally, it has been reported that in mice with a clock gene mutation, the absorption of sugar, triglyceride, and cholesterol from intestinal contents was higher and the absorption of peptides was lower. In addition to intestinal epithelial cells, enteroendocrine cells, such as ghrelin-producing cells, are also regulated by clock genes such as Bmal1 and Per1/2. For example, in *Bmal1*-deficient mice, no diurnal variation in ghrelin nor diurnal variation in feeding was observed [9, 10]. It has also been reported that a circadian rhythm is observed in the expression of toll-like receptors in the small intestine, which is involved in intestinal immunity [11]. Since diurnal rhythms in the function of the intestine were first observed, it was assumed that they may affect the intestinal microbiota in the intestinal lumen. Recent findings have revealed that the intestinal microbiota plays a pivotal role in the regulation of host homeostasis [12–16]. Importantly, several groups have reported diurnal oscillations of intestinal microbiota [17–19]. The bacteria belonging to Clostridiales and Lactobacillaceae showed diurnal variation, and at the species level, *Lactobacillus reuteri* decreased and *Dehalobacterium* increased in the dark phase. Along with the diurnal changes in the composition of intestinal bacteria, diurnal fluctuations are also observed in the functions of the microbiota, such as vitamin and nucleic acid metabolism by the bacteria. The functions of DNA repair, cell proliferation, and mucin degradation were dominant in the dark phase, whereas bacterial motility and sensing pathways were dominant in the light phase. The diurnal rhythm in intestinal microbiota was also examined in humans, and it was found that *Parabacteroides* and *Bulleidia* were increased in the daytime and decreased at night, while *Lachnospira* decreased in the daytime and increased in the nighttime. This is consistent with the findings in mice and suggests that there are diurnal rhythms in protein synthesis as it primarily occurs in the daytime.

These findings demonstrate that peripheral organs, including intestinal microbiota, have circadian rhythms and systemically modulate energy homeostasis and metabolism.

## 3. The nutritional stimuli and circadian rhythms

Metabolic homeostasis is modulated by circadian rhythms, as mentioned above, but nutritional stimuli affect circadian rhythms and vice versa.

Importantly, the circadian rhythm found in gene expression is tissue-specific, and the type and number of oscillating genes differ depending on the type of tissue or cell [20]. Transcriptional factors can define tissue specificities and result in the diversity of chromatin structures, but an oscillation has been reported to be reconstructed by various nutritional stimuli [6, 21–23]. Notably, the molecular mechanism by which metabolic alterations affect circadian rhythms has been investigated intensively. For example, the transcriptional factors SREBP1 and PPARs, which are related to lipid metabolism, are activated periodically by the intake of a high-fat diet, thereby driving the specific oscillation of gene expression [24, 25]. It has also been shown that fluctuations in energy metabolites are deeply involved in transcriptional regulation. Acetyl-CoA is used as an acetylating substrate for histones and clock genes, and NAD modulates the oscillation of gene expression by acting as a coenzyme for sirtuins that deacetylate proteins [26, 27]. The acetylation of histones is also conducted by S-adenosylmethionine (SAM) by the transfer of a methyl donor from SAM. S-adenosylhomocysteine (SAH) is produced from SAM by methyltransferases. Interestingly, the SAH hydrolyzing enzyme binds to clock genes and contributes to the interaction among methionine metabolism, clock gene expression, and chromatin remodeling [28]. These findings indicate the adaptability and plasticity of transcriptional regulation of clock genes, which flexibly respond to metabolic changes, and imply the existence of a circuit in which transcriptional and metabolic rhythms regulate each other.

The impact of the timing of the nutritional stimuli has also been investigated. The exposure of the intestine to the nutrients is fundamental, but bile acids in the intestine secreted from the liver are also reported to be important regulators to elicit circadian rhythms [29]. Importantly, time-restricted feeding (TRF), which limits feeding time, has been reported to be a good method for restoring circadian rhythms by modulating nutritional stimuli. Even when the food had the same amount of energy in this model, if the feeding time was limited to less than nine hours a day (TRF) in comparison with the mice fed ad libitum for 24 h, the suppression of body fat accumulation and

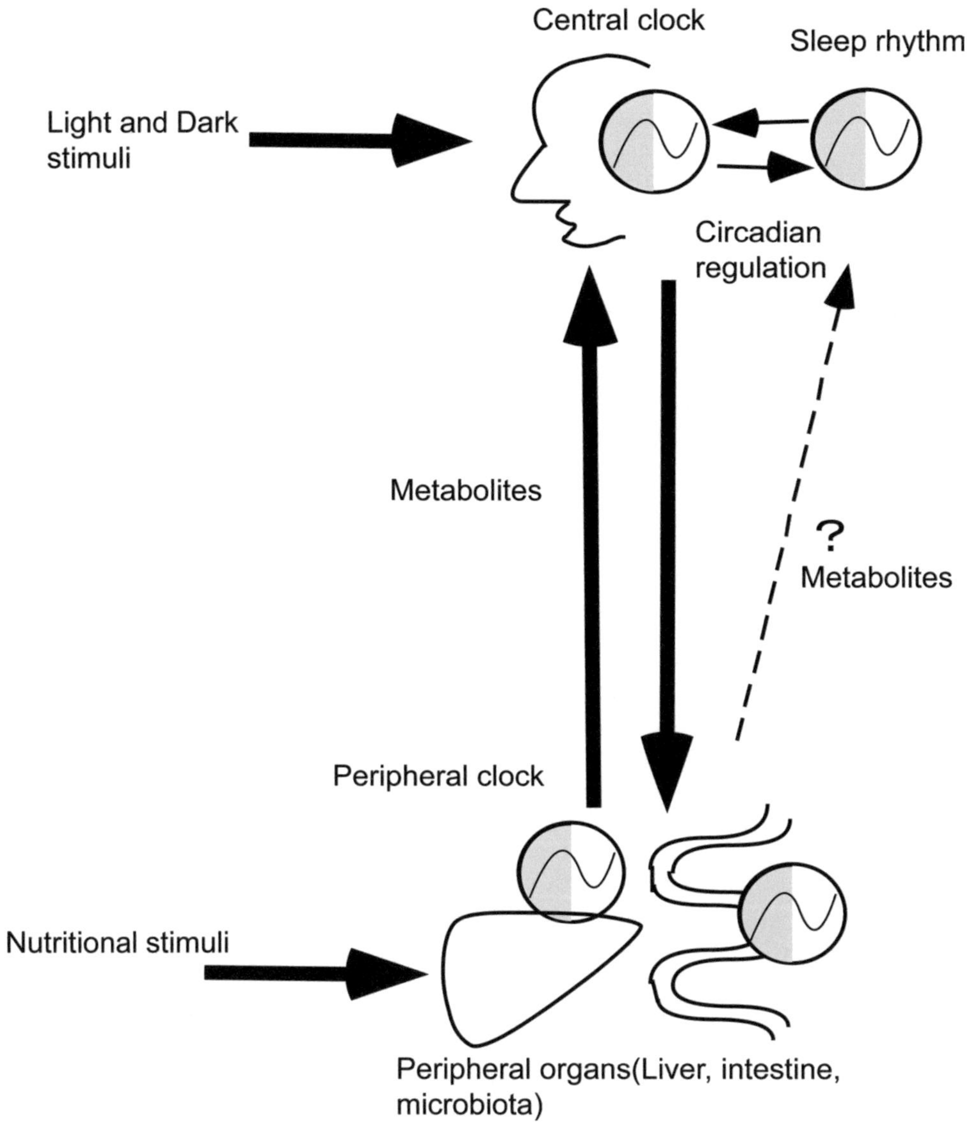


**Figure 1.**
*The interaction between the circadian rhythm in the central nervous system (CNS), peripheral organs, and sleep. The central clock in the hypothalamus is the master keeper of circadian rhythm and is primarily entrained by light and dark stimuli, while feeding-fasting rhythm, that is, nutritional stimuli, entrains peripheral clocks in peripheral organs such as the liver and intestine. Sleep rhythm is evoked mainly by the central clock, and disturbed sleep affects the circadian rhythm in the CNS. The rhythm in peripheral organs that is regulated by nutritional stimuli may modulate sleep rhythm.*

the improvement of glucose intolerance were observed [30, 31]. In addition, TRF improved the metabolic disarrangement found in various organs, and the circadian rhythm of intestinal bacteria and functions recovered. These findings indicate that nutritional stimuli. That is, diet is an important regulator of circadian rhythm and systemic metabolism (**Figure 1**).

## 4. The sleep, circadian rhythm, and the intestine

The sleep-wake cycle is a good example of the circadian rhythms found in living organisms that are regulated by many biological and environmental factors.

In humans, sleep regulation is governed by homeostatic mechanisms and circadian rhythms, that is, a two-process model [32, 33]. In this model, sleep is regulated by sleep homeostasis (process S) and circadian rhythm (process C; circadian rhythm) (**Figure 2**). Sleep controlled through homeostasis means that sleep debt increases during wakefulness and decreases with sleep; thus, when the sleep debt reaches the sleep threshold, humans fall asleep and when it reaches the lower limit, humans awaken. It is believed that this threshold is dominated by the circadian rhythm, and diurnal variation is observed (process C). This idea is that daytime awakening and nighttime sleep are determined by the sleep debt that accumulates by continuing to stay awake and drowsiness that is induced by the biological clock. It is understood to be a system that compensates for sleep time in response to changes in the environment while physiologically promoting sleep *via* circadian rhythm.

When mammals sleep, rapid eye movement (REM) sleep and non-rapid eye movement sleep (non-REM sleep) occur in a cycle of about 90 min. When you fall asleep, non-REM sleep appears first. Subsequently, light REM sleep appears. REM sleep is accompanied by rapid eye movements, and the body is in a resting state with relaxed skeletal muscles, but the brain is active and awake. The cerebral cortex is more active than during wakefulness, and electroencephalography (EEG) shows mainly theta waves from 4 to 7 Hz and exhibits an amplitude close to that during awakening. Sleep without REM is called non-REM sleep, and the brain is in the so-called state of deep sleep. Low-frequency, high-amplitude brain waves called delta waves ranging from 1-4 Hz are observed in brain waves, and non-REM sleep is characterized as slow-wave sleep based on EEG findings. However, the molecular mechanism(s) underlying the cyclical changes that occur in non-REM sleep and REM sleep are not yet clear.

Sleep disturbances deteriorate the circadian rhythms across various organs. For example, when mice were subjected to sleep disturbances in which the light and dark phases were changed weekly, the circadian rhythm of *Per2* expression in the large intestine disappeared, and the intestinal microbiota was altered, with increased Firmicutes and decreased Bacteroidetes at the phylum level [34]. Other sleep disorders have been reported to increase intestinal permeability and blood LPS levels [35]. In addition, the effects of interventions that cause sleep disorders using tactile stimulation without changing the cycle of light and dark phases have also been investigated, in which the cycle of light stimulation is

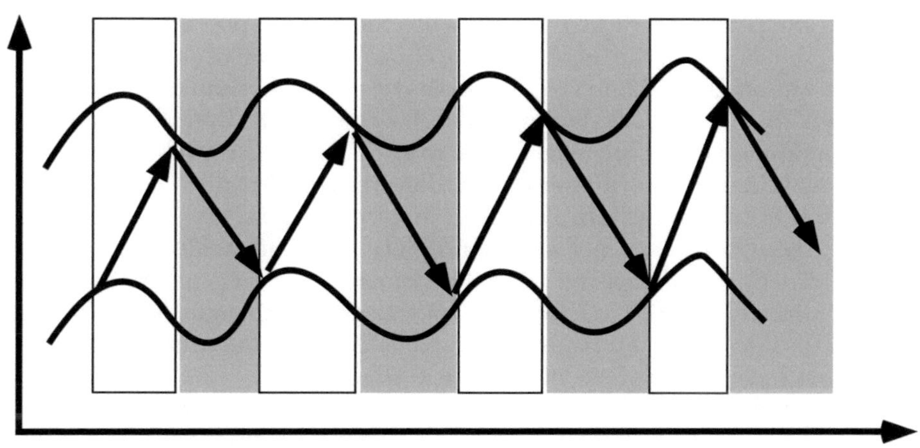

**Figure 2.**
*A two-process model of sleep. Sleep debt accumulates during awakening, and sleep is encouraged when the sleep threshold is reached. Sleep reduces sleep debt and awakens when the wake threshold is reached. Sleep debt increases during awakening and decreases during sleep (process S). The sleep-wake threshold fluctuates diurnal (process C).*

periodic. An increase in Lachnospiraceae and Ruminococcaceae and a decrease in Lactobacillaceae and Bifidobacteriaceae were observed after a 4-week sleep disturbance [36]. Furthermore, the intestinal contents, such as propionate and citrate, changed after the intervention, indicating functional changes in the intestinal microbiota. When intestinal bacteria from sleep-disturbed mice were transplanted into germ-free mice, the blood levels of inflammatory cytokines, such as IL-6, increased and insulin resistance was exacerbated in the recipient mice. The blood concentration of lipopolysaccharide-binding protein (LBP), which transports LPS to the CD14-TLR4-MD2 complex on the cell membrane of macrophages, was also increased in sleep-disordered mice. The effects of sleep disturbance without alteration of meals and motions in life were also examined in humans. A randomized crossover study was conducted in which nine healthy subjects slept for about 4 h for two days and about 8 h for two days with equal daily activities other than sleep. A short sleep for two days increased Firmicutes, and decreased Bacteroidetes in the intestine as well as worsened insulin resistance and glucose tolerance [37]. These findings demonstrate that sleep disturbances deteriorate the central and peripheral circadian rhythms, leading to metabolic disorders.

## 5. The stimuli from the intestine, circadian rhythm, and sleep

From the abovementioned examination of sleep disturbances in animals and humans, it was shown that sleep disturbances distort circadian rhythms in the central nervous system and peripheral organs. As mentioned above, the circadian rhythm in the intestine is regulated by the central and peripheral clocks as well as nutritional stimuli, that is, dietary intake. Therefore, the possibility of recovery of the host's circadian rhythm and the control of sleep *via* the intestine is being investigated. In fact, even in Per1/2-deficient mice, diurnal oscillation in the intestinal microbiota was observed by feeding them in a timely fashion.

Recently, Leone et al. compared the expression of clock genes Bmal1 and Clock in the medial basal hypothalamus and liver of germ-free mice with that of control mice and found that circadian rhythms diminished in the germ-free mice [19]. The mechanism by which intestinal bacteria regulate the circadian rhythm of the liver and hypothalamus has also been investigated, and butyric acid, a metabolite of intestinal bacteria, was found to be a key molecule in tuning the circadian rhythm in the CNS and peripheral organs. In fact, when butyric acid was administered to hepatic organoids *in vitro*, an increase in the circadian rhythm of Per2 and Bmal1 expression was observed. Moreover, when butyric acid was injected into germ-free mice every 12 h, the circadian rhythm of the clock gene in the liver reappeared, and the amplitude of the clock gene tended to be enhanced in the medial basal hypothalamus. Consistent with this report, the circadian rhythm of Bmal1 and Cry1 in the intestinal epithelium disappears in mice in which intestinal bacteria are reduced by the administration of a set of antibiotics [38]. Bile acids deconjugated by intestinal bacteria are an important signal for tuning the clock genes in the intestine by dietary stimuli [12, 39]. Therefore, it is considered that changing the circadian rhythm of the intestine by nutritional stimuli could change the circadian rhythm in other organs, including the CNS, and may also affect sleep.

In terms of the stimuli from the intestine to modulate sleep, various modulations have been examined. The muramyl peptide derived from the cell wall of bacteria, LPS, and inflammatory cytokines such as IL-1b, TNF-a, and IL-18 have been reported to promote sleep [40, 41]. These microbial products prolonged and increased non-REM sleep and reduced REM sleep in model animals. In humans without infectious diseases, the levels of serum IL-1b and TNF-a showed a circadian rhythm, which peaked at night and troughed at dawn, implying that these molecules may be a trigger for falling asleep [42]. Studies on sleep have also been conducted using antibiotic agents to modulate stimuli from the intestine. For example, one study administered a single dose of 200 mg of minocycline or 500 mg of ampicillin to 19 healthy men and found that administration of minocycline significantly reduced the proportion of non-REM sleep, an effect that lasted for two days. No effect was observed on REM sleep, and ampicillin did not affect either non-REM sleep or REM sleep [43]. These findings imply that changes in the gut microbiota may lead to improved sleep quantity and quality. Considering that long-term administration of antibiotics is not realistic in clinics, prebiotics and probiotics have been intensively investigated. It was reported that administration of *Lactobacillus brevis* to mice increased physical activity, prolonged waking hours, and reduced non-REM sleep [44]. Similarly, the administration of prebiotics containing lactoferrin to rats prevented the expected decrease in non-REM sleep due to electric shock [45]. In humans, many clinical trials have been conducted to evaluate the effects of prebiotics and probiotics on sleep. For example, the daily administration of *Lactobacillus gasseri* CP2305 for five weeks was reported to improve sleep quality in healthy volunteers, with a reduction in the amount of intestinal Enterobacteriaceae [46, 47]. Additionally, administration of a probiotic mixture of *Lactobacillus fermentum*, *L. rhamnosus*, *L. plantarum*, and *Bifidobacterium longum* for six weeks was reported to improve sleep quality [48]. Nevertheless, more studies are needed to conclude that modulation of nutritional stimuli from the intestine changes circadian rhythm and sleep quality.

## 6. Conclusions

The mechanisms by which circadian rhythm and sleep regulate systemic metabolism and nutritional stimuli from the intestine modulate circadian rhythm and sleep were summarized and discussed dietary therapies could be a novel treatment strategy for both metabolic and sleep disorders, although future studies are needed to validate these strategies.

## Acknowledgements

This work was supported in part by the Japan Society for the Promotion of Science (JSPS) KAKENHI Grant-in-Aid (C) 16K09374 and the Japan Agency for Medical Research and Development (Grant JP21gm1010007s0505).

## Author details

Junichiro Irie[1,2]

1 Division of Endocrinology, Metabolism, and Nephrology, Department of Internal Medicine, Keio University School of Medicine, Tokyo, Japan

2 Japan Agency for Medical Research and Development-Core Research for Evolutionary Medical Science and Technology (AMED-CREST), Japan Agency for Medical Research and Development, Tokyo, Japan

*Address all correspondence to: j-irie@z8.keio.jp

## References

[1] Huang W, Ramsey KM, Marcheva B, Bass J. Circadian rhythms, sleep, and metabolism. The Journal of Clinical Investigation. 2011;**121**:2133-2141

[2] Schibler U, Sassone-Corsi P. A web of circadian pacemakers. Cell. 2002;**111**:919-922

[3] Aras E, Ramadori G, Kinouchi K, Liu Y, Ioris RM, Brenachot X, et al. Light entrains diurnal changes in insulin sensitivity of skeletal muscle via ventromedial hypothalamic neurons. Cell Reports. 2019;**27**:2385-2398 e2383

[4] Asher G, Sassone-Corsi P. Time for food: The intimate interplay between nutrition, metabolism, and the circadian clock. Cell. 2015;**161**:84-92

[5] Reppert SM, Weaver DR. Coordination of circadian timing in mammals. Nature. 2002;**418**:935-941

[6] Pastore N, Vainshtein A, Herz NJ, Huynh T, Brunetti L, Klisch TJ, et al. Nutrient-sensitive transcription factors TFEB and TFE3 couple autophagy and metabolism to the peripheral clock. EMBO Journal. 2019;**38**:e101347

[7] Konturek PC, Brzozowski T, Konturek SJ. Gut clock: Implication of circadian rhythms in the gastrointestinal tract. Journal of Physiology and Pharmacology. 2011;**62**:139-150

[8] Pan X, Hussain MM. Clock is important for food and circadian regulation of macronutrient absorption in mice. Journal of Lipid Research. 2009;**50**:1800-1813

[9] Laermans J, Vancleef L, Tack J, Depoortere I. Role of the clock gene Bmal1 and the gastric ghrelin-secreting cell in the circadian regulation of the ghrelin-GOAT system. Scientific Reports. 2015;**5**:16748

[10] LeSauter J, Hoque N, Weintraub M, Pfaff DW, Silver R. Stomach ghrelin-secreting cells as food-entrainable circadian clocks. Proceedings of the National Academy of Sciences of the United States of America. 2009;**106**: 13582-13587

[11] Froy O, Chapnik N. Circadian oscillation of innate immunity components in mouse small intestine. Molecular Immunology. 2007;**44**: 1954-1960

[12] Kusumoto Y, Irie J, Iwabu K, Tagawa H, Itoh A, Kato M, et al. Bile acid binding resin prevents fat accumulation through intestinal microbiota in high-fat diet-induced obesity in mice. Metabolism. 2017;**71**:1-6

[13] Yoshifuji A, Wakino S, Irie J, Tajima T, Hasegawa K, Kanda T, et al. Gut Lactobacillus protects against the progression of renal damage by modulating the gut environment in rats. Nephrology, Dialysis, Transplantation. 2016;**31**:401-412

[14] Irie J, Kanno Y, Kikuchi R, Yoshida T, Murai S, Watanabe M, et al. L-Carnitine improves gastrointestinal disorders and altered the intestinal microbiota in hemodialysis patients. Bioscience of Microbiota, Food and Health. 2017;**36**:11-16

[15] Kikuchi R, Irie J, Yamada-Goto N, Kikkawa E, Seki Y, Kasama K, et al. The impact of laparoscopic sleeve gastrectomy with duodenojejunal bypass on intestinal microbiota differs from that of laparoscopic sleeve gastrectomy in Japanese patients with obesity. Clinical Drug Investigation. 2018;**38**:545-552

[16] Kimura I, Miyamoto J, Ohue-Kitano R, Watanabe K, Yamada T, Onuki M, et al. Maternal gut microbiota in pregnancy influences offspring

metabolic phenotype in mice. Science. 2020;**367**:eaaw8429

[17] Thaiss CA, Zeevi D, Levy M, Zilberman-Schapira G, Suez J, Tengeler AC, et al. Transkingdom control of microbiota diurnal oscillations promotes metabolic homeostasis. Cell. 2014;**159**:514-529

[18] Liang X, Bushman FD, FitzGerald GA. Rhythmicity of the intestinal microbiota is regulated by gender and the host circadian clock. Proceedings of the National Academy of Sciences of the United States of America. 2015;**112**:10479-10484

[19] Leone V, Gibbons SM, Martinez K, Hutchison AL, Huang EY, Cham CM, et al. Effects of diurnal variation of gut microbes and high-fat feeding on host circadian clock function and metabolism. Cell Host & Microbe. 2015;**17**:681-689

[20] Zhang R, Lahens NF, Ballance HI, Hughes ME, Hogenesch JB. A circadian gene expression atlas in mammals: Implications for biology and medicine. Proceedings of the National Academy of Sciences of the United States of America. 2014;**111**:16219-16224

[21] Tognini P, Samad M, Kinouchi K, Liu Y, Helbling JC, Moisan MP, et al. Reshaping circadian metabolism in the suprachiasmatic nucleus and prefrontal cortex by nutritional challenge. Proceedings of the National Academy of Sciences of the United States of America. 2020;**117**:29904-29913

[22] Tognini P, Murakami M, Liu Y, Eckel-Mahan KL, Newman JC, Verdin E, et al. Distinct circadian signatures in liver and gut clocks revealed by ketogenic diet. Cell Metabolism. 2017;**26**:523-538 e525

[23] Kinouchi K, Magnan C, Ceglia N, Liu Y, Cervantes M, Pastore N, et al. Fasting imparts a switch to alternative daily pathways in liver and muscle. Cell Reports. 2018;**25**:3299-3314 e3296

[24] Eckel-Mahan KL, Patel VR, de Mateo S, Orozco-Solis R, Ceglia NJ, Sahar S, et al. Reprogramming of the circadian clock by nutritional challenge. Cell. 2013;**155**:1464-1478

[25] Guan D, Xiong Y, Borck PC, Jang C, Doulias PT, Papazyan R, et al. Diet-induced Circadian enhancer remodeling synchronizes opposing hepatic lipid metabolic processes. Cell. 2018;**174**: 831-842 e812

[26] Doi M, Hirayama J, Sassone-Corsi P. Circadian regulator CLOCK is a histone acetyltransferase. Cell. 2006;**125**: 497-508

[27] Ramsey KM, Yoshino J, Brace CS, Abrassart D, Kobayashi Y, Marcheva B, et al. Circadian clock feedback cycle through NAMPT-mediated NAD+ biosynthesis. Science. 2009;**324**: 651-654

[28] Greco CM, Cervantes M, Fustin JM, Ito K, Ceglia N, Samad M, et al. S-adenosyl-l-homocysteine hydrolase links methionine metabolism to the circadian clock and chromatin remodeling. Science Advances. 2020;**6**

[29] Yang Y, Zhang J. Bile acid metabolism and circadian rhythms. American Journal of Physiology. Gastrointestinal and Liver Physiology. 2020;**319**:G549-G563

[30] Zarrinpar A, Chaix A, Yooseph S, Panda S. Diet and feeding pattern affect the diurnal dynamics of the gut microbiome. Cell Metabolism. 2014;**20**:1006-1017

[31] Hatori M, Vollmers C, Zarrinpar A, DiTacchio L, Bushong EA, Gill S, et al. Time-restricted feeding without reducing caloric intake prevents metabolic diseases in mice fed a high-fat diet. Cell Metabolism. 2012;**15**:848-860

[32] Borbely AA. A two process model of sleep regulation. Human Neurobiology. 1982;**1**:195-204

[33] Daan S, Beersma DG, Borbely AA. Timing of human sleep: Recovery process gated by a circadian pacemaker. The American Journal of Physiology. 1984;**246**:R161-R183

[34] Voigt RM, Forsyth CB, Green SJ, Mutlu E, Engen P, Vitaterna MH, et al. Circadian disorganization alters intestinal microbiota. PLoS One. 2014;**9**:e97500

[35] Summa KC, Voigt RM, Forsyth CB, Shaikh M, Cavanaugh K, Tang Y, et al. Disruption of the Circadian clock in mice increases intestinal permeability and promotes alcohol-induced hepatic pathology and inflammation. PLoS One. 2013;**8**:e67102

[36] Poroyko VA, Carreras A, Khalyfa A, Khalyfa AA, Leone V, Peris E, et al. Chronic sleep disruption alters gut microbiota, Induces Systemic and Adipose Tissue Inflammation and Insulin Resistance in Mice. Scientific Reports. 2016;**6**:35405

[37] Benedict C, Vogel H, Jonas W, Woting A, Blaut M, Schurmann A, et al. Gut microbiota and glucometabolic alterations in response to recurrent partial sleep deprivation in normal-weight young individuals. Molecular Metabolism. 2016;**5**:1175-1186

[38] Mukherji A, Kobiita A, Ye T, Chambon P. Homeostasis in intestinal epithelium is orchestrated by the circadian clock and microbiota cues transduced by TLRs. Cell. 2013;**153**:812-827

[39] Govindarajan K, MacSharry J, Casey PG, Shanahan F, Joyce SA, Gahan CG. Unconjugated bile acids influence expression of circadian genes: A potential mechanism for microbe-host crosstalk. PLoS One. 2016;**11**: e0167319

[40] Krueger JM, Bacsik J, Garcia-Arraras J. Sleep-promoting material from human urine and its relation to factor S from brain. The American Journal of Physiology. 1980;**238**:E116-E123

[41] Krueger JM, Pappenheimer JR, Karnovsky ML. The composition of sleep-promoting factor isolated from human urine. The Journal of Biological Chemistry. 1982;**257**:1664-1669

[42] Galland L. The gut microbiome and the brain. Journal of Medicinal Food. 2014;**17**:1261-1272

[43] Nonaka K, Nakazawa Y, Kotorii T. Effects of antibiotics, minocycline and ampicillin, on human sleep. Brain Research. 1983;**288**:253-259

[44] Miyazaki K, Itoh N, Yamamoto S, Higo-Yamamoto S, Nakakita Y, Kaneda H, et al. Dietary heat-killed Lactobacillus brevis SBC8803 promotes voluntary wheel-running and affects sleep rhythms in mice. Life Sciences. 2014;**111**:47-52

[45] Thompson RS, Roller R, Mika A, Greenwood BN, Knight R, Chichlowski M, et al. Dietary prebiotics and bioactive milk fractions improve NREM sleep, enhance REM sleep rebound and attenuate the stress-induced decrease in diurnal temperature and gut microbial alpha diversity. Frontiers in Behavioral Neuroscience. 2016;**10**:240

[46] Nishida K, Sawada D, Kawai T, Kuwano Y, Fujiwara S, Rokutan K. Para-psychobiotic Lactobacillus gasseri CP2305 ameliorates stress-related symptoms and sleep quality. Journal of Applied Microbiology. 2017;**123**: 1561-1570

[47] Sawada D, Kawai T, Nishida K, Kuwano Y, Fujiwara S, Rokutan K. Daily intake of Lactobacillus gasseri CP2305 improves mental, physical, and sleep

quality among Japanese medical students enrolled in a cadaver dissection course. Journal of Functional Foods. 2017;**31**:188-197

[48] Marotta A, Sarno E, Del Casale A, Pane M, Mogna L, Amoruso A, et al. Effects of probiotics on cognitive reactivity, mood, and sleep quality. Frontiers in Psychiatry. 2019;**10**:164

Section 2

# Diabetes Mellitus and Disorders of the Metabolism

Chapter 5

# ER Stress Response Failure and Steatohepatitis Comorbid with Diabetes

*Takayoshi Sasako and Kohjiro Ueki*

## Abstract

Dynamic metabolic changes occur in the liver during the transition between fasting and eating, which is mainly mediated by insulin, a hormone to promote anabolism and suppress catabolism. In obesity and diabetes, insulin resistance is induced via various mechanisms, and among them is endoplasmic reticulum (ER) stress. We recently reported that eating induces transient ER stress and consequent ER stress response in the liver. During eating, expression of Sdf2l1, an ER-resident molecule involved in ER stress-associated degradation, is induced as a part of ER stress response. XBP-1s regulates expression of Sdf2l1 at the transcription level, and Sdf2l1 terminates eating-induced ER stress in the liver, consequently regulating glucose and lipid metabolism. In obesity and diabetes, however, ER stress response is impaired, partly because insulin-mediated translocation of XBP-1s to the nucleus is suppressed, which results in further excessive ER stress. Induction of Sdf2l1 by XBP-1s is highly down-regulated, but restoration of Sdf2l1 ameliorates glucose intolerance and fatty liver. In diabetic patients, hepatic insulin resistance induces enhanced ER stress and ER stress response failure in the liver, which in turn promote hepatic fibrosis and contribute to the development of steatohepatitis comorbid with diabetes.

**Keywords:** liver, insulin signaling, insulin resistance, diabetes mellitus, feeding, endoplasmic reticulum stress, stromal cell-derived factor 2 like 1, X-box binding protein 1, fatty liver

## 1. Introduction

Organisms need to take in nutrients from outside for biological activities and survival, and deprivation of nutrients is a heavy burden for organisms. However, various responses are induced even during eating, in order to cope with the rapid influx of nutrients. The liver plays pivotal roles in the maintenance of systemic nutritional homeostasis depending on the feeding conditions, and dynamic changes are induced during the transition between fasting and feeding, or eating. During fasting, the liver releases glucose by glycogenolysis and gluconeogenesis, and ketone bodies by fatty acid oxidation, while during feeding, it stores excessive nutrition derived from food by synthesizing glycogen and fatty acids. Conversely, dysregulation of these processes may lead to metabolic disorders, such as insulin resistance and fatty liver disease [1].

In this chapter, we are going to discuss physiological and patho-physiological aspects of stress response during eating, by reviewing the insulin signaling cascade first, then endoplasmic reticulum (ER) stress, which is becoming an emerging player in the regulation of metabolism in the liver, and finally the roles of ER stress response failure in the development of steatohepatitis comorbid with diabetes.

## 2. Insulin action and downstream molecules

Insulin is the major regulator of metabolism which is secreted from pancreatic beta cells, and it promotes anabolism and suppresses catabolism in the targeted tissues including the liver [2–5].

In the early 1980s, tyrosine kinase activity of insulin receptor was first reported [6], and the whole cascade of the signaling has been uncovered in the past 40 years. In brief, in the presence of insulin, IR (insulin receptor) phosphorylates IRSs (insulin receptor substrates). Among the isoforms of IRSs, IRS-1 and IRS-2 are the major ones, and they activate two main signaling pathways: the PI3K (phosphatidylinositol 3-kinase)-Akt/PKB (protein kinase B) pathway and the Ras–MAPK (mitogen-activated protein kinase) pathway. The former is mainly responsible for metabolic actions of insulin, and the latter mainly regulates cell growth and differentiation [5] (**Figure 1**).

In obesity and diabetes, however, the insulin signaling cascade is impaired by various mechanisms despite normal or high concentrations of insulin, which is called insulin resistance. It is generally thought that serine/threonine kinases, such as PKC (protein kinase C), JNK (c-jun N-terminal kinases), IKKβ (inhibitor of nuclear factor kappa-B kinase subunit β), and PP2A (protein phosphatase 2A), are activated in obesity via lipotoxicity, inflammation, hyperglycemia, mitochondrial dysfunction and subsequent oxidative stress, and ER stress, which is reviewed in the following subsection. Serine/threonine kinases thus activated in

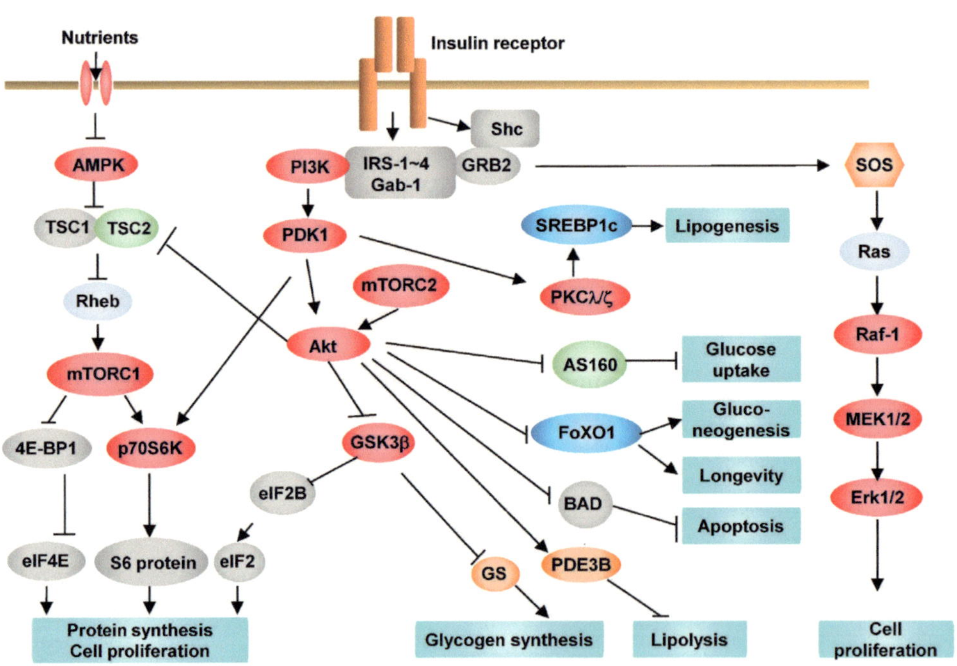


**Figure 1.**
*Insulin signaling pathways (adapted from [7]).*

turn causes inhibitory phosphorylation of insulin receptor, IRSs, and Akt [8, 9]. Hyperinsulinemia also down-regulates expression of IRS-2 via suppression of a transcription factor, FoxO1 (forkhead box protein O1), in the liver, contributing to the induction of insulin resistance [10, 11].

## 3. ER stress and ER stress response

### 3.1 Overview of ER stress response cascade

The ER is an organelle involved in synthesis of secretory proteins and membrane proteins. In the ER, unfolded proteins, immediately after translation and entrance into the organelle, are matured through modification, such as folding, formation of disulfide bonds, and initiation of glycosylation. Under ER stress, in which unfolded or misfolded proteins accumulate in the ER due to increased protein synthesis or chaperone dysfunction, various kinds of ER stress response are induced, and some of them are cytoprotective and others are cytotoxic [12].

Among the numerous molecules involved in ER stress response, also called UPR (unfolded protein response), BiP (binding immunoglobulin protein), also known as GRP78 (glucose-regulated protein 78), is a chaperone with an ATPase domain, which plays pivotal roles in ER stress response mainly via interaction with ERdjs (ER-localized DnaJ family members) [13]. BiP binds to unfolded or misfolded proteins in the ER and promotes folding by consuming ATP. Moreover, BiP binds to ER stress sensor molecules, IRE1-alpha (inositol-requiring enzyme 1 alpha), ATF6 (activating transcription factor 6), and PERK (PKR-like endoplasmic reticulum kinase), and prevent them from activation. Under ER stress, however, BiP is mainly engaged in increased unfolded or misfolded proteins and dissociates from the ER stress sensors, resulting in phosphorylation of IRE1-alpha and PERK, as well as cleavage of ATF6 followed by nuclear translocation to the nucleus [12, 14].

It is well known that phosphorylated IRE1-alpha splices Xbp1 (X-box binding protein 1) mRNA [15]. XBP-1 s protein induces chaperones, including BiP and XBP-1 s itself, as a transcription factor by binding to motifs called ERSEs (ER stress response elements). XBP-1 s also promotes ERAD (ER-associated degradation) by binding to motifs called UPRs (UPR response elements), and attenuates translation via mRNA degradation. nATF6 (nuclear ATF6) also works as a transcription factor to induce chaperones by binding to ERSEs. Phosphorylated PERK phosphorylates eIF2 alpha (eukaryotic initiation factor-2 alpha), which suppresses translation and lowers protein loading. Overall, these responses are protective against ER stress, by suppressing protein synthesis, inducing chaperones, and promoting protein degradation.

Sustained ER stress is, however, known to induce rather cytotoxic responses. Phosphorylated IRE1-alpha activates JNK, resulting in inflammation, oxidative stress and apoptosis. Phosphorylated eIF-2 alpha also induces CHOP (CCAAT-enhancer-binding protein homologous protein), a transcription factor involved in apoptosis, as well as oxidative stress and inflammation, via another transcription factor, ATF4 [12, 14].

It is difficult to detect unfolded/misfolded proteins in the ER of mammals directly, but activation of the upstream ER stress sensors is considered to be a good marker to reflect ER stress. Activation or expression of the downstream molecules involved in ER stress response are also frequently used as ER stress markers, but we are going to discuss the discrepancy between the upstream sensors and the downstream effectors, which we call ER stress response failure, in subsections below (**Figure 2**).

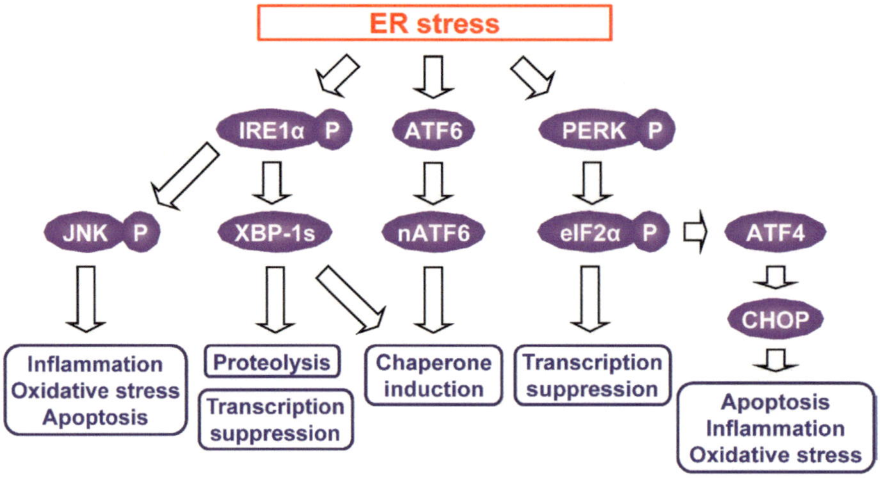


**Figure 2.**
*Schematic description of the cascade of ER stress response.*

### 3.2 ER stress and metabolic disorders

In the field of metabolism, ER stress causes metabolic disorders in various tissues and, in the liver, ER stress is considered to be involved in the development of insulin resistance and fatty liver disease [16]. It was first reported that ER stress markers were enhanced in the liver of mouse models of obesity and diabetes [17, 18]. Systemic Xbp1 knockout mice are a well-known model of impaired ER stress response, which shows elevated ER stress, impaired insulin signaling, and glucose intolerance [17]. Moreover, administration of chemical chaperones improves not only insulin resistance and hyperglycemia but also fatty liver [19]. Similarly, suppressed activation of the PERK branch of the ER stress response cascade, by dephosphorylation of eIF2 alpha, also improves hepatosteatosis as well as glucose tolerance [20]. Thus generally, impaired responses to chronic ER stress or excessive chronic ER stress in the liver are considered to result in hepatic insulin resistance and fatty liver disease, although these phenotypes were not necessarily replicated in other models [21, 22], and XBP-1 s protein was also reported to up-regulate lipogenic genes [23].

However, some years later, ER stress response was reported to be suppressed, contrary to the earlier reports, and a controversy was thus raised about whether ER stress and ER stress response are enhanced or suppressed in obesity and diabetes. Activity of nATF6 is suppressed in the liver of mouse models of obesity and diabetes [24]. Moreover, binding with p85, one of the key downstream molecules of insulin signaling, is required for XBP-1 s protein to be translocated to the nucleus and exert its activity as a transcription factor in the liver. In model mice of obesity and diabetes, however, insulin-mediated nuclear translocation of XBP-1 s protein is impaired due to insulin resistance [25, 26]. A similar insulin signaling-mediated nuclear translocation of XBP-1 s protein was recently reported in other tissues as well [27]. Interestingly, XBP-1 s protein regulates gluconeogenesis rather directly, via ubiquitination and consequent proteasome-mediated degradation of FoxO1, a transcription factor involved in the induction of gluconeogenic enzymes in the liver [28] (**Figure 3**).

Taken together, insulin signaling appears not only to promote protein synthesis, but also to be involved in quality control of synthesized proteins. Moreover, XBP-1 s is a multi-talented molecule which is closely associated with regulation of not only ER stress response but also glucose and lipid metabolism.

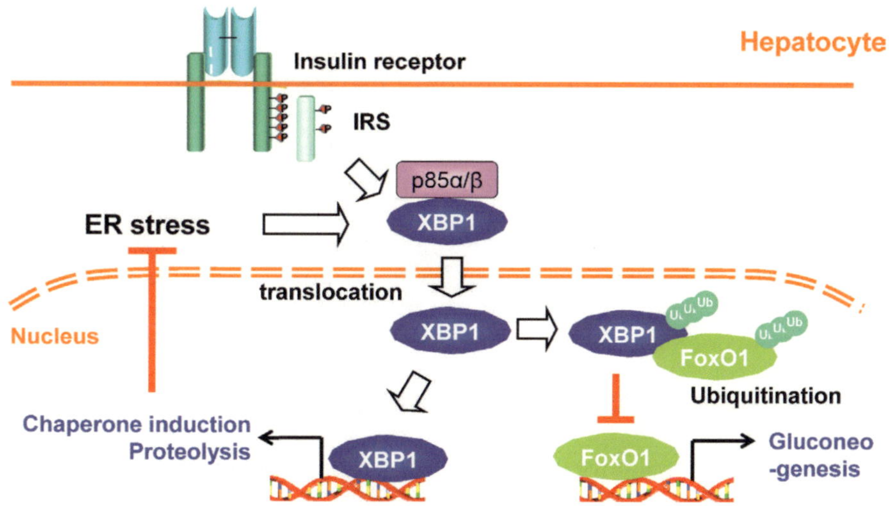


**Figure 3.**
*XBP-1s protein in the regulation of glucose metabolism: insulin-mediated nuclear translocation and regulation of gluconeogenesis.*

### 3.3 ER stress in the liver and diseases in humans

In humans, some ER stress markers are known to be affected by insulin resistance and nonalcoholic steatohepatitis (NASH). NASH is associated with phosphorylation of JNK and lower XBP-1 s protein levels [29]. Expression of sXBP1 and BiP mRNA is not correlated with insulin resistance [30], but is lowered by gastric bypass surgery [31]. We and colleagues previously reported that IRS-1 expression in the liver is negatively correlated with fibrosis [32], suggesting the protective role of insulin signaling against the development of NASH. These reports, however, did not distinguish ER stress and ER stress response or NASH in diabetic patients and NASH in non-diabetic patients.

## 4. Roles of Sdf2l1 in the regulation of ER stress and metabolism

### 4.1 Feeding induces ER stress response in the liver

Recently, we reported that a chaperone, Sdf2l1 (stromal cell-derived factor 2 like 1), plays crucial roles in the termination of feeding-induced ER stress in the liver and consequently in the maintenance of glucose and lipid metabolism. We propose that ER stress response failure, including suppressed induction of Sdf2l1 by XBP-1 s, is a key link between insulin resistance and steatohepatitis comorbid with diabetes [33].

Our first finding was that ER stress is induced transiently during feeding in the liver, based on the microarray data using murine liver samples comparing the fasting and refeeding conditions in the public domain [34]. We were particularly interested in Sdf2l1 among the genes highly up-regulated by refeeding, which showed a large increase in expression. Sdf2l1 had been reported to be induced by ER stress [35], and to function as a component of the ER chaperone complex including BiP [36–39]. Besides, the orthologs in yeast, Pmt1p and Pmt2p, are *O*-mannosyltransferases and known to enhance ubiquitination of unfolded proteins as an initiation of ERAD [40–42]. Little is known, however, of roles of Sdf2l1 in the regulation of glucose and lipid metabolism.

Indeed, the cascade of ER stress response is activated during feeding in the liver: phosphorylation, expression, and nuclear localization of the downstream ER stress marker proteins, as well as expression of ER stress marker genes, are elevated (**Figure 4**) [33].

Therefore, although major attention had been focused on the chronic and pathophysiological aspects of ER stress and ER stress response in the field of metabolism, transient ER stress and consequent ER stress response (just for a few hours) are induced in the liver by the physiological stimulation of feeding, or eating, even in lean nondiabetic mice. Such induction of ER stress during feeding is attributed to protein intake and insulin signaling [33], both of which reach the liver during feeding and promote protein synthesis [3, 5, 43].

### 4.2 Regulation and function of Sdf2l1 as an ER stress response

We explored the regulatory mechanism underlying the induction of Sdf2l1, and found that Sdf2l1, as well as BiP, is regulated by transcription factors, XBP-1 s and nATF6 by not only chemically induced ER stress but also refeeding in the liver. XBP-1 s and nATF6 binds to an 11-bp motif responsible for the induction of Sdf2l1 upstream in the promotor region [33], which is similar to ERSEs targeted by XBP-1 s and nATF6 with nuclear factor Y as a co-factor [12].

We further explored the function of Sdf2l1 in ER stress response, and found that knocking down of Sdf2l1 leads to accumulation of exogenously expressed $Ins2^{C96Y}$, a mutant insulin found in Akita mice as a model of misfolded protein degraded by ERAD [44], showing that Sdf2l1 modulates ER stress via regulating ERAD. Although Sdf2l1 had been known to interact with BiP [36–38], knocking down of BiP did not affect such accumulation, suggesting the existence of some other counterparts of Sdf2l1. Then, based on the results of mass spectrometric analysis of microsomal fractions, we focused on TMED10 (transmembrane emp24-like trafficking protein 10), a membrane protein known to regulate protein transportation from the ER to the Golgi apparatus [45]. Indeed, knocking down of either Sdf2l1 or TMED10 results in increased accumulation of misfolded protein and enhanced ER stress, showing that TMED10 is the major counterpart of Sdf2l1 to regulate ERAD and consequently ER stress. Interestingly, in yeast, p24, the ortholog of TMED10, interacts with Pmt1/2p and promotes ER export of unfolded proteins for ERAD

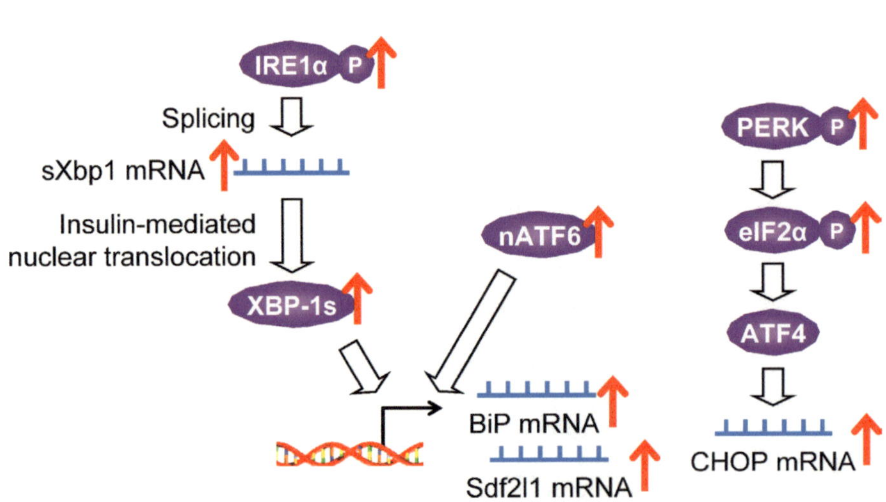


**Figure 4.**
*Schematic description of the ER stress response cascade in the liver during feeding (adapted from [33]).*

[41], and now the orthologs in mice turns out to interact with each other to regulate ERAD to cope with ER stress [33].

### 4.3 Sdf2l1 modulates ER stress response and metabolism

We then assessed the physiological and pathophysiological roles of Sdf2l1 *in vivo*. Adenovirus-mediated knocking down and knocking out of Sdf2l1 specifically in the liver of adult mice both result in enhanced ER stress during refeeding, impaired insulin signaling in the liver, systemic insulin resistance, glucose intolerance, and markedly increased triglyceride contents in the liver.

Thus, impaired induction of Sdf2l1 results in sustained ER stress, leading to insulin resistance and increased triglyceride contents, even with a normal-chow diet, indicating that dysregulation of ER stress by suppression of Sdf2l1 is a causal factor of metabolic disorders. Together with the previous reports showing that ablation of key molecules in ER stress response links impaired glucose and lipid metabolism in mice fed on a high-fat diet or a high-fructose diet [17, 21, 22], our data strongly suggest that an appropriate transient response to ER stress is induced physiologically during feeding, or eating, and terminated by Sdf2l1, and that this process may be important for the maintenance of nutrient homeostasis [33].

### 4.4 Impaired ER stress response in obesity and diabetes

Then we explored the roles of ER stress response in the development of insulin resistance and fatty liver in obesity and diabetes. **Figure 5** summarizes the changes in the ER stress response cascade observed in a mouse model, *db/db* mice. The ER stress sensors are activated, suggesting excessive ER stress in the liver possibly due to hyperinsulinemia and over-nutrition. However, downstream molecules of the cascade that are expected to cope with ER stress are suppressed in expression or insufficiently activated. Among those, Sdf2l1 is highly down-regulated, and chromatin immunoprecipitation (ChIP) assay revealed that the down-regulation of Sdf2l1 is attributed to suppressed activity of XBP-1 s, not of ATF6 [33], presumably due to the decreased insulin action to promote the translocation of XBP-1 s to the nucleus by binding to p85 [25, 26].

We call it ER stress 'response failure', which results in further excessive ER stress, forming a vicious cycle. It is known that activation of the ER stress sensors

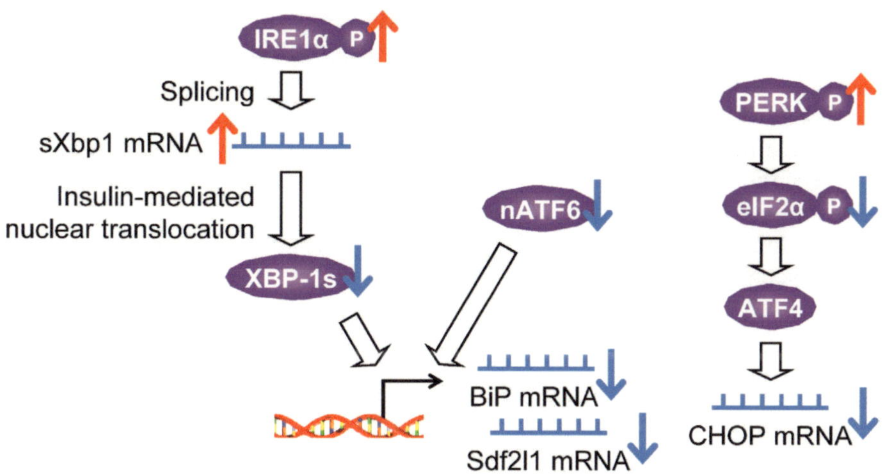


**Figure 5.**
*Schematic description of the ER stress response cascade in the liver in obesity and diabetes (adapted from [33]).*

is attenuated during prolonged ER stress, resulting in only insufficient activation or induction of downstream molecules involved in ER stress response [46]. Suppression of the whole cascade of ER stress response might be called ER stress 'sensing failure', which draws clear contrast with ER stress 'response failure' [33], and this novel concept is now gaining publicity [47].

In order to rescue ER stress response failure, over-expression of the upstream XBP-1 s protein does not show full recovery of expression of downstream chaperones and consequently insulin resistance. On the other hand, restoration of suppressed expression of a downstream chaperone, Sdf2l1, does improve insulin signaling in the liver, systemic insulin resistance, glucose intolerance, and fatty liver. Moreover, larger beneficial effects come from co-restoration of Sdf2l1 and BiP, and in accordance with the findings *in vitro*, we conclude that Sdf2l1 improves insulin sensitivity independently of BiP, at least in part [33].

### 4.5 ER stress and ER stress response in humans

Lastly, we assessed whether impaired ER stress response could be associated with progression of human diseases by examining data from male subjects with suspected NAFLD (nonalcoholic fatty liver disease) who underwent liver biopsy after oral glucose tolerance test early in the morning, partially mimicking the fed state. In diabetic subjects, expression of the upstream sXBP1 mRNA is elevated in subjects with insulin resistance, but the downstream-to-upstream ratio, the SDF2L1/sXBP1 ratio, is lower in subjects with insulin resistance. Similarly, in those with diabetes, sXBP1 is positively, but the SDF2L1/sXBP1 ratio is negatively, correlated with stage or fibrosis of NASH. These changes and correlations are not observed in nondiabetic subjects, showing that impaired response to ER stress, as well as enhanced ER stress, are associated with the progression of insulin resistance and steatohepatitis, which is unique to patients with diabetes (**Table 1**) [33].

In the 'two-hit hypothesis' on the development of NASH, accumulation of lipids or steatosis is promoted by the first 'hit', whereas the further progression to steatohepatitis requires the presence of the second 'hit(s)' [48]. Given that ER stress is one of the major potential second hits (and others are inflammation, oxidative stress, autophagy failure, and mitochondria dysfunction), our data show that not only ER stress but also ER stress response failure serve as the second hits in the progression from NAFLD to NASH. Moreover, insulin resistance is one of the major potential first hits, but diabetes is a disease in which insulin resistance fails to be compensated and insulin action is impaired. Decompensated insulin resistance leads to insufficient induction of ER stress response via suppressed nuclear translocation of XBP-1 s protein to the nucleus [25, 26]. Thus, our data show that insulin-mediated nuclear translocation of XBP-1 s protein links the first and second hits, and the SDF2L1/sXBP1 ratio is a promising biomarker [33]. It is also implied that mechanisms underlying NASH in diabetic patients and those underlying NASH in non-diabetic patients could be different and should be elucidated separately (**Figure 6**).

| | **Insulin resistance** | **Stage (fibrosis)** |
|---|---|---|
| sXBP1 mRNA (upstream) | Elevated | Positively correlated |
| SDF2L1/sXBP1 mRNA ratio (downstream-to-upstream ratio) | Lowered | Negatively correlated |

**Table 1.**
*Summary of ER stress and ER stress response in diabetic patients (adapted from [33]).*

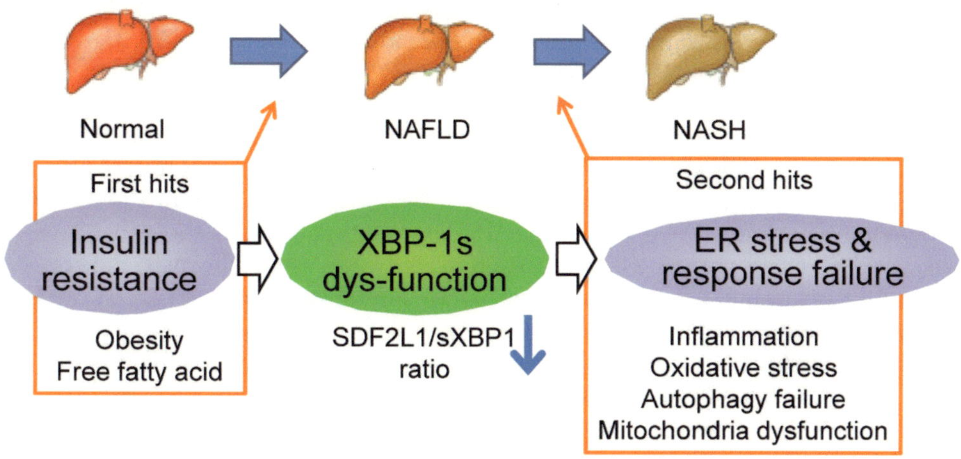


**Figure 6.**
*Schematic description of ER stress and ER stress response in the 'two-hit hypothesis' on the development of NASH comorbid with diabetes (adapted from [33]).*

These findings could account for the therapeutic effects of insulin sensitizers against not only diabetes but also NASH [49], although insulin signaling itself promotes anabolism of lipids [1]. Moreover, it may be useful to identify the effectors downstream of Sdf2l1 to regulate ERAD more directly, when we consider development of more effective drugs for these diseases by shutting down the vicious cycle due to ER stress response failure [33].

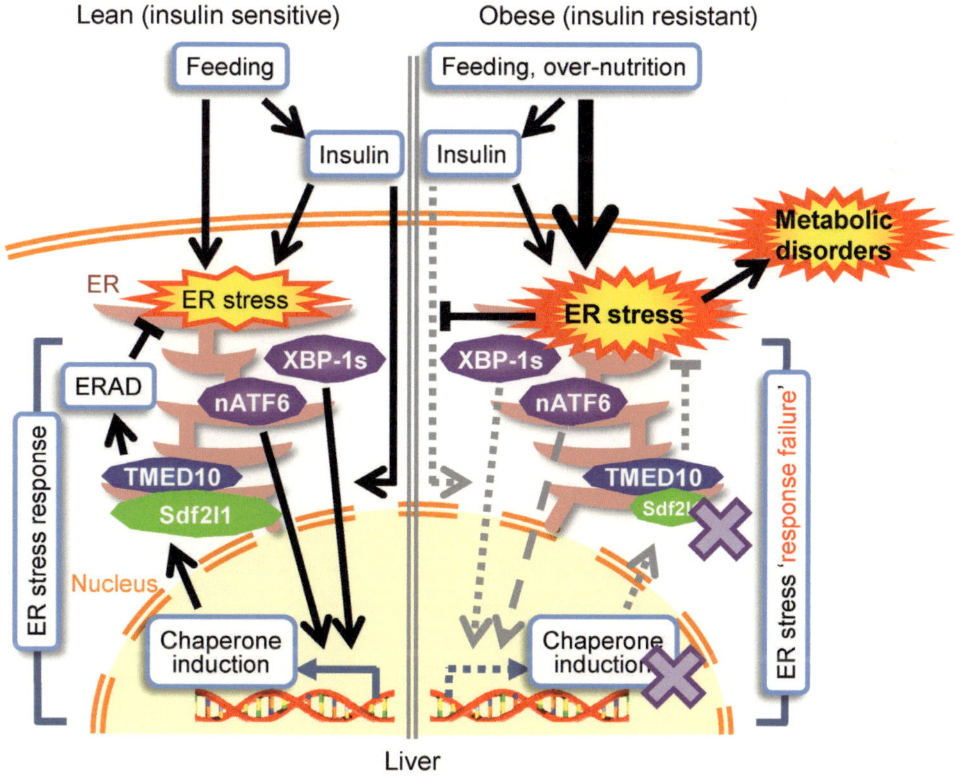


**Figure 7.**
*Schematic description of our hypothesis on physiological and pathophysiological roles of Sdf2l1-centered ER stress response in the liver [33].*

Recently, a novel concept of metabolic dysfunction-associated fatty liver disease, or MAFLD, was proposed [50, 51], a broader concept than NAFLD, which was proposed in the 1980s [52]. The roles of insulin resistance are considered to be increasingly important [53], and ER stress response failure is expected to contribute also to the development of steatohepatitis in patients with diabetes and MAFLD.

Most recently, Fib-4 index, a marker of hepatic fibrosis, was reported to be a good prognostic factor for the development of hepatocellular carcinoma in diabetic patients, in a nationwide survey in Japan [54]. Given that our data show that ER stress and ER stress response failure are associated with hepatic fibrosis, improvement of ER stress and ER stress response failure might be protective against carcinogenesis as well.

Overall, feeding, or eating, induces physiological and transient ER stress in the liver, and induced Sdf2l1 appropriately terminates ER stress, in cooperation with TMED10, and contributes to normal glucose and lipid metabolism. In obesity and diabetes, impaired ER stress termination signals, including the down-regulation of Sdf2l1 that is caused by decreased insulin signaling, sustains ER stress and exacerbates insulin resistance, creating a vicious cycle. Thus, Sdf2l1 is expected to be a therapeutic target and a sensitive biomarker in obesity-associated diseases (**Figure 7**).

## 5. Conclusions

We reveal that eating induces physiological and transient ER stress and ER stress response, including up-regulation of Sdf2l1, in the liver. In obesity and diabetes, however, ER stress response failure, including down-regulation of Sdf2l1, results in sustained ER stress, which links insulin resistance and the development of steatohepatitis comorbid with diabetes.

## Acknowledgements

We thank the co-workers, especially Dr. Naoto Kubota (The University of Tokyo), Prof. Kazuyuki Tobe (The University of Toyama), Prof. Kazuhiko Koike (The University of Tokyo), and Prof. Takashi Kadowaki (The University of Tokyo; Toranomon Hospital).

## Conflict of interest

The authors declare no conflict of interest.

*DOI: http://dx.doi.org/10.5772/intechopen.100054*

## Author details

Takayoshi Sasako[1,2]* and Kohjiro Ueki[2]

1 Department of Diabetes and Metabolic Diseases, Graduate School of Medicine, The University of Tokyo, Tokyo, Japan

2 Diabetes Research Center, National Center for Global Health and Medicine, Tokyo, Japan

*Address all correspondence to: tsasako-tky@umin.ac.jp

## References

[1] Gribble FM. Metabolism: a higher power for insulin. Nature. 2005;434(7036):965-966.

[2] Cross DA, Alessi DR, Cohen P, Andjelkovich M, Hemmings BA. Inhibition of glycogen synthase kinase-3 by insulin mediated by protein kinase B. Nature. 1995;378(6559):785-789.

[3] Ueki K, Yamamoto-Honda R, Kaburagi Y, Yamauchi T, Tobe K, Burgering BM, et al. Potential role of protein kinase B in insulin-induced glucose transport, glycogen synthesis, and protein synthesis. J Biol Chem. 1998;273(9):5315-5322.

[4] Brunet A, Bonni A, Zigmond MJ, Lin MZ, Juo P, Hu LS, et al. Akt promotes cell survival by phosphorylating and inhibiting a Forkhead transcription factor. Cell. 1999;96(6):857-868.

[5] Taniguchi CM, Emanuelli B, Kahn CR. Critical nodes in signalling pathways: insights into insulin action. Nat Rev Mol Cell Biol. 2006;7(2):85-96.

[6] Kasuga M, Karlsson FA, Kahn CR. Insulin stimulates the phosphorylation of the 95,000-dalton subunit of its own receptor. Science. 1982;215(4529): 185-187.

[7] Kadowaki T, Ueki K, Yamauchi T, Kubota N. SnapShot: Insulin signaling pathways. Cell. 2012;148(3):624, e1.

[8] Boucher J, Kleinridders A, Kahn CR. Insulin receptor signaling in normal and insulin-resistant states. Cold Spring Harb Perspect Biol. 2014;6(1).

[9] Czech MP. Insulin action and resistance in obesity and type 2 diabetes. Nat Med. 2017;23(7):804-814.

[10] Kubota N, Kubota T, Itoh S, Kumagai H, Kozono H, Takamoto I, et al. Dynamic functional relay between insulin receptor substrate 1 and 2 in hepatic insulin signaling during fasting and feeding. Cell Metab. 2008;8(1): 49-64.

[11] Kubota N, Kubota T, Kajiwara E, Iwamura T, Kumagai H, Watanabe T, et al. Differential hepatic distribution of insulin receptor substrates causes selective insulin resistance in diabetes and obesity. Nat Commun. 2016;7:12977.

[12] Ji C, Kaplowitz N. ER stress: can the liver cope? J Hepatol. 2006;45(2): 321-333.

[13] Pobre KFR, Poet GJ, Hendershot LM. The endoplasmic reticulum (ER) chaperone BiP is a master regulator of ER functions: Getting by with a little help from ERdj friends. J Biol Chem. 2019;294(6): 2098-2108.

[14] Malhi H, Kaufman RJ. Endoplasmic reticulum stress in liver disease. J Hepatol. 2011;54(4):795-809.

[15] Yoshida H, Matsui T, Yamamoto A, Okada T, Mori K. XBP1 mRNA is induced by ATF6 and spliced by IRE1 in response to ER stress to produce a highly active transcription factor. Cell. 2001;107(7):881-891.

[16] Cnop M, Foufelle F, Velloso LA. Endoplasmic reticulum stress, obesity and diabetes. Trends Mol Med. 2012;18(1):59-68.

[17] Ozcan U, Cao Q, Yilmaz E, Lee AH, Iwakoshi NN, Ozdelen E, et al. Endoplasmic reticulum stress links obesity, insulin action, and type 2 diabetes. Science. 2004;306(5695): 457-461.

[18] Nakatani Y, Kaneto H, Kawamori D, Yoshiuchi K, Hatazaki M, Matsuoka TA, et al. Involvement of endoplasmic reticulum stress in insulin resistance and

diabetes. J Biol Chem. 2005;280(1):847-851.

[19] Ozcan U, Yilmaz E, Ozcan L, Furuhashi M, Vaillancourt E, Smith RO, et al. Chemical chaperones reduce ER stress and restore glucose homeostasis in a mouse model of type 2 diabetes. Science. 2006;313(5790):1137-1140.

[20] Oyadomari S, Harding HP, Zhang Y, Oyadomari M, Ron D. Dephosphorylation of translation initiation factor 2alpha enhances glucose tolerance and attenuates hepatosteatosis in mice. Cell Metab. 2008;7(6):520-532.

[21] Ye R, Jung DY, Jun JY, Li J, Luo S, Ko HJ, et al. Grp78 heterozygosity promotes adaptive unfolded protein response and attenuates diet-induced obesity and insulin resistance. Diabetes. 2010;59(1):6-16.

[22] Jurczak MJ, Lee AH, Jornayvaz FR, Lee HY, Birkenfeld AL, Guigni BA, et al. Dissociation of inositol-requiring enzyme (IRE1alpha)-mediated c-Jun N-terminal kinase activation from hepatic insulin resistance in conditional X-box-binding protein-1 (XBP1) knock-out mice. J Biol Chem. 2012;287(4):2558-2567.

[23] Lee AH, Scapa EF, Cohen DE, Glimcher LH. Regulation of hepatic lipogenesis by the transcription factor XBP1. Science. 2008;320(5882):1492-1496.

[24] Dentin R, Hedrick S, Xie J, Yates J, 3rd, Montminy M. Hepatic glucose sensing via the CREB coactivator CRTC2. Science. 2008;319(5868):1402-1405.

[25] Park SW, Zhou Y, Lee J, Lu A, Sun C, Chung J, et al. The regulatory subunits of PI3K, p85alpha and p85beta, interact with XBP-1 and increase its nuclear translocation. Nat Med. 2010;16(4):429-437.

[26] Winnay JN, Boucher J, Mori MA, Ueki K, Kahn CR. A regulatory subunit of phosphoinositide 3-kinase increases the nuclear accumulation of X-box-binding protein-1 to modulate the unfolded protein response. Nat Med. 2010;16(4):438-445.

[27] Winnay JN, Solheim MH, Sakaguchi M, Njolstad PR, Kahn CR. Inhibition of the PI 3-kinase pathway disrupts the unfolded protein response and reduces sensitivity to ER stress-dependent apoptosis. FASEB J. 2020;34(9):12521-12532.

[28] Zhou Y, Lee J, Reno CM, Sun C, Park SW, Chung J, et al. Regulation of glucose homeostasis through a XBP-1-FoxO1 interaction. Nat Med. 2011;17(3):356-365.

[29] Puri P, Mirshahi F, Cheung O, Natarajan R, Maher JW, Kellum JM, et al. Activation and dysregulation of the unfolded protein response in nonalcoholic fatty liver disease. Gastroenterology. 2008;134(2):568-576.

[30] Kumashiro N, Erion DM, Zhang D, Kahn M, Beddow SA, Chu X, et al. Cellular mechanism of insulin resistance in nonalcoholic fatty liver disease. Proc Natl Acad Sci USA. 2011;108(39):16381-16385.

[31] Gregor MF, Yang L, Fabbrini E, Mohammed BS, Eagon JC, Hotamisligil GS, et al. Endoplasmic reticulum stress is reduced in tissues of obese subjects after weight loss. Diabetes. 2009;58(3):693-700.

[32] Enooku K, Kondo M, Fujiwara N, Sasako T, Shibahara J, Kado A, et al. Hepatic IRS1 and ss-catenin expression is associated with histological progression and overt diabetes emergence in NAFLD patients. J Gastroenterol. 2018.

[33] Sasako T, Ohsugi M, Kubota N, Itoh S, Okazaki Y, Terai A, et al. Hepatic

Sdf2l1 controls feeding-induced ER stress and regulates metabolism. Nat Commun. 2019;10(1):947.

[34] Musso G, Cassader M, Paschetta E, Gambino R. Thiazolidinediones and Advanced Liver Fibrosis in Nonalcoholic Steatohepatitis: A Meta-analysis. JAMA Intern Med. 2017;177(5):633-640.

[35] Fukuda S, Sumii M, Masuda Y, Takahashi M, Koike N, Teishima J, et al. Murine and human SDF2L1 is an endoplasmic reticulum stress-inducible gene and encodes a new member of the Pmt/rt protein family. Biochem Biophys Res Commun. 2001;280(1):407-414.

[36] Meunier L, Usherwood YK, Chung KT, Hendershot LM. A subset of chaperones and folding enzymes form multiprotein complexes in endoplasmic reticulum to bind nascent proteins. Mol Biol Cell. 2002;13(12):4456-4469.

[37] Bies C, Blum R, Dudek J, Nastainczyk W, Oberhauser S, Jung M, et al. Characterization of pancreatic ERj3p, a homolog of yeast DnaJ-like protein Scj1p. Biol Chem. 2004;385(5):389-395.

[38] Tiwari A, Schuiki I, Zhang L, Allister EM, Wheeler MB, Volchuk A. SDF2L1 interacts with the ER-associated degradation machinery and retards the degradation of mutant proinsulin in pancreatic beta-cells. J Cell Sci. 2013;126(Pt 9):1962-1968.

[39] Fujimori T, Suno R, Iemura SI, Natsume T, Wada I, Hosokawa N. Endoplasmic reticulum proteins SDF2 and SDF2L1 act as components of the BiP chaperone cycle to prevent protein aggregation. Genes Cells. 2017;22(8):684-698.

[40] Nakatsukasa K, Okada S, Umebayashi K, Fukuda R, Nishikawa S, Endo T. Roles of O-mannosylation of aberrant proteins in reduction of the load for endoplasmic reticulum chaperones in yeast. J Biol Chem. 2004;279(48):49762-49772.

[41] Goder V, Melero A. Protein O-mannosyltransferases participate in ER protein quality control. J Cell Sci. 2011;124 (Pt 1):144-153.

[42] Xu C, Wang S, Thibault G, Ng DT. Futile protein folding cycles in the ER are terminated by the unfolded protein O-mannosylation pathway. Science. 2013;340(6135):978-981.

[43] Yoshizawa F. Translational regulation of protein synthesis in the liver and skeletal muscle of mice in response to refeeding. J Nutr Biochem. 1995;6:130-136.

[44] Allen JR, Nguyen LX, Sargent KE, Lipson KL, Hackett A, Urano F. High ER stress in beta-cells stimulates intracellular degradation of misfolded insulin. Biochem Biophys Res Commun. 2004;324(1):166-170.

[45] Fujita M, Watanabe R, Jaensch N, Romanova-Michaelides M, Satoh T, Kato M, et al. Sorting of GPI-anchored proteins into ER exit sites by p24 proteins is dependent on remodeled GPI. J Cell Biol. 2011;194(1):61-75.

[46] Lin JH, Li H, Yasumura D, Cohen HR, Zhang C, Panning B, et al. IRE1 signaling affects cell fate during the unfolded protein response. Science. 2007;318(5852):944-949.

[47] Bhattarai KR, Chaudhary M, Kim HR, Chae HJ. Endoplasmic Reticulum (ER) Stress Response Failure in Diseases. Trends Cell Biol. 2020;30(9):672-675.

[48] Day CP, James OF. Steatohepatitis: a tale of two "hits"? Gastroenterology. 1998;114(4):842-845.

[49] Ratziu V, Goodman Z, Sanyal A. Current efforts and trends in the

treatment of NASH. J Hepatol. 2015;62(1S):S65-S75.

[50] Eslam M, Sanyal AJ, George J, International Consensus P. MAFLD: A Consensus-Driven Proposed Nomenclature for Metabolic Associated Fatty Liver Disease. Gastroenterology. 2020;158(7):1999-2014 e1.

[51] Eslam M, Newsome PN, Sarin SK, Anstee QM, Targher G, Romero-Gomez M, et al. A new definition for metabolic dysfunction-associated fatty liver disease: An international expert consensus statement. J Hepatol. 2020;73(1): 202-209.

[52] Ludwig J, Viggiano TR, McGill DB, Oh BJ. Nonalcoholic steatohepatitis: Mayo Clinic experiences with a hitherto unnamed disease. Mayo Clin Proc. 1980;55(7):434-438.

[53] Sakurai Y, Kubota N, Yamauchi T, Kadowaki T. Role of Insulin Resistance in MAFLD. Int J Mol Sci. 2021;22(8).

[54] Tateishi R, Matsumura T, Okanoue T, Shima T, Uchino K, Fujiwara N, et al. Hepatocellular carcinoma development in diabetic patients: a nationwide survey in Japan. J Gastroenterol. 2021;56(3):261-273.

Chapter 6

# The Effect of Glycation Stress on Skeletal Muscle

*Tatsuro Egawa, Kohei Kido, Takumi Yokokawa, Mami Fujibayashi, Katsumasa Goto and Tatsuya Hayashi*

## Abstract

Glycation stress (glycative stress) is a general concept of biological stress caused by a series of non-enzymatic glycation reactions, including advanced glycation end products (AGEs) formation, AGEs accumulation, glycation-associated dysfunction of proteins and cellular signaling, inflammation, oxidation, and/or tissue damage. There has been increasing evidence supporting a profound effect of AGEs on human diseases such as type 2 diabetes, cardiovascular disease, cancer, Alzheimer's disease, osteoporosis, and dementia, as well as aging process itself. In addition, dietary AGEs intake has also been suggested to contribute to tissue dysfunction and development of the diseases. Skeletal muscle is the largest organ in the human body and important responsibility for maintaining our health as not only locomotor system but also metabolic and endocrine systems. Especially in past decades, numerous studies have suggested the contribution of glycation stress to skeletal muscle dysfunctions (e.g. muscle atrophy, reducing contractile property, and insulin resistance). In this chapter, we provide current evidence on the potential role of glycation stress in the impairment of skeletal muscle functions.

**Keywords:** glycative stress, skeletal muscle dysfunction, skeletal muscle atrophy, advanced glycation end products, AGEs

## 1. Introduction

Skeletal muscle is the largest organ in the human body, accounting for approximately 40% of body weight. A primary characteristic of skeletal muscle is its ability to contract and cause movement. In addition, skeletal muscle is a metabolic organ of high metabolic activity regarding nutrient (glucose, lipid, and protein) storage and supply. It has also recently been found that skeletal muscle is a secretary organ that produces and releases cytokines and other peptides, which is known as myokine, that function in manner similar to hormones [1]. Thus, skeletal muscle has an important responsibility for maintaining our health as not only locomotor system but also metabolic and endocrine systems [2]. After the age of 50, approximately 1–2% of muscle mass and 1.5–5% of muscle strength are lost per year [3]. These reductions in muscle mass, strength, and function, the so-called sarcopenia, link to numerous adverse consequences including frailty, disability, morbidity, and mortality [2].

Over the last few decades, there has been increasing evidence supporting a profound effect of advanced glycation end products (AGEs) on human diseases,



IntechOpen

including type 2 diabetes, cardiovascular disease, cancer, Alzheimer's disease, osteoporosis, and dementia, as well as the aging process itself [4, 5]. Especially in past decades, many epidemiological studies have suggested the contribution of glycation stress (also called as glycative stress) from AGEs to sarcopenia [6–17]. In this chapter, we provide current evidence on the potential role of glycation stress in the impairment of skeletal muscle functions.

## 2. Glycation stress

Glycation stress is a general concept of biological stress caused by a series of glycation reactions, including AGEs formation, AGEs accumulation, glycation-associated dysfunction of proteins and cellular signaling, inflammation, oxidation, and/or tissue damage (**Figure 1**).

Protein glycation is a complex series of sequential reactions collectively called the Maillard reaction, which is named after the French chemist Louis Camilli Maillard. The Maillard reaction is divided into three stages, early (the formation of reversible Schiff base and rearrangement to Amadori products), intermediate (the formation of unstable AGEs precursors), and late (the formation of irreversible AGEs products). At the early stage, the carbonyl group of the reducing sugar reacts with the α-amino group at the N-terminal of protein or the ε-amino group of lysine or arginine residue, resulting in a formation of Schiff-base intermediates, followed by a rearrangement to Amadori products, relatively stable ketoamine. Amadori products in the living body include hemoglobin A1c and glycoalbumin. At the intermediate stage, the reaction proceeds and produces highly reactive dicarbonyl intermediates such as 3-deoxyglucosone and methylglyoxal. These intermediates are up to 20,000 times more reactive than glucose in glycation reactions [18]. At the late stage, the intermediates undergo complex reactions such as oxidation, dehydration, condensation, and cleavage to form stable AGEs, with a variety of physicochemical characteristics such as brown color, fluorescence, and cross-linking. Glycation of protein is a post-translational modification that progresses non-enzymatically, unlike enzymatic glycosylation, phosphorylation, acetylation, and glycosylation. Among more than 20 types of AGEs identified in vivo, methylglyoxal-derived hydroimidazolone (MG-H1) and Nε-carboxymethyllysine (CML) are likely the most abundant [19, 20].

Intracellular protein glycation can cause changes in the protein structure due to covalent cross-linking, resulting in the formation of protein misfolding and aggregation [21]. Although these unfunctional proteins are usually degraded through

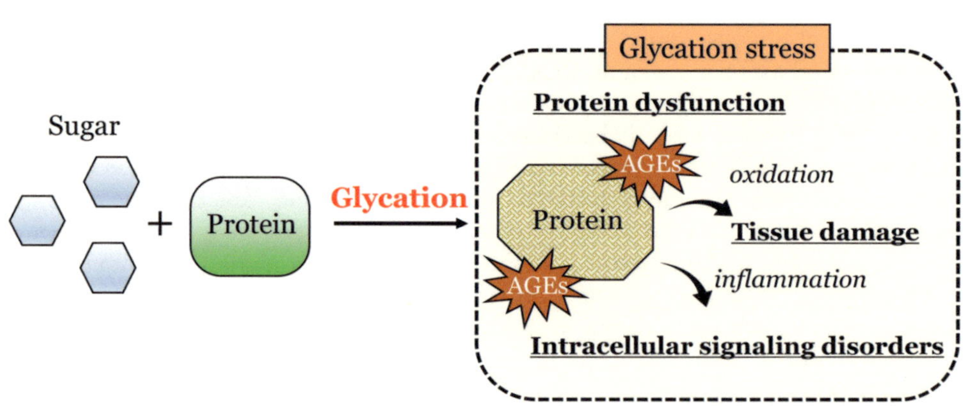


**Figure 1.**
*Conceptual diagram of glycation stress.*

ubiquitin-proteasome system, AGEs-modified protein is the lack of free lysine residue needed for ubiquitin conjugation, preventing protein ubiquitination and subsequent its degradation by proteasome [22]. In addition, enzymes present in the ubiquitin-proteasome system and lysosomal proteolytic system are also undergone glycation [23]. Thus, intracellular glycation disrupts proteostasis, inducing cell apoptosis, and thereby increasing the risk of disorders.

On the other hand, extracellular AGEs stimulate several signaling pathways by a series of cell surface receptors. The most studied of which is receptor for AGEs (RAGE), a multi-ligand member of the immunoglobulin superfamily [24]. The activation of AGEs-RAGE axis causes the onset of several diseases, including diabetic complications, cardiovascular disease, Alzheimer's disease, and osteoporosis, by inducing inflammation and the production of reactive oxygen species [25–28]. RAGE is widely expressed in various cells and organs, can be upregulated under pathological conditions where AGEs are increased, and participate in those aging-related pathophysiologies [29]. On the other hand, other groups of cell-surface receptors of AGEs with opposite functions to RAGE, including AGE-R1/Oligosaccharyltransferase 48 KDa Subunit, AGE-R2/protein kinase C substrate 80 K-H, and AGE-R3/galectin-3, and scavenger receptor families act as regulators of endocytosis and clearance of AGEs [30, 31]. These receptors can suppress AGEs-RAGE interaction, but their expressions and functions are impaired during aging and under higher levels of oxidative stress [30]. There is an inverse relationship between AGE-R1 expression and AGEs toxicity [30].

## 3. Dietary AGEs

AGEs are not only produced endogenously; we ingested them from diet. AGEs content of food depends on the content of protein, fat, and sugar and the types of processing and cooking methods, predominantly on the temperature and duration of preparation [32]. High temperatures during various processes like baking, roasting, frying and grilling promote glycation in food. Scheijen et al. [33] analyzed the content of CML, Nε-carboxyethyllysine (CEL), MG-H1 in the protein fraction of the 190 food items by UPLC-MS/MS, and they showed that CML and CEL were contained in <7 mg/100 g in high-content foods such as fried bacon, chocolate, and peanut butter. The content of MG-H1 was higher compared to those of CML and CEL, and it was <65 mg/100 g in high-content foods such as black pudding, peanut butter, cereals, and biscuit.

Proteins are digested into amino acids and small peptide in the gastrointestinal tract. Therefore, dietary AGEs are expected to be absorbed in the circulation mostly in the form of free AGEs and AGEs-modified peptides. The amount of AGEs absorbed in the circulation was estimated to be 10% in healthy people; 1/3 of the absorbed AGEs are excreted in urine within 48 hours and 2/3 remained in the body [34]. For healthy people, a daily AGEs intake of around 9,000–23,000 kU/day was determined [32]; one AGE Unit was defined as the amount of antibody-reactive material that was equivalent to that in 1 μg of an AGEs-BSA standard. The AGEs content of major meals [35] is listed in **Table 1**.

A cross-sectional study revealed that higher levels of dietary AGEs were associated with higher levels of free plasma and urinary AGEs [36]. In addition, a tracer study using $^{13}C_2$-CML found that dietary CML was accumulated in kidney, ileum, colon, lung, brain, testis, heart muscle, skeletal muscle, and liver, but not in fat [37], suggesting the contribution of dietary AGEs to tissue dysfunction and development of diseases. In fact, a meta-analysis of 13 randomized controlled trials showed a decrease in metabolic parameters including body weight, insulin resistance, total

| Meal | AGEs kU/serving | Calory kcal/serving |
|---|---|---|
| Carbonara spaghetti (280 g) | 27,033 | 1,043 |
| Sirloin steak (200 g) | 26,843 | 1,003 |
| Mixed pizza (1/2 piece) | 21,783 | 1,211 |
| Seafood pizza (1/2 piece) | 19,676 | 1,211 |
| Beef cutlet curry (450 g) | 17,337 | 1,407 |
| Hamburger steak (220 g) | 11,170 | 453 |
| Roasted dumplings (10 pieces) | 8,668 | 627 |
| Fried chicken (130 g) | 7,997 | 532 |
| Fried shrimp (245 g) | 7,290 | 588 |
| Deep-fried tofu (155 g) | 6,063 | 204 |
| Salt-grilled saury (130 g) | 6,032 | 315 |
| Hamburger (1 piece) | 5,851 | 302 |
| Soy sauce ramen (270 g) | 5,377 | 476 |
| Fried egg (2 pieces) | 4,304 | 257 |
| Fried potato (160 g) | 4,099 | 448 |
| Cream puff (1 piece) | 3,799 | 123 |
| Fried noodles (190 g) | 3,628 | 512 |
| Strawberry sponge cake (1 cut) | 2,998 | 539 |
| Toast with butter (1 piece) | 2,447 | 259 |
| Spaghetti with meat sauce (280 g) | 2,063 | 616 |
| Tofu with soy sauce (118 g) | 624 | 73 |
| Boiled egg (2 pieces) | 382 | 211 |
| Potato salad (140 g) | 249 | 372 |
| Miso soup (1 cup) | 227 | 39 |
| Raw egg (2 pieces) | 164 | 211 |
| Udon noodles (130 g) | 71 | 339 |
| Strawberry (120 g) | 52 | 96 |
| Banana (90 g) | 51 | 78 |
| Boiled spinach (30 g) | 30 | 9 |
| White rice (150 g) | 16 | 252 |

**Table 1.**
*AGEs content in meals.*

cholesterol, low-density lipoprotein, and leptin and an increase in adiponectin levels after consumption of low AGEs diets compared to high AGEs diets [38, 39]. This study indicates that the restriction of AGEs from food can be effective in reducing the incidence of chronic metabolic diseases and promoting health.

## 4. The effect of AGEs on skeletal muscle

### 4.1 AGEs accumulation and skeletal muscle dysfunction

In this about 10 years, epidemiological studies have reported the relationship between AGEs level in the body and skeletal muscle functions. The first report by

Dalal et al. [6] found an association between elevated serum CML level and poor grip strength in 559 older women with physical disability (≥ 65 years old). A similar result was observed in the InCHIANTI study, which is a population-based prospective cohort study conducted in the Chianti region in Italy. The study showed that elevated plasma CML level was at high risk of slow walking speed (odds ratio 1.56, 95% confidence interval 1.02–2.38, P = 0.04) in 944 older community-dwelling adults (≥ 65 years old) [7]. Sun et al. [9] also reported that elevated serum CML level was a risk factor for developing severe walking disability. In the study, which had a 30-month follow-up in 394 older women (≥ 65 years old), it was shown that compared with the group of lower three quartiles of CML, the patients in the group of highest quartile of CML were more likely to develop severe walking disability (hazard ratio 1.54, 95% confidence interval 1.04–2.29, P = 0.03). A community-based cross-sectional study by Yang et al. [16] showed that urinary CML level was negatively associated with grip strength among 41 older women but not 63 older men (≥ 65 years old). Furthermore, the joint association of urinary CML level and mobility function was correlated with the risk of developing sarcopenia among older adults (odds ratio 13.76, 95% confidence interval 1.03–183.83, P < 0.05). In addition to CML, increased serum pentosidine, a well-known AGEs found in the plasma and tissues of diabetic and uremic subjects [40], was shown to be negatively associated with skeletal muscle mass in 133 postmenopausal women with type 2 diabetes (mean age 66.8 years) [10] and in 70 elderly women with or without sarcopenia (≥ 53 years old) [17].

These findings are also supported by studies using non-invasive AGEs measurement methods. Because several AGEs have characteristic fluorescence, the measurement of skin autofluorescence (SAF) is often adopted to assess the level of AGEs in the body. Momma et al. [8] investigated the relationship between SAF and muscle strength and power in 232 adult men (median age 46.0 years) and found that participants with higher SAF had lower grip strength and leg extension power. Kato et al. [11] also reported that SAF was significantly higher in the low skeletal muscle index group compared with the normal skeletal muscle index group among 132 elderly people (mean age 59.0 years). Moreover, SAF was shown to be an independent factor associated with low skeletal muscle index (odds ratio 15.7, 95% confidence interval 1.85–133.01, P = 0.012). The negative association between SAF and muscle mass (odds ratio 1.48, 95% confidence interval 1.23–1.78, P < 0.001), grip strength (odds ratio 1.98, P = 0.003), hip flexion strength (odds ratio 1.50, P = 0.012), and hip abduction strength (odds ratio 1.78, P = 0.001) was found among 9,203 participants (mean age 57.8 years) in the Nagahama study, which is a large-scale population-based cohort study in Japan [13]. Another large population-based cohort study in the Netherlands, the Lifelines study also demonstrated the relationship between SAF and poor physical functioning among 5,624 participants (≥ 65 years old) [14]. In a study of diabetic patients, Mori et al. [12] reported that knee extension power was negatively correlated with SAF among 36 patients with type 1 diabetes (mean age 55.7 years). They subsequently reported that SAF was the independent determinant for skeletal muscle mass index (odds ratio 6.38, 95% confidence interval 1.93–21.08, P < 0.05), grip strength (odds ratio 3.55, 95% confidence interval 1.57–8.00, P < 0.05), knee extension power (odds ratio 3.68, 95% confidence interval 1.87–7.23, P < 0.05), and sarcopenia (odds ratio 7.73, 95% confidence interval 2.13–28.02, P < 0.05) among 166 patients with type 2 diabetes (mean age 63.2 years) [15]. Collectively, accumulation of AGEs may be a better predictor of skeletal muscle dysfunctions during aging process. Furthermore, recent our preliminary study found that SAF was negatively associated with leg extension power in 20 health young men (mean age 19.0 years) (**Figure 2**). Therefore, glycation stress may affect muscle strength even in young people, and it is considered

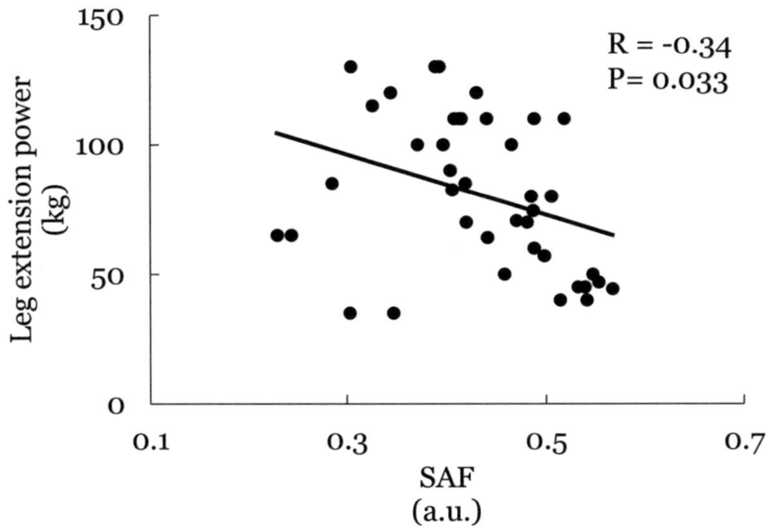


**Figure 2.**
*Correlation between skin autofluorescence (SAF) and leg extension power. The subjects were 20 healthy young men, and after measuring the subcutaneous glycation state with an AGEs sensor (RQ-AG01J, Sharp Life Sciences, Hyogo, Japan), the maximum lift weight of leg extension was measured. Statistical significance was assessed using Pearson's correlation.*

that grasping the glycation stress state not only from the elderly but also from the young age can contribute to the prevention of future muscle dysfunctions.

### 4.2 AGEs modification of contractile proteins in skeletal muscle

Decreased skeletal muscle quantity is deemed a crucial cause of aging-associated muscle dysfunctions. However, recent evidence suggests that the quality of muscle tissue is more functionally relevant than its quantity. Muscle contractile properties are identified as an important determinant of functional limitations in older adults [41]. In this context, several studies have focused on the effect of intracellular glycation on protein structure and function in skeletal muscle. Syrovy and Hodny [42] first reported in 1993 that incubation of myofibrils with ribose promoted the glycation of myofibrillar proteins such as myosin heavy chain, α-actinin, actin, and tropomyosin, accompanied by reduced ATPase activity. The decrease in ATPase activity associated with the glycation is supported by several subsequent studies [43–45]. A major component of skeletal muscle, myosin contains 201 lysine residues and offers numerous potential sites for glycation. In fact, Ramamurthy et al. [46] demonstrated that glucose exposure to rodent skeletal muscle fiber induced myosin structural change and reduction of shortening velocity of myosin. The study is the first report to show the glycation-induced protein structural and functional changes in skeletal muscle. Furthermore, some researchers have found that actin and connective tissues were also modified with AGEs in skeletal muscle of old rats [47] and human [48]. Structural or chemical changes in actin, myosin, and extracellular matrix are likely to deteriorate muscle function by affecting actomyosin ATPase activity or stiffness [49, 50]. Our preliminary experiment also found that 45 AGEs-modified proteins were increased in skeletal muscle of old mice (24-month age) compared with that of young adult mice (6-month age) (unpublished data). These intracellular or extracellular AGEs modifications of skeletal muscle proteins may be a potent factor of aging-associated skeletal muscle dysfunctions.

### 4.3 AGEs and insulin resistance in skeletal muscle

In skeletal muscle, the initial insulin signaling events include insulin binding to the extracellular α-subunit of the insulin receptor, rapid phosphorylation of the receptor (auto-phosphorylation) and insulin receptor substrate (IRS)-1 on tyrosine residues, and recruitment and activation of class IA phosphatidylinositol 3-kinase. These lead to the generation of the critical second messenger PI-3,4,5-triphosphate, which in turn triggers the activation of Akt [51]. TBC1 domain (TBC1D) family member 1 and TBC1D4 act as downstream mediators of Akt. TBC1D1 and TBC1D4 contain a Rab-GTPase-activating protein domain that prevents glucose transporter 4 (GLUT4) translocation by inactivating Rab proteins. TBC1D1 and TBC1D4 dissociate from GLUT4 vesicles in the phosphorylated state, and thereby facilitating GLUT4 translocation and glucose transport [52, 53].

Many evidence have shown that AGEs impair insulin signaling transduction and induce insulin resistance in skeletal muscle. Miele et al. [54] showed that exposure of glycated albumin (0.1–0.2 mg/ml) to skeletal muscle cells for 24 hours impaired insulin-stimulated 2-deoxyglucose uptake, accompanied by reduced IRS-1 tyrosine phosphorylation, Akt activity, but not insulin receptor kinase activity, suggesting that AGEs affect factors downstream from insulin receptor. AGEs-induced inhibition of glucose transport was supported by the work of Wu et al. [55] that exposure of glyoxal-derived AGEs (0.1 mg/ml) to skeletal muscle cells for 8–48 hours completely abolished 2-deoxyglucose uptake. Their subsequent research found that AGEs-induced impairment of insulin action might be mediated by the formation of multimolecular complex among RAGE/IRS-1/src and protein kinase C [56]. Animal study by Rai et al. [57] demonstrated that fructose intake (20% in drinking water) for 16 weeks decreased insulin-stimulated Akt phosphorylation accompanied by elevated serum and muscle AGEs level and RAGE mRNA level in rat skeletal muscle. However, these changes were suppressed by co-ingestion of AGEs inhibitor aminoguanidine (100 mg/kg). Pinto-Junior et al. [58] showed that injection of glycolaldehyde-derived AGEs (20 mg/kg/day) to rat for 12 weeks led to whole-body insulin resistance and decreased GLUT4 mRNA and protein levels in skeletal muscle. Furthermore, they demonstrated that exposure of glycolaldehyde-derived AGEs (1.0 mg/ml) to skeletal muscle cells for 2.5 hours increased nuclear factor (NF)-κB expression and nuclear protein binding activity into a GLUT4 gene promoter NF-κB binding site, suggesting that AGEs reduce GLUT4 transcription through NF-κB signaling. These AGEs-induced aggravating effect on insulin signaling may induce skeletal muscle insulin resistance, and thereby contributing to impairment of whole-body glucose homeostasis with aging or diabetes.

### 4.4 The effect of AGEs on myogenesis, development, atrophy of skeletal muscle

As described above, AGEs are a crucial factor affecting skeletal muscle functions, especially skeletal muscle mass. Considering the formation process of AGEs derived from sugar, it has been initially investigated the effects of AGEs on diabetic muscle atrophy. Snow et al. [59] observed distribution patterns of AGEs in skeletal muscle of diabetic rats and found the presence of CML intracellularly and at sites along the muscle fiber periphery. However, there was no difference in muscle fiber cross-sectional area between AGEs-positive and -negative fibers in both control and diabetic rats, indicating the indirect effect of intracellular AGEs on muscle size. Alternatively, a more detailed study by Chiu et al. [60] demonstrated that decreased muscle mass and fiber cross-sectional area in diabetic rats was attenuated by the 4-week treatment with AGEs inhibitor, alagebrium chloride, accompanied by decreased AGEs and RAGE expressions. They also investigated the direct effect of AGEs on muscle atrophy and found that exposure of glucose-derived AGEs (0.025–0.2 mg/ml) to human primary skeletal muscle cells for 48 hours induced myotube atrophy via RAGE, 5'AMP-activated protein kinase, and Akt signaling-mediated upregulation of ubiquitin-proteasome system.

Our recent study supports the involvement of RAGE in skeletal muscle atrophy. In addition to diabetes, muscle disuse due to injury, casting, and bedrest is a potent inducer of muscle mass loss [61]. However, there was no evidence that glycation stress was involved in disuse-induced skeletal muscle atrophy. Therefore, we investigated the contribution of RAGE to disuse-induced skeletal muscle atrophy [62]. Our study showed that 1-week hindlimb suspension procedure to mice led to muscle atrophy accompanied by intracellular MG-H1 and CML accumulations. However, treatment with RAGE antagonist during the suspension attenuated the atrophic response (**Figure 3**), and muscle mass inversely correlated with the accumulation of MG-H1 and CML in skeletal muscle (**Figure 4**). RAGE inhibition also suppressed the atrophy-associated expression of proinflammatory cytokines and activation of ubiquitin-proteasome system. These findings suggest the contribution of RAGE to

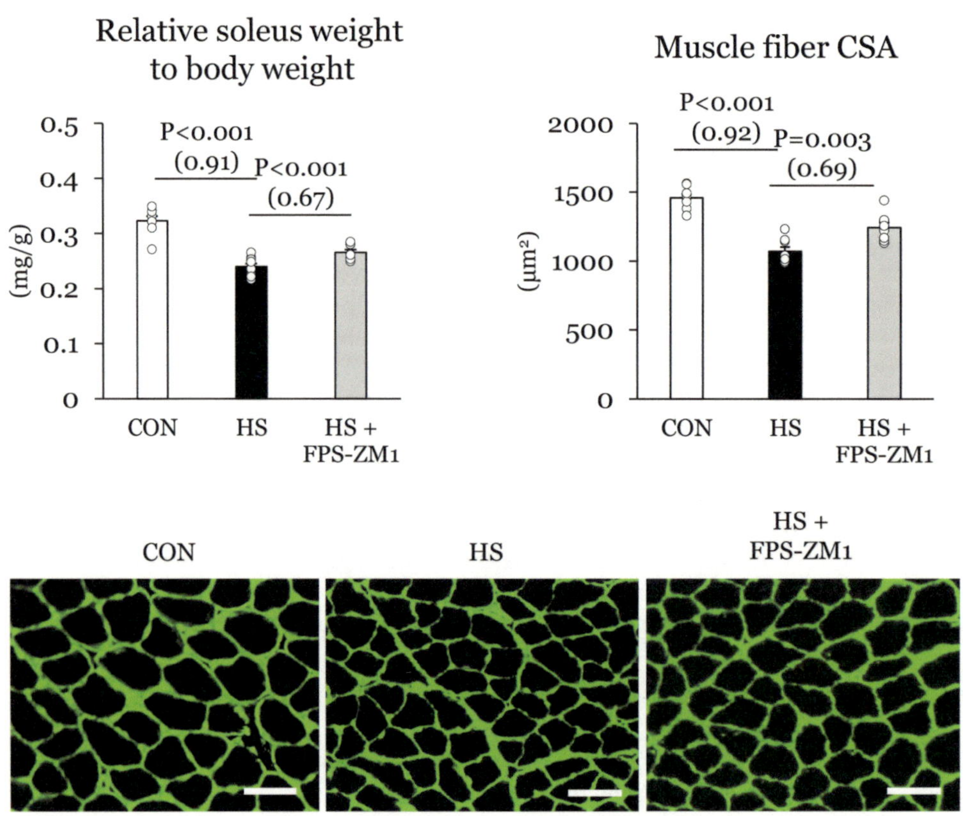


**Figure 3.**
*Soleus weight normalized to body weight and muscle fiber cross sectional area (CSA) after hindlimb suspension and/or receptor for AGEs (RAGE) antagonist treatment. Mice in the HS group were subjected to continuous hindlimb suspension for 1 week. Age-matched mice that did not undergo hindlimb suspension were used as controls (CON). Mice in the HS + FPS-ZM1 group were injected daily intraperitoneally with 1 mg/kg FPS-ZM1, a RAGE antagonist, during hindlimb suspension. Data are expressed as means ± SE; n = 7–9 per group. Individual data points are indicated on the bar graph. Representative images of immunofluorescence are shown. Scale bars, 50 μm. The value of effect size is listed in parentheses. Statistical significance was analyzed using Tukey–Kramer multiple comparison tests. This figure was adapted from Egawa et al. [62] with permission from the publisher.*

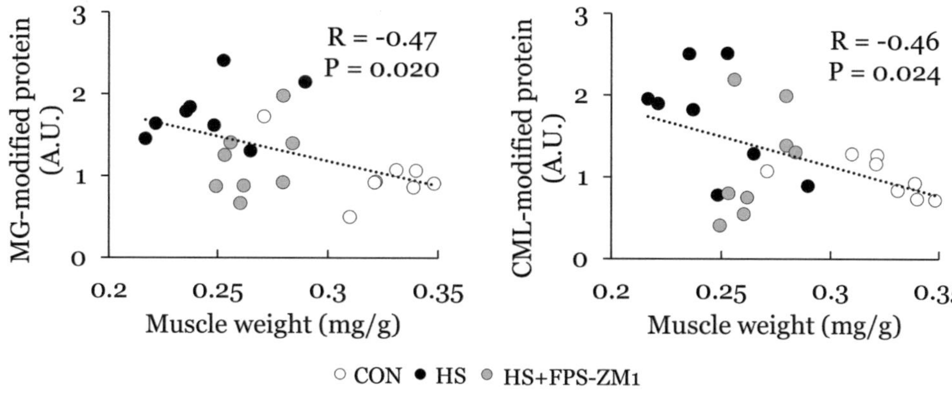


**Figure 4.**
*The correlation between methylglyoxal (MG)- or Nε-(carboxymethyl) lysine (CML)-modified protein level and muscle weight. For the quantification of MG-modified and CML-modified proteins, the signal intensity of full-molecular-weight was quantified after western blotting. n = 8 per group. Statistical significance was assessed using Pearson's correlation. This figure was adapted from Egawa et al. [62] with permission from the publisher.*

disuse-induced skeletal muscle atrophy. Furthermore, in this study, RAGE expression was increased in response to suspension, and this was limited to atrophied soleus and plantaris muscles but not unatrophied extensor digitorum longus muscle. Therefore, muscle disuse itself but not systemic mediators may regulate RAGE expression.

The effect of glycation stress on muscle growth was first reported in our research [63]. We evaluated the differences in muscle mass, contractile properties and molecular responses between mice that received a diet containing high-AGEs and low-AGEs for 16 weeks [63]. As a result, exposure to a high-AGEs promoted CML accumulation in skeletal muscle, suppressed muscle growth, and induced skeletal muscle dysfunctions including suppression of muscle strength, fatigue resistance, and force production (**Figure 5**). In addition, the expression of myogenic factors and phosphorylation of p70 s6 kinase, an enzyme playing a key role in the regulation of protein synthesis, were decreased in the high-AGEs treated group. These results suggest that exposure to AGEs impairs postnatal growth and muscle development.

To clarify the underlying mechanism of AGEs-induced inhibition of muscle growth, we next carried out the comprehensive analysis of protein phosphorylation status by using the reverse phase protein array method [64]. In the study, the average level of phosphorylation of skeletal muscle cells exposed to various kinds of AGEs (glyoxylic-, pyruvate, glycolaldehyde, and glucose-derived AGEs, 0.1 mg/ml) was increased at eight phosphorylation sites and decreased at 64. The most upregulated phosphorylation sites were signal transducer and activator of transcription 3 (STAT3) $Tyr^{705}$. The most downregulated phosphorylation sites were extracellular signal-regulated kinase (ERK) $Thr^{202}/Tyr^{204}$. Almost all of the phosphorylation sites related to insulin/insulin-like growth factor 1 (IGF-1) signaling were also downregulated by AGEs (**Figure 6**). Increased STAT3 $Tyr^{705}$ phosphorylation and decreased ERK $Thr^{202}/Tyr^{204}$ phosphorylation were also confirmed in the skeletal muscles of mice treated with a diet high in AGEs for 16 weeks. These results suggest that systemic AGEs modulate cellular signaling transduction pathways, such as STAT3 and insulin/IGF-1 signaling, and thereby contribute to the impairment of skeletal muscle growth and development. Accordingly, Adachi et al. demonstrated that IGF-1 treatment protected AGEs-induced deterioration of myogenic differentiation in skeletal muscle cells [65].

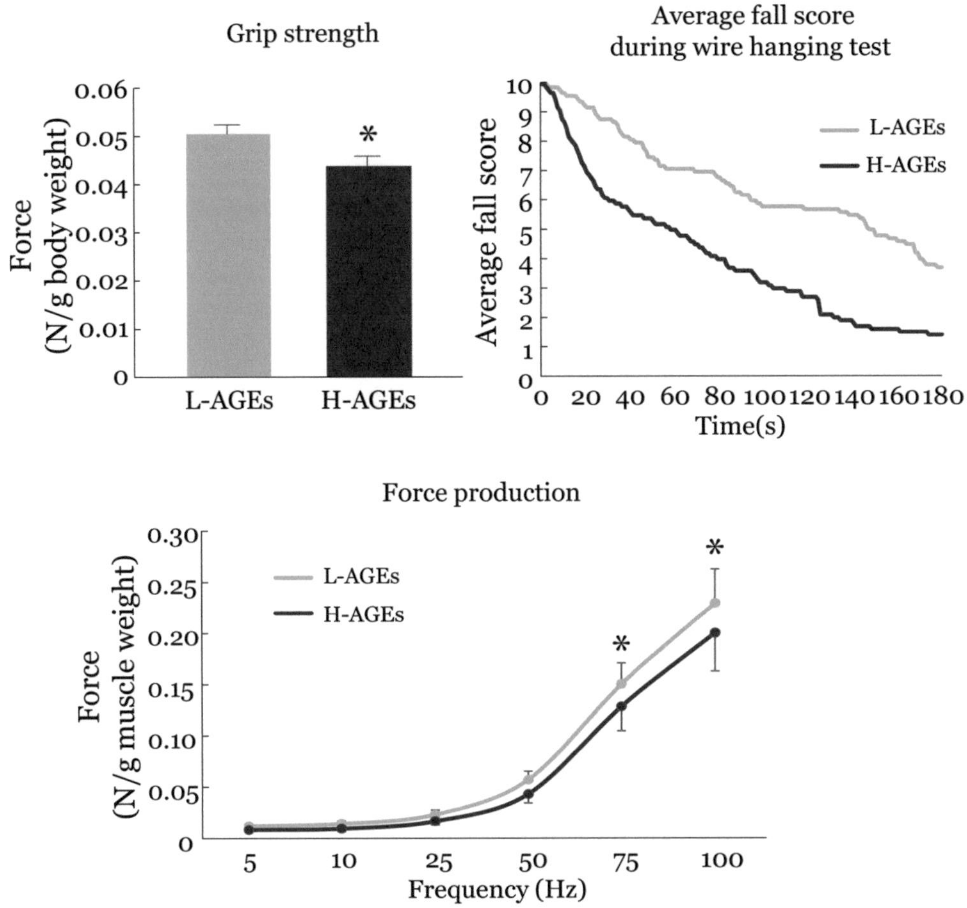


**Figure 5.**
*The grip strength test, wire-hanging test, and in vitro force production of plantaris muscles in mice fed a diet low in AGEs (L-AGEs) or a diet high in AGEs (H-AGEs). The grip strength test and wire-hanging test was conducted 5 and 4 days before the end of the 16-week study, respectively. For measuring in vitro forth production, isolated plantaris muscle was allowed to rest for 30 min and the muscle was tetanically contracted at frequencies of 0, 5, 10, 25, 50, 75, and 100 Hz with a 2 min rest between contractions. Data are expressed as mean ± SE, $n = 10$ per group. *$P < 0.05$ vs. L-AGEs mice. Statistical significance was analyzed using Student's t test or Tukey–Kramer multiple comparisons tests. This figure was adapted from Egawa et al. [63] with permission from the publisher.*

## 5. Therapeutic perspectives for AGEs-induced skeletal muscle dysfunctions

AGEs-RAGE axis seems to be the most contributor to skeletal muscle dysfunctions under glycation stress condition [66]. Recently, Chiappalupi et al. [67] demonstrated that cancer cachexia-induced muscle wasting and inflammatory responses were prevented in RAGE-null mice. In this regard, several RAGE antagonists were used for preclinical and clinical studies [68, 69]. For example, FPS-ZM1, which was identified by screening 5,000 compounds for their ability to inhibit RAGE and amyloid-β interaction, can block amyloid-β-induced cellular stress [70]. Azeliragon, which is an orally-active small-molecule antagonist of RAGE, improves cognitive function in Alzheimer disease patients by inhibiting inflammation and amyloid-β accumulation [71]. As our study showed, RAGE inhibition by FPS-ZM1 could prevent disuse-induced muscle atrophy [62]. Potentially, these RAGE inhibitors might be useful for various skeletal muscle atrophy.

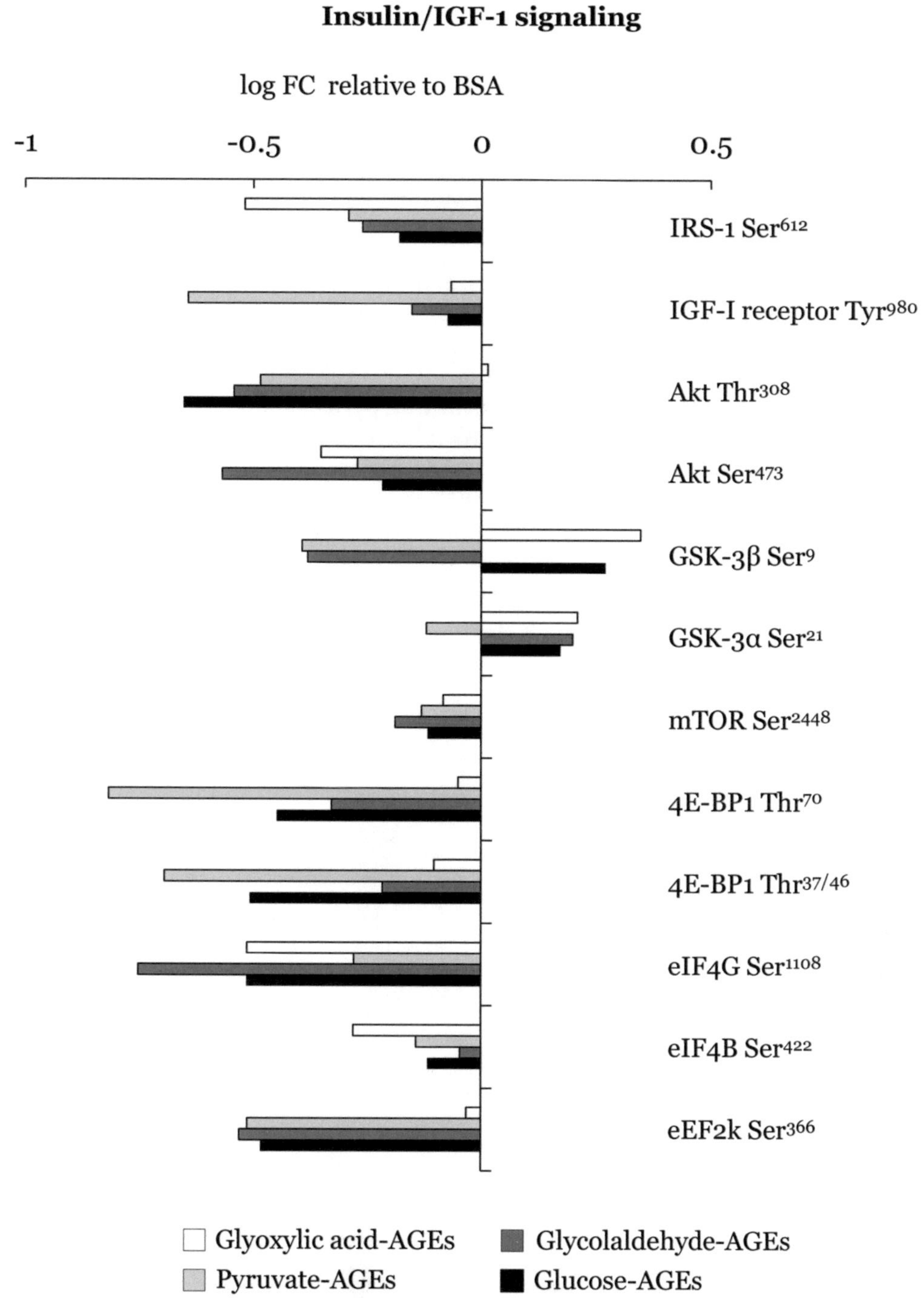


**Figure 6.**
*The phosphoproteins related to insulin/insulin-like growth factor-1 (IGF-1) signaling. C2C12 myotubes on day 4 of differentiation were incubated with glyoxylic acid-derived AGEs, pyruvate- derived AGEs, glycolaldehyde- derived AGEs, glucose- derived AGEs, or BSA at 0.1 mg/mL for 24 h. After that, reverse phase protein array analysis was performed. The phosphoproteins related to insulin/IGF-1 signaling are represented as the relative log fold-change (FC) values. This figure was adapted from Egawa et al. [64] with permission from the publisher. IRS-1, insulin receptor substrate-1; IGF-1, insulin-like growth factor-1; GSK, glycogen synthase kinase; mTOR, mammalian target of rapamycin; 4E-BP1, eukaryotic translation initiation factor 4E binding protein- 1; eIF, eukaryotic translation initiation factor; eEF2k, eukaryotic elongation factor- 2 kinase.*

Plant-derived phytochemicals are also potentially beneficial for maintaining muscle functions. Screening of 536 kinds of plants has confirmed anti-glycation activity in more than 100 kinds of materials [72]. Recent our study [73] found that propolis, a natural resinous substance produced by honeybees, has an inhibitory effect on AGEs formation. Furthermore, propolis intake (0.1%-containing diet) for 20 weeks under glycation stress conditions from methylglyoxal exposure prevented intracellular MG-H1 accumulation and inflammatory cytokine expressions in mouse skeletal muscle (**Figure 7**).

In addition to phytochemicals, organic compound with anti-glycation effect, pyridoxamine has been shown to inhibit diabetes-related muscle dysfunctions. Muellenbach et al. [74] first showed that treatment with pyridoxamine (60 mg/kg i.p. injection) for 6 weeks improved insulin-stimulated glucose transport in the skeletal muscle of obese Zucker rats. In a study by Hagiwara et al. [75] using a high-fat diet fed rats, it was shown that 12-week treatment with pyridoxamine (300 mg/kg/day in drinking water) attenuated reductions in Akt phosphorylation and GLUT4 expression in the plasma membrane of skeletal muscle. Mastrocola et al. [76] demonstrated that pyridoxamine treatment to rats fed a high-fructose diet (60% of calories) for 12 weeks suppressed CML accumulation, RAGE upregulation, sirtuin-1 reduction, mitochondrial dysfunction, and contractile dysfunction in skeletal muscle. These

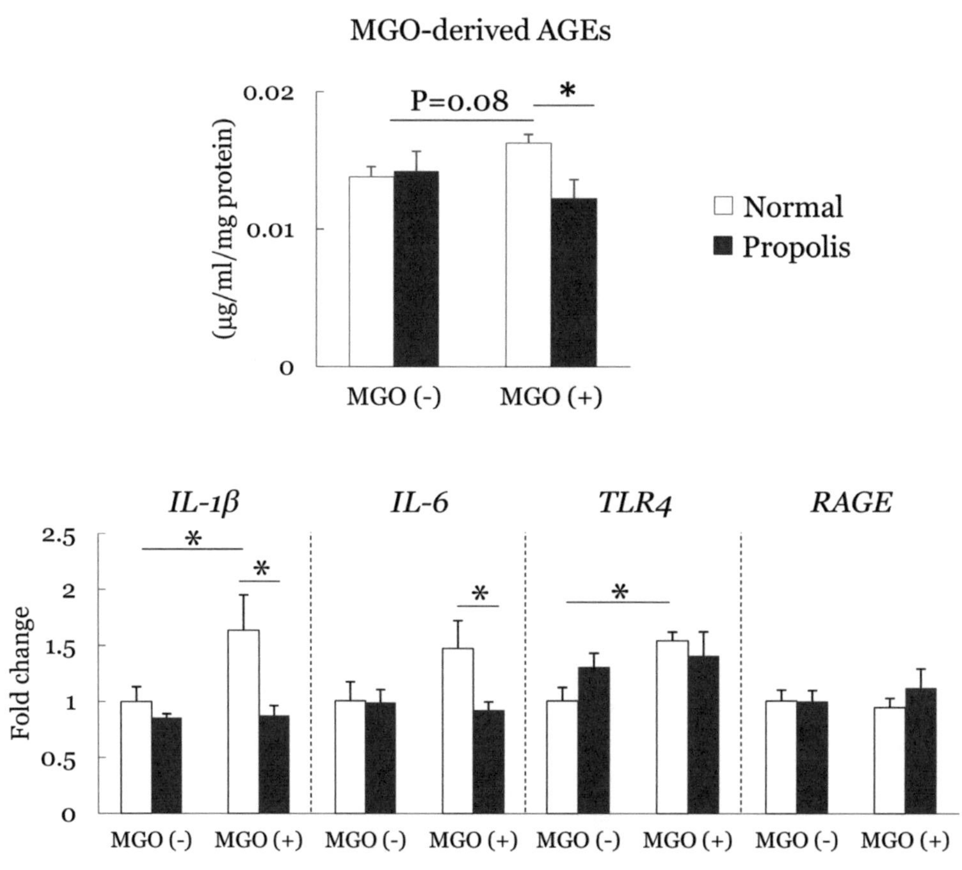


**Figure 7.**
*The content of methylglyoxal (MGO)-derived AGEs and mRNA expression of interleukin (IL)-1β, IL-6, toll-like receptor 4 (TLR4), and receptor for AGEs (RAGE) in the extensor digitorum longus muscles. The muscles were dissected from mice treated with or without propolis (0.1%)-containing diet or MGO (0.1%)-containing drinking water for 20 weeks. Data are expressed as means ± SE; n = 3–6 per group. * P < 0.05 between the groups. Statistical significance was analyzed using Tukey–Kramer multiple comparisons tests. This figure was adapted from Egawa et al. [73] with permission from the publisher.*

results suggest that even in situations where glycation stress increase such as high-AGEs diet intake, skeletal muscle dysfunctions can be prevented by simultaneously ingesting compounds and foods that have anti-glycation effects.

## 6. Conclusion

Glycation stress is a potential factor that reduces physical functions, which has become attention in recent years as well as oxidative stress. Glycation stress is mainly caused by intracellular AGEs formation and accumulation in the body, and also by ingestion from food products. Exposure to AGEs on skeletal muscle cells leads to skeletal muscle dysfunctions including reductions of mass, contractile function, insulin sensitivity. These dysfunctions seem to be attributed to RAGE-induced inflammatory responses and deteriorations of cellular signaling transduction, including insulin/IGF-1 signaling. However, some therapeutic strategies, such as treatment with RAGE antagonists, AGEs inhibitors, phytochemicals can overcome the aggravating effects. Glycation research on skeletal muscle has not been sufficiently carried out, and further studies in the future, especially the elucidation of the effect of glycation stress on skeletal muscle and its underlying molecular mechanism, and the development of strategies on preventing the accumulation of AGEs in skeletal muscle, are desired.

## Acknowledgements

This work was supported, in part, by JSPS KAKENHI Grant Number 18H03148, 19 K22806 (TE), 19 K20007 (KK), 19 K24330, 20 K19498 (TY), 18H03160, 19 K22825, 19KK0254 (KG), 19 K11520 (TH), and research grants from the Descente Foundation for the Promotion of Sports Science, the Uehara Memorial Foundation (TE), and the Graduate School of Health Sciences, Toyohashi SOZO University (KG).

## Conflict of interest

The authors declare no conflict of interest.

## Author details

Tatsuro Egawa[1*], Kohei Kido[2,3], Takumi Yokokawa[4], Mami Fujibayashi[5], Katsumasa Goto[6] and Tatsuya Hayashi[7]

1 Laboratory of Health and Exercise Sciences, Graduate School of Human and Environmental Studies, Kyoto University, Kyoto, Japan

2 Faculty of Sports and Health Science, Fukuoka University, Fukuoka, Japan

3 Institute for Physical Activity, Fukuoka University, Fukuoka, Japan

4 Division of Food Science and Biotechnology, Graduate School of Agriculture, Kyoto University, Kyoto, Japan

5 Faculty of Agriculture, Setsunan University, Osaka, Japan

6 Department of Physiology, Graduate School of Health Sciences, Toyohashi SOZO University, Aichi, Japan

7 Laboratory of Sports and Exercise Medicine, Graduate School of Human and Environmental Studies, Kyoto University, Kyoto, Japan

*Address all correspondence to: egawa.tatsuro.4u@kyoto-u.ac.jp

## References

[1] Hoffmann C, Weigert C: Skeletal Muscle as an Endocrine Organ: The Role of Myokines in Exercise Adaptations. Cold Spring Harbor Perspectives in Medicine. 2017;7. DOI: 10.1101/cshperspect.a029793

[2] Argiles JM, Campos N, Lopez-Pedrosa JM, Rueda R, Rodriguez-Manas L: Skeletal Muscle Regulates Metabolism via Interorgan Crosstalk: Roles in Health and Disease. Journal of the American Medical Directors Association. 2016;17:789-796. DOI: 10.1016/j.jamda.2016.04.019

[3] Keller K, Engelhardt M: Strength and muscle mass loss with aging process. Age and strength loss. Muscles Ligaments Tendons J. 2013;3:346-350. DOI:

[4] Chaudhuri J, Bains Y, Guha S, Kahn A, Hall D, Bose N, et al.: The Role of Advanced Glycation End Products in Aging and Metabolic Diseases: Bridging Association and Causality. Cell Metabolism. 2018;28:337-352. DOI: 10.1016/j.cmet.2018.08.014

[5] Fournet M, Bonte F, Desmouliere A: Glycation Damage: A Possible Hub for Major Pathophysiological Disorders and Aging. Aging and Disease. 2018;9:880-900. DOI: 10.14336/AD.2017.1121

[6] Dalal M, Ferrucci L, Sun K, Beck J, Fried LP, Semba RD: Elevated serum advanced glycation end products and poor grip strength in older community-dwelling women. Journals of Gerontology Series A: Biological Sciences and Medical Sciences. 2009;64:132-137. DOI: 10.1093/gerona/gln018

[7] Semba RD, Bandinelli S, Sun K, Guralnik JM, Ferrucci L: Relationship of an advanced glycation end product, plasma carboxymethyl-lysine, with slow walking speed in older adults: the InCHIANTI study. European Journal of Applied Physiology. 2010;108:191-195. DOI: 10.1007/s00421-009-1192-5

[8] Momma H, Niu K, Kobayashi Y, Guan L, Sato M, Guo H, et al.: Skin advanced glycation end product accumulation and muscle strength among adult men. European Journal of Applied Physiology. 2011;111:1545-1552. DOI: 10.1007/s00421-010-1779-x

[9] Sun K, Semba RD, Fried LP, Schaumberg DA, Ferrucci L, Varadhan R: Elevated Serum Carboxymethyl-Lysine, an Advanced Glycation End Product, Predicts Severe Walking Disability in Older Women: The Women's Health and Aging Study I. Journal of Aging Research. 2012;2012:586385. DOI: 10.1155/2012/586385

[10] Tanaka K, Kanazawa I, Sugimoto T: Elevated Serum Pentosidine and Decreased Serum IGF-I Levels are Associated with Loss of Muscle Mass in Postmenopausal Women with Type 2 Diabetes Mellitus. Experimental and Clinical Endocrinology and Diabetes. 2016;124:163-166. DOI: 10.1055/s-0035-1565103

[11] Kato M, Kubo A, Sugioka Y, Mitsui R, Fukuhara N, Nihei F, et al.: Relationship between advanced glycation end-product accumulation and low skeletal muscle mass in Japanese men and women. Geriatr Gerontol Int. 2017;17:785-790. DOI: 10.1111/ggi.12787

[12] Mori H, Kuroda A, Araki M, Suzuki R, Taniguchi S, Tamaki M, et al.: Advanced glycation end-products are a risk for muscle weakness in Japanese patients with type 1 diabetes. J Diabetes Investig. 2017;8:377-382. DOI: 10.1111/jdi.12582

[13] Tabara Y, Ikezoe T, Yamanaka M, Setoh K, Segawa H, Kawaguchi T, et al.:

Advanced Glycation End Product Accumulation Is Associated With Low Skeletal Muscle Mass, Weak Muscle Strength, and Reduced Bone Density: The Nagahama Study. Journals of Gerontology Series A: Biological Sciences and Medical Sciences. 2019;74:1446-1453. DOI: 10.1093/gerona/gly233

[14] Drenth H, Zuidema SU, Krijnen WP, Bautmans I, Smit AJ, van der Schans C, et al.: Advanced Glycation End Products Are Associated With Physical Activity and Physical Functioning in the Older Population. Journals of Gerontology Series A: Biological Sciences and Medical Sciences. 2018;73:1545-1551. DOI: 10.1093/gerona/gly108

[15] Mori H, Kuroda A, Ishizu M, Ohishi M, Takashi Y, Otsuka Y, et al.: Association of accumulated advanced glycation end-products with a high prevalence of sarcopenia and dynapenia in patients with type 2 diabetes. J Diabetes Investig. 2019;10:1332-1340. DOI: 10.1111/jdi.13014

[16] Yang CW, Li CI, Liu CS, Lin CH, Lin WY, Li TC, et al.: Relationship among urinary advanced glycation-end products, skeletal muscle mass and physical performance in community-dwelling older adults. Geriatr Gerontol Int. 2019;19:1017-1022. DOI: 10.1111/ggi.13762

[17] Eguchi Y, Toyoguchi T, Inage K, Fujimoto K, Orita S, Suzuki M, et al.: Advanced glycation end products are associated with sarcopenia in older women: aging marker dynamics. J Women Aging. 2019:1-13. DOI: 10.1080/08952841.2019.1697161

[18] Thornalley PJ: Dicarbonyl intermediates in the maillard reaction. Annals of the New York Academy of Sciences. 2005;1043:111-117. DOI: 10.1196/annals.1333.014

[19] Teichert T, Hellwig A, Pessler A, Hellwig M, Vossoughi M, Sugiri D, et al.: Association between Advanced Glycation End Products and Impaired Fasting Glucose: Results from the SALIA Study. PloS One. 2015;10:e0128293. DOI: 10.1371/journal.pone.0128293

[20] Ahmed N, Babaei-Jadidi R, Howell SK, Thornalley PJ, Beisswenger PJ: Glycated and oxidized protein degradation products are indicators of fasting and postprandial hyperglycemia in diabetes. Diabetes Care. 2005;28:2465-2471. DOI: 10.2337/diacare.28.10.2465

[21] Haque E, Kamil M, Hasan A, Irfan S, Sheikh S, Khatoon A, et al.: Advanced glycation end products (AGEs), protein aggregation and their cross talk: new insight in tumorigenesis. Glycobiology. 2019;30:49-57. DOI: 10.1093/glycob/cwz073

[22] Sun F, Suttapitugsakul S, Xiao H, Wu R: Comprehensive Analysis of Protein Glycation Reveals Its Potential Impacts on Protein Degradation and Gene Expression in Human Cells. J Am Soc Mass Spectrom. 2019;30:2480-2490. DOI: 10.1007/s13361-019-02197-4

[23] Goh SY, Cooper ME: Clinical review: The role of advanced glycation end products in progression and complications of diabetes. J Clin Endocrinol Metab. 2008;93:1143-1152. DOI: 10.1210/jc.2007-1817

[24] Ramasamy R, Yan SF, Herold K, Clynes R, Schmidt AM: Receptor for advanced glycation end products: fundamental roles in the inflammatory response: winding the way to the pathogenesis of endothelial dysfunction and atherosclerosis. Annals of the New York Academy of Sciences. 2008;1126:7-13. DOI: 10.1196/annals.1433.056

[25] Yan SF, Ramasamy R, Schmidt AM: The receptor for advanced glycation endproducts (RAGE) and cardiovascular disease. Expert Reviews

in Molecular Medicine. 2009;11:e9. DOI: 10.1017/S146239940900101X

[26] Srikanth V, Maczurek A, Phan T, Steele M, Westcott B, Juskiw D, et al.: Advanced glycation endproducts and their receptor RAGE in Alzheimer's disease. Neurobiology of Aging. 2011;32:763-777. DOI: 10.1016/j.neurobiolaging.2009.04.016

[27] Yamagishi S: Role of advanced glycation end products (AGEs) and receptor for AGEs (RAGE) in vascular damage in diabetes. Experimental Gerontology. 2011;46:217-224. DOI: 10.1016/j.exger.2010.11.007

[28] Yamagishi S: Role of advanced glycation end products (AGEs) in osteoporosis in diabetes. Current Drug Targets. 2011;12:2096-2102. DOI: 10.2174/138945011798829456

[29] Wautier MP, Guillausseau PJ, Wautier JL: Activation of the receptor for advanced glycation end products and consequences on health. Diabetes & Metabolic Syndrome. 2017;11:305-309. DOI: 10.1016/j.dsx.2016.09.009

[30] Ott C, Jacobs K, Haucke E, Navarrete Santos A, Grune T, Simm A: Role of advanced glycation end products in cellular signaling. Redox Biol. 2014;2:411-429. DOI: 10.1016/j.redox.2013.12.016

[31] Shen CY, Lu CH, Wu CH, Li KJ, Kuo YM, Hsieh SC, et al.: The Development of Maillard Reaction, and Advanced Glycation End Product (AGE)-Receptor for AGE (RAGE) Signaling Inhibitors as Novel Therapeutic Strategies for Patients with AGE-Related Diseases. Molecules. 2020;25. DOI: 10.3390/molecules25235591

[32] Nowotny K, Schroter D, Schreiner M, Grune T: Dietary advanced glycation end products and their relevance for human health. Ageing Res Rev. 2018;47:55-66. DOI: 10.1016/j.arr.2018.06.005

[33] Scheijen J, Clevers E, Engelen L, Dagnelie PC, Brouns F, Stehouwer CDA, et al.: Analysis of advanced glycation endproducts in selected food items by ultra-performance liquid chromatography tandem mass spectrometry: Presentation of a dictary AGE database. Food Chemistry. 2016;190:1145-1150. DOI: 10.1016/j.foodchem.2015.06.049

[34] Koschinsky T, He CJ, Mitsuhashi T, Bucala R, Liu C, Buenting C, et al.: Orally absorbed reactive glycation products (glycotoxins): an environmental risk factor in diabetic nephropathy. Proceedings of the National Academy of Sciences of the United States of America. 1997;94:6474-6479. DOI: 10.1073/pnas.94.12.6474

[35] Yamagishi S. exAGE handbook [Translated from Japanese.]. Fukuoka, Japan: AGE Reseach Association; 2015. 96 p.

[36] Scheijen J, Hanssen NMJ, van Greevenbroek MM, Van der Kallen CJ, Feskens EJM, Stehouwer CDA, et al.: Dietary intake of advanced glycation endproducts is associated with higher levels of advanced glycation endproducts in plasma and urine: The CODAM study. Clinical Nutrition. 2018;37:919-925. DOI: 10.1016/j.clnu.2017.03.019

[37] Tessier FJ, Niquet-Leridon C, Jacolot P, Jouquand C, Genin M, Schmidt AM, et al.: Quantitative assessment of organ distribution of dietary protein-bound (13) C-labeled N(varepsilon) -carboxymethyllysine after a chronic oral exposure in mice. Molecular Nutrition & Food Research. 2016;60:2446-2456. DOI: 10.1002/mnfr.201600140

[38] Sohouli MH, Sharifi-Zahabi E, Lari A, Fatahi S, Shidfar F: The impact

of low advanced glycation end products diet on obesity and related hormones: a systematic review and meta-analysis. Scientific Reports. 2020;10:22194. DOI: 10.1038/s41598-020-79216-y

[39] Sohouli MH, Fatahi S, Sharifi-Zahabi E, Santos HO, Tripathi N, Lari A, et al.: The Impact of Low Advanced Glycation End Products Diet on Metabolic Risk Factors: A Systematic Review and Meta-Analysis of Randomized Controlled Trials. Advances in Nutrition. 2020. DOI: 10.1093/advances/nmaa150

[40] Sell DR, Nagaraj RH, Grandhee SK, Odetti P, Lapolla A, Fogarty J, et al.: Pentosidine: a molecular marker for the cumulative damage to proteins in diabetes, aging, and uremia. Diabetes/Metabolism Reviews. 1991;7:239-251. DOI: 10.1002/dmr.5610070404

[41] Reid KF, Fielding RA: Skeletal muscle power: a critical determinant of physical functioning in older adults. Exerc Sport Sci Rev. 2012;40:4-12. DOI: 10.1097/JES.0b013e31823b5f13

[42] Syrovy I, Hodny Z: In vitro non-enzymatic glycosylation of myofibrillar proteins. International Journal of Biochemistry. 1993;25:941-946. DOI: 10.1016/0020-711x(93)90251-9

[43] Patterson MF, Stephenson DG, Kemp JG, Stephenson GM: Ca2+-activation characteristics of single fibres from chemically skinned rat muscle incubated with glucose-6-phosphate. Pflügers Archiv European Journal of Physiology. 2000;439:845-852. DOI: 10.1007/s004249900245

[44] Lal S, Chithra P, Chandrakasan G: The possible relevance of autoxidative glycosylation in glucose mediated alterations of proteins: an in vitro study on myofibrillar proteins. Molecular and Cellular Biochemistry. 1996;154:95-100. DOI: 10.1007/BF00226776

[45] Syrovy I: Glycation of myofibrillar proteins and ATPase activity after incubation with eleven sugars. Physiological Research. 1994;43:61-64.

[46] Ramamurthy B, Hook P, Jones AD, Larsson L: Changes in myosin structure and function in response to glycation. FASEB Journal. 2001;15:2415-2422. DOI: 10.1096/fj.01-0183com

[47] Snow LM, Fugere NA, Thompson LV: Advanced glycation end-product accumulation and associated protein modification in type II skeletal muscle with aging. Journals of Gerontology Series A: Biological Sciences and Medical Sciences. 2007;62:1204-1210. DOI: 10.1093/gerona/62.11.1204

[48] Haus JM, Carrithers JA, Trappe SW, Trappe TA: Collagen, cross-linking, and advanced glycation end products in aging human skeletal muscle. J Appl Physiol (1985). 2007;103:2068-2076. DOI: 10.1152/japplphysiol.00670.2007

[49] Thompson LV: Age-related muscle dysfunction. Experimental Gerontology. 2009;44:106-111. DOI: 10.1016/j.exger.2008.05.003

[50] Pavan P, Monti E, Bondi M, Fan C, Stecco C, Narici M, et al.: Alterations of Extracellular Matrix Mechanical Properties Contribute to Age-Related Functional Impairment of Human Skeletal Muscles. International Journal of Molecular Sciences. 2020;21. DOI: 10.3390/ijms21113992

[51] Hayashi T, Wojtaszewski JF, Goodyear LJ: Exercise regulation of glucose transport in skeletal muscle. American Journal of Physiology. 1997;273:E1039-1051. DOI:

[52] Miinea CP, Sano H, Kane S, Sano E, Fukuda M, Peranen J, et al.: AS160, the Akt substrate regulating GLUT4 translocation, has a functional Rab GTPase-activating protein domain.

Biochemical Journal. 2005;391:87-93. DOI: 10.1042/BJ20050887

[53] Roach WG, Chavez JA, Miinea CP, Lienhard GE: Substrate specificity and effect on GLUT4 translocation of the Rab GTPase-activating protein Tbc1d1. Biochemical Journal. 2007;403:353-358. DOI: 10.1042/BJ20061798

[54] Miele C, Riboulet A, Maitan MA, Oriente F, Romano C, Formisano P, et al.: Human glycated albumin affects glucose metabolism in L6 skeletal muscle cells by impairing insulin-induced insulin receptor substrate (IRS) signaling through a protein kinase C alpha-mediated mechanism. Journal of Biological Chemistry. 2003;278:47376-47387. DOI: 10.1074/jbc.M301088200

[55] Wu CH, Huang HW, Huang SM, Lin JA, Yeh CT, Yen GC: AGE-induced interference of glucose uptake and transport as a possible cause of insulin resistance in adipocytes. J Agric Food Chem. 2011;59:7978-7984. DOI: 10.1021/jf201271y

[56] Cassese A, Esposito I, Fiory F, Barbagallo AP, Paturzo F, Mirra P, et al.: In skeletal muscle advanced glycation end products (AGEs) inhibit insulin action and induce the formation of multimolecular complexes including the receptor for AGEs. Journal of Biological Chemistry. 2008;283:36088-36099. DOI: 10.1074/jbc.M801698200

[57] Rai AK, Jaiswal N, Maurya CK, Sharma A, Ahmad I, Ahmad S, et al.: Fructose-induced AGEs-RAGE signaling in skeletal muscle contributes to impairment of glucose homeostasis. Journal of Nutritional Biochemistry. 2019;71:35-44. DOI: 10.1016/j.jnutbio.2019.05.016

[58] Pinto-Junior DC, Silva KS, Michalani ML, Yonamine CY, Esteves JV, Fabre NT, et al.: Advanced glycation end products-induced insulin resistance involves repression of skeletal muscle GLUT4 expression. Scientific Reports. 2018;8:8109. DOI: 10.1038/s41598-018-26482-6

[59] Snow LM, Lynner CB, Nielsen EM, Neu HS, Thompson LV: Advanced glycation end product in diabetic rat skeletal muscle in vivo. Pathobiology. 2006;73:244-251. DOI: 10.1159/000098210

[60] Chiu CY, Yang RS, Sheu ML, Chan DC, Yang TH, Tsai KS, et al.: Advanced glycation end-products induce skeletal muscle atrophy and dysfunction in diabetic mice via a RAGE-mediated, AMPK-down-regulated, Akt pathway. Journal of Pathology. 2016;238:470-482. DOI: 10.1002/path.4674

[61] Rudrappa SS, Wilkinson DJ, Greenhaff PL, Smith K, Idris I, Atherton PJ: Human Skeletal Muscle Disuse Atrophy: Effects on Muscle Protein Synthesis, Breakdown, and Insulin Resistance-A Qualitative Review. Frontiers in Physiology. 2016;7:361. DOI: 10.3389/fphys.2016.00361

[62] Egawa T, Kido K, Yokokawa T, Fujibayashi M, Goto K, Hayashi T: Involvement of receptor for advanced glycation end products in microgravity-induced skeletal muscle atrophy in mice. Acta Astronautica. 2020;176:332-340. DOI: 10.1016/j.actaastro.2020.07.002

[63] Egawa T, Tsuda S, Goto A, Ohno Y, Yokoyama S, Goto K, et al.: Potential involvement of dietary advanced glycation end products in impairment of skeletal muscle growth and muscle contractile function in mice. British Journal of Nutrition. 2017;117:21-29. DOI: 10.1017/S0007114516004591

[64] Egawa T, Ohno Y, Yokoyama S, Goto A, Ito R, Hayashi T, et al.: The effect of advanced glycation end products on cellular signaling molecules in skeletal muscle. Journal of Physical Fitness and Sports Medicine.

2018;7:229-238. DOI: 10.7600/jpfsm.7.229

[65] Adachi N, Kanazawa I, Tanaka KI, Takeno A, Notsu M, Tanaka S, et al.: Insulin-Like Growth Factor-I Protects Against the Detrimental Effects of Advanced Glycation End Products and High Glucose in Myoblastic C2C12 Cells. Calcified Tissue International. 2019;105:89-96. DOI: 10.1007/s00223-019-00537-w

[66] Riuzzi F, Sorci G, Sagheddu R, Chiappalupi S, Salvadori L, Donato R: RAGE in the pathophysiology of skeletal muscle. J Cachexia Sarcopenia Muscle. 2018;9:1213-1234. DOI: 10.1002/jcsm.12350

[67] Chiappalupi S, Sorci G, Vukasinovic A, Salvadori L, Sagheddu R, Coletti D, et al.: Targeting RAGE prevents muscle wasting and prolongs survival in cancer cachexia. J Cachexia Sarcopenia Muscle. 2020;11:929-946. DOI: 10.1002/jcsm.12561

[68] Bongarzone S, Savickas V, Luzi F, Gee AD: Targeting the Receptor for Advanced Glycation Endproducts (RAGE): A Medicinal Chemistry Perspective. Journal of Medicinal Chemistry. 2017;60:7213-7232. DOI: 10.1021/acs.jmedchem.7b00058

[69] Hudson BI, Lippman ME: Targeting RAGE Signaling in Inflammatory Disease. Annual Review of Medicine. 2018;69:349-364. DOI: 10.1146/annurev-med-041316-085215

[70] Deane R, Singh I, Sagare AP, Bell RD, Ross NT, LaRue B, et al.: A multimodal RAGE-specific inhibitor reduces amyloid beta-mediated brain disorder in a mouse model of Alzheimer disease. Journal of Clinical Investigation. 2012;122:1377-1392. DOI: 10.1172/JCI58642

[71] Burstein AH, Grimes I, Galasko DR, Aisen PS, Sabbagh M, Mjalli AM: Effect of TTP488 in patients with mild to moderate Alzheimer's disease. BMC Neurology. 2014;14:12. DOI: 10.1186/1471-2377-14-12

[72] Yagi M, Takabe W, S. M, A. S, Maruyama T, Yonei Y: Screening and selection of anti-glycative materials: Kuromoji (Lindera umbellata). Glycative Stress Research. 2017;4:317-328. DOI: 10.24659/gsr.4.4_317

[73] Egawa T, Ohno Y, Yokoyama S, Yokokawa T, Tsuda S, Goto K, et al.: The Protective Effect of Brazilian Propolis against Glycation Stress in Mouse Skeletal Muscle. Foods. 2019;8. DOI: 10.3390/foods8100439

[74] Muellenbach EA, Diehl CJ, Teachey MK, Lindborg KA, Archuleta TL, Harrell NB, et al.: Interactions of the advanced glycation end product inhibitor pyridoxamine and the antioxidant alpha-lipoic acid on insulin resistance in the obese Zucker rat. Metabolism. 2008;57:1465-1472. DOI: 10.1016/j.metabol.2008.05.018

[75] Hagiwara S, Gohda T, Tanimoto M, Ito T, Murakoshi M, Ohara I, et al.: Effects of pyridoxamine (K-163) on glucose intolerance and obesity in high-fat diet C57BL/6J mice. Metabolism. 2009;58:934-945. DOI: 10.1016/j.metabol.2009.02.033

[76] Mastrocola R, Nigro D, Chiazza F, Medana C, Dal Bello F, Boccuzzi G, et al.: Fructose-derived advanced glycation end-products drive lipogenesis and skeletal muscle reprogramming via SREBP-1c dysregulation in mice. Free Radical Biology and Medicine. 2016;91:224-235. DOI: 10.1016/j.freeradbiomed.2015.12.022

Chapter 7

# Metabolic Responses to Energy-Depleted Conditions

*Tomohiro Suzuki, Tetsuro Komatsu, Hiroshi Shibata and Takeshi Inagaki*

## Abstract

Dietary intervention is one of the most important approaches for the treatment of metabolic diseases such as diabetes mellitus. Fasting and caloric restriction have profound effects on systemic metabolism. The energy source-producing organs, such as the liver, and peripheral tissues rewire their metabolism to meet the energy demands of the whole body. Glycogenolysis, fatty acid oxidation, and ketone body production are characteristic metabolic changes that occur during fasting and caloric restriction. These metabolic changes are regulated by various signaling cascades including PPARα and FGF21. Moderate fasting and caloric restriction have also been implicated in extending the lifespan in a variety of organisms from nematodes to vertebrates. Intensive research has unveiled several regulatory mechanisms of longevity including metabolic regulators such as mTOR and sirtuins. The epigenome has been attracting attention as a mechanism underlying metabolic diseases and longevity. The epigenome is the concept that involves covalent modifications of DNA, histones, and RNA, which are mediated by the action of epigenetic enzymes. The activity of these enzymes is regulated by energy states, i.e. metabolites including ketone bodies and intermediates of various metabolic pathways. Thus, energy states are recorded in cells as an epigenetic memory, which may cause future onset of metabolic diseases and affect lifespan.

**Keywords:** Fasting, caloric restriction, diabetes mellitus, obesity, glycolysis, the TCA cycle, fatty acid oxidation, ketone body, PPARα, FGF21, insulin, glucagon, longevity, metabolites, and epigenome

## 1. Introduction

For the treatment of diabetes mellitus, dietary intervention is one of the most important basic approaches along with exercise therapy. Since dietary guidance for diabetes is often based on limiting caloric intake, it is important to understand the effects of fasting and caloric restriction on systemic metabolism. Furthermore, the effects of the Mediterranean diet and the pros and cons of carbohydrate-restricted diets have recently attracted attention, and it is now widely recognized that the proportion of certain nutrients in the diet and the order in which they are eaten can affect nutrient absorption and systemic metabolism. In countries where excessive food supply has caused obesity and the associated diseases, many people have adopted fasting and caloric restriction for weight control. Academic studies have shown that moderate caloric restriction has a positive effect on those diseases and contributes to longevity through anti-aging effects and prevention of age-related diseases. However, given that excessive fasting or caloric restriction can lead to malnutrition, it is important to accurately understand the effects on systemic metabolism.

During fasting, carbohydrates, fats, and proteins are utilized as energy sources in many organs. However, since the brain cannot directly utilize fatty acids derived from lipolysis, the insight into energy metabolism in the brain is essential to understand the systemic metabolism during fasting. In the early stages of fasting, glucose is provided to the brain by glycogenolysis (**Figure 1A**). In the case of prolonged fasting, gluconeogenesis is activated in the liver to produce glucose from pyruvate and lactate, as well as from glycerol produced by lipolysis and from amino acids produced by proteolysis (**Figure 1B**) [1]. When fasting is further prolonged, glucose is supplied by renal gluconeogenesis, and ketone bodies produced by fatty acid oxidation (or β-oxidation), and acetate are used as energy sources for the brain and skeletal muscles (**Figure 1A**) [2, 3]. Thus, brain activity is maintained by glucose and ketone bodies from the multiple sources. Of note, most of gluconeogenesis takes place in the liver and to a lesser extent in the proximal tubules of the kidney, and ketone bodies are mainly produced in the liver.

It has long been known that fasting and caloric restriction are associated with an extended lifespan in many organisms. Longevity is regulated by several factors such as mechanistic target of rapamycin (mTOR), sirtuins (SIRTs), AMP-activated protein kinase (AMPK), forkhead box protein O (FOXO), and growth hormone (GH)/insulin-like growth factor-1 (IGF-1), but the mechanism by which these factors extend lifespan in humans is not yet fully understood. One possible hypothesis is that fasting and caloric restriction are memorized in the epigenome of cells. More specifically, metabolites produced during fasting serve as inhibitors or substrates of epigenetic enzymes. For example, ketone bodies mainly inhibit class I histone deacetylases (HDACs) to promote histone acetylation. In addition, acetyl-CoA, produced by fatty acid oxidation, and α-ketoglutarate (α-KG, also known as 2-oxoglutarate), an intermediate metabolite of the tricarboxylic acid (TCA) cycle (also known as the citric acid cycle or the Krebs cycle), are substrates for histone acetyltransferases and epigenetic demethylases, respectively. Thus, the states of energy metabolism, including fasting, are recorded in cells as epigenomic memories, which may cause the development of future diseases.

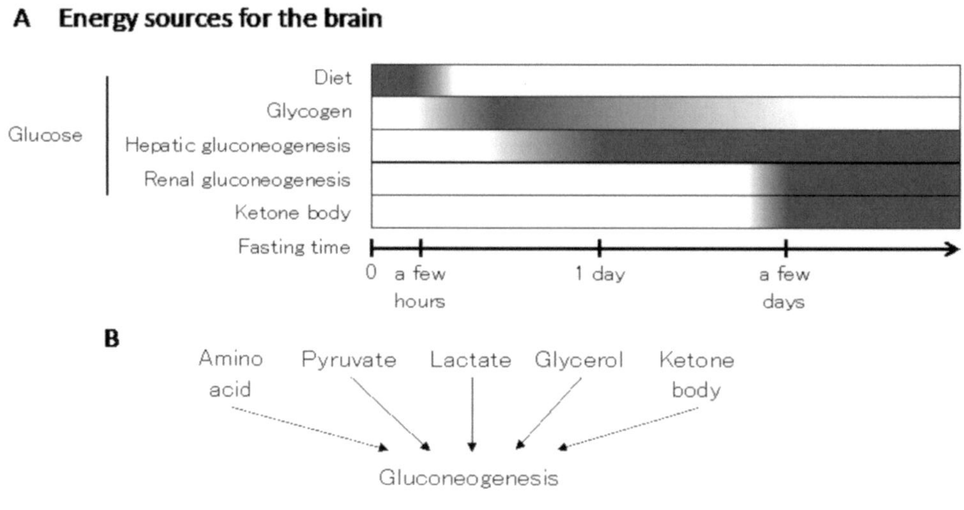


**Figure 1.**
*The brain energy sources under the fasting condition. A. Energy sources for the brain, B. Energy sources for gluconeogenesis.*

## 2. Energy storage in the body

Under normal metabolic conditions, some of the excess glucose is stored as glycogen, mainly in the liver and muscles, and further excess energy is stored as fat mainly in the adipose tissue. Fat in the body consists of triglycerides (TGs), which are transported to the adipose tissue in the form of chylomicrons from the intestine, and also produced from excess glucose in the adipose tissue and the liver. Under the feeding conditions, glucose is metabolized mainly in adipocytes and hepatocytes via glycolysis to produce pyruvate, which is then converted to acetyl-CoA and combined with oxaloacetate to enter the TCA cycle as citrate in mitochondria. Excess citrate is transported to the cytoplasm and converted to acetyl-CoA, which is then used as a substrate for fatty acids synthesis via malonyl CoA produced by the rate-limiting enzyme, acetyl-CoA carboxylase. Fatty acids are esterified with glycerol to produce triglycerides and stored in the adipose tissue.

## 3. Energy supply under fasting conditions

The liver, muscles, adipose tissues, and brain are all closely involved in energy metabolism and are important organs for understanding whole body metabolism in the fasting state. The brain cannot directly utilize fat because it is not capable of fatty acid oxidation unlike many other organs. Therefore, during prolonged fasting, glucose is supplied to the brain from multiple sources to maintain its functions. In addition, ketone bodies are produced as an energy source for the brain during extremely long fasting. The reason why the brain is unable to oxidize fatty acids remains controversial, but it is thought to be because fatty acids cannot cross the blood–brain barrier and the brain does not have the enzymes necessary for β-oxidation.

In the normal state of energy metabolism under feeding conditions, dietary sugar is commonly used as an energy source in all organs. Glucose is oxidized via glycolysis to eventually yield two molecules of pyruvate. In the presence of oxygen, pyruvate enters the TCA cycle, and it is completely oxidized to produce six molecules of carbon dioxide. At this step, $NAD^+$ and FAD are reduced to produce NADH and $FADH_2$, respectively, and are transported to the respiratory chain of mitochondria to produce energy in the form of ATP.

In the early stage of fasting, stored glycogen, a branched polymer of glucose, is degraded to provide glucose via glucose 6-phosphate (**Figure 2**). Glycogen-derived glucose is used for energy supply by the glycolytic pathway and the TCA cycle in most of organs except the liver, muscles, and adipose tissue. However, the amount of energy stored as glycogen is consumed in a day of fasting, and hepatic glycogen is almost completely depleted after two to three days of starvation. The degradation of glycogen proceeds as phosphorylase sequentially removes glucose monomers by cleaving the $\alpha$-($1 \rightarrow 4$) bond in a phosphate-dependent manner. At the branched end of glycogen, when degradation proceeds to four glucose residues near the $\alpha$-($1 \rightarrow 6$) bond, three glucose molecules at the branching end are transferred to the other chain end by a group of glycogen debranching enzymes. The remaining glucose molecules are then hydrolyzed to remove them, and further degradation by phosphorylases continues. The glucose 1-phosphate produced by phosphorylase is converted to glucose 6-phosphate by phosphoglucomutase and enters the glycolytic pathway (**Figure 2**). Glucose 6-phosphate is converted to glucose by the action of glucose 6-phosphatase (G6Pase) in the liver, and then released into the bloodstream via Glut2 to supply glucose to the brain and other organs. On the other hand, G6Pase is not expressed in the muscles, so stored glycogen is used only for local energy production.

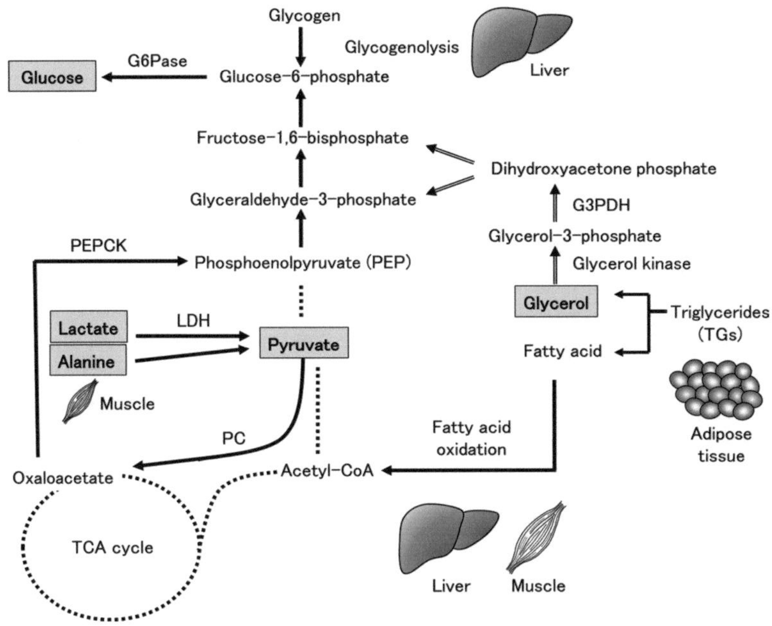


**Figure 2.**
*Gluconeogenesis under the fasting condition.*

During fasting, TGs in the adipose tissue are also degraded and used for fatty acid oxidation (**Figures 2** and **3**). TGs are broken down into fatty acids and glycerol by hormone-sensitive lipase (HSL) and a rate-limiting enzyme, adipose triglyceride lipase (ATGL). Fatty acids are bound to albumin and transported to the liver and muscles, where they are taken up by facilitated transport for fatty acid oxidation. Long-chain fatty acids taken up by the cells pass through the mitochondrial membrane to the matrix. Fatty acids are converted to acyl-CoA by acyl-CoA synthase and then conjugated with carnitine to form acyl-carnitine by carnitine palmitoyltransferase (CPT1) on mitochondrial outer membrane (CPT1a: mainly in the liver, CPT1b: mainly in the skeletal muscle and brown fat) and pass through mitochondrial inner membrane to the matrix via carnitine-acylcarnitine translocase (CACT). Fatty acids are then released from carnitine through the action of CPT2 on mitochondrial inner membrane (**Figure 3**). In mitochondrial matrix, fatty acids are continuously oxidized via FAD-dependent acyl-CoA dehydrogenase to produce $FADH_2$, $NADH+H^+$, and acetyl-CoA (**Figure 3**). Although fatty acid-derived acetyl-CoA enters the TCA cycle for energy production, it does not contribute to gluconeogenesis because two carbon atoms derived from the acetyl-CoA are removed in the TCA cycle. In contrast, the glycerol produced by lipolysis can be used as a substrate for gluconeogenesis (**Figure 2**).

When fasting persists, glucose is supplied to multiple organs via gluconeogenesis in the liver. Gluconeogenesis is particularly important to provide glucose as an energy source for the brain, which is unable to oxidize fatty acids. In the liver, gluconeogenesis is carried out from amino acids, pyruvate, lactate, glycerol, and ketone bodies (**Figures 1B** and **2**). During several weeks of starvation, about 80 grams of glucose is produced daily via gluconeogenesis, of which 15–20 grams is derived from amino acids, mainly alanine, 35–40 grams from pyruvate and lactate, 20 grams from glycerol from fat, and 10 grams from ketone bodies [1]. Amino acids are supplied by degradation of proteins in the muscles during fasting. Alanine is transported to the liver via the bloodstream, and is then converted to pyruvate for gluconeogenesis (**Figure 2**). Pyruvate is metabolized to oxaloacetate by pyruvate carboxylase (PC)

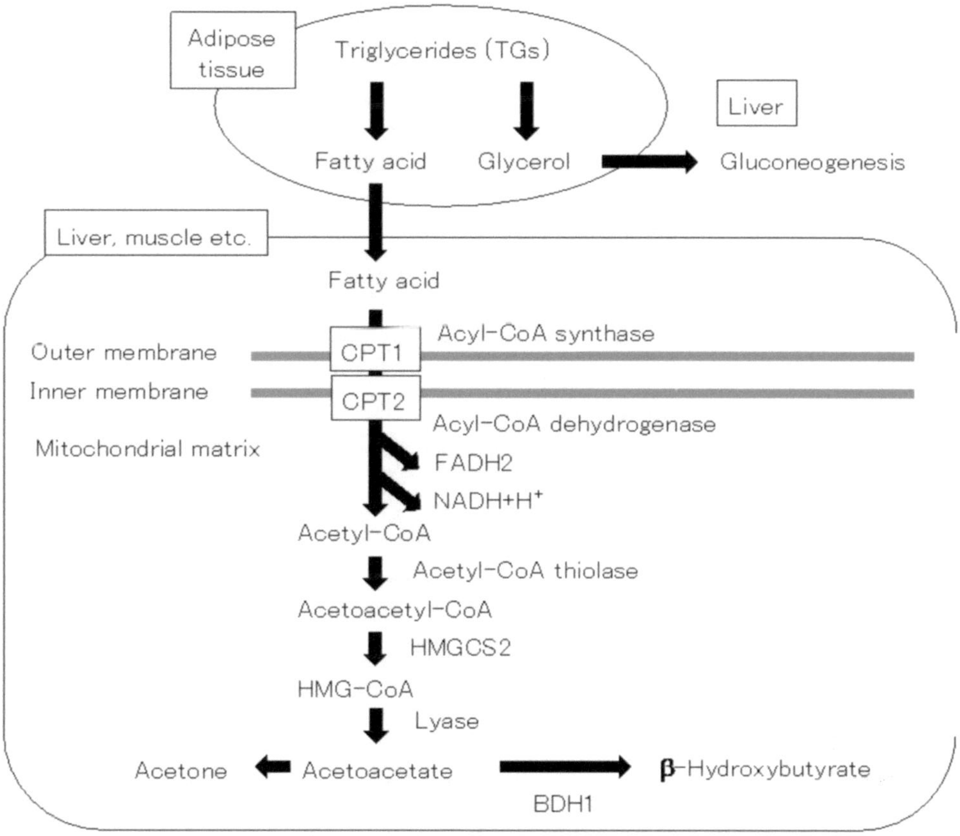


**Figure 3.**
*Lipid metabolism and ketone body production during fasting.*

and then decarboxylated by phosphoenolpyruvate carboxykinase (PEPCK) to produce phosphoenolpyruvate (PEP) (**Figure 2**). PEP is an intermediate product of the glycolytic pathway, and the following gluconeogenic process utilizes the glycolytic enzymes except for the step of fructose-1,6-bisphosphate to fructose-6-phosphate which requires fructose-1,6-bisphosphatase [4] and the step of glucose-6-phosphate to glucose mediated by G6Pase. Lactic acid is converted to pyruvate by lactate dehydrogenase (LDH) for gluconeogenesis (**Figure 2**). Glycerol is phosphorylated by glycerol kinase in the liver to produce glycerol 3-phosphate, which is then oxidized by glycerol 3-phosphate dehydrogenase (G3PDH) to dihydroxyacetone phosphate, an intermediate of the glycolytic pathway. Dihydroxyacetone phosphate undergoes gluconeogenesis via glyceraldehyde 3-phosphate or fructose 1,6-diphosphate (**Figure 2**). Furthermore, under long-term starvation for several days or a week where water, vitamins, salt, and other minerals are supplied, glucose production occurs not only in the liver but also in the renal cortex, which is responsible for about 40% of total body glucose production [1].

Gluconeogenesis is tightly regulated by the products of fatty acid oxidation such as NADH+$H^+$, acetyl-CoA, and ATP (**Figure 4**). In normal glucose metabolism, pyruvate enters the TCA cycle via acetyl-CoA by the action of pyruvate dehydrogenase (PDH). However, during fasting, pyruvate is converted to oxaloacetate by PC for gluconeogenesis as described above (**Figure 4**). The activity of PC is stimulated by acetyl-CoA. In addition, NADH+$H^+$, acetyl-CoA, and ATP inhibit PDH activity (**Figure 4**). Furthermore, NADH+$H^+$ inhibits isocitrate dehydrogenase (IDH), one of the enzymes responsible for the TCA cycle (**Figure 4**). Thus, NADH+$H^+$,

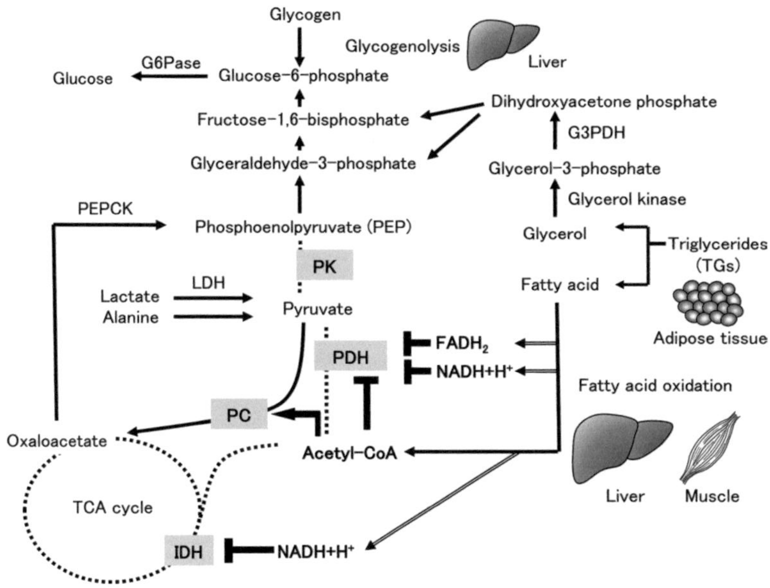


**Figure 4.**
*Fatty acid oxidation and gluconeogenesis during fasting.*

acetyl-CoA, and ATP, which are generated by fatty acid oxidation, regulate the activities of enzymes in the gluconeogenesis pathway, and these regulatory mechanisms ensure a consistent flow of metabolites for energy supply through gluconeogenesis and fatty acid oxidation during fasting. Since PEP produced by PEPCK is an intermediate product of the glycolytic pathway, it could theoretically be converted to pyruvate and re-enter the TCA cycle. However, because pyruvate kinase (PK) in the liver is inhibited by alanine and inactivated by protein kinase A (PKA), which is activated by glucagon, PEP produced during fasting is used for gluconeogenesis but not glycolysis. In other words, gluconeogenesis and amino acid metabolism are consistently regulated under fasting conditions. In addition, nitrogen sources stored in the muscles are used for gluconeogenesis in the renal cortex under prolonged fasting. Glutamine and alanine are metabolized from branched-chain amino acids such as leucine, isoleucine, and valine in the muscles, and released into the bloodstream. Glutamine is then primarily used for gluconeogenesis via the TCA cycle in the renal cortex. This indicates that diet therapies that focus primarily on fasting result not only in burning of stored fat but also loss of muscle mass.

## 4. Ketone body as an energy source during long-term fasting

Under glucose-depleted conditions during fasting, the brain and muscles use ketone bodies and acetate as energy sources other than glucose (**Figure 1B**) [3, 5]. These energy sources are critical to sustain function of the brain because it cannot directly metabolize fatty acids. A human study investigated the energy sources of the brain under long-term starvation for 5–6 weeks. When only water, vitamins, and minerals such as salt are supplied, urinary nitrogen excretion, an indicator of amino acid-derived gluconeogenesis, dropped to about 4–5 grams per day, and two-thirds of the energy source of the brain comes from β-hydroxybutyrate and acetoacetate [1].

The metabolic systems that use ketone bodies as an energy source can be traced back to bacteria, archaea, and protozoa. In humans, most ketone bodies are produced in the liver. During fasting, the most part of acetyl-CoA produced by fatty acid oxidation is used for ketone body production, while only the limited amount enters the TCA cycle (**Figure 3**). At the first step of the TCA cycle, acetyl-CoA is conjugated to oxaloacetate through the action of citrate synthase to produce citrate. However, oxaloacetate is relatively scarce during fasting because it is consumed by glucose production. As a result, excess acetyl-CoA produced by fatty acid oxidation is used exclusively for ketone body production. In addition, NADH+H$^+$, acetyl-CoA, and ATP, which are produced by fatty acid oxidation, regulate gluconeogenesis-related enzymes to stimulate gluconeogenesis. In addition, NADH+H$^+$ suppresses the activity of IDH in the TCA cycle, which in turn suppresses the TCA cycle and directs fatty acid-derived acetyl-CoA toward ketone body production.

Ketone bodies are produced in mitochondria in the following reactions: two molecules of acetyl-CoA are combined by acetoacetyl-CoA thiolase to produce acetoacetyl-CoA, and an additional molecule of acetyl-CoA is conjugated by HMG-CoA synthase 2 (HMGCS2) to produce HMG-CoA, which is then cleaved by lyase to form acetoacetate (**Figures 3** and **5**). Acetoacetate can be converted to acetone through spontaneous non-enzymatic decarboxylation or to β-hydroxybutyrate (D-3-hydroxybutyrate) by 3-hydroxybutyrate dehydrogenase (BDH1) (**Figure 3**). β-Hydroxybutyrate is the most abundant ketone body in the blood. Here, the irreversible reaction by HMGCS2 is a key reaction for ketone body production, and the activity of BDH1 is increased by NADH+H$^+$.

The basal level of β-hydroxybutyrate in humans is at the level of a few μM under feeding conditions, and the blood concentration increases to 200–300 μM after 12–16 hours of fasting, 1–2 mM after 2 days of fasting, and as high as 6–8 mM after prolonged fasting [6]. Ketone bodies also reach more than 2 mM with a ketogenic diet that excludes most carbohydrates, and intense exercise for about 90 minutes also increases ketone bodies to 1–2 mM. In neonates, the production and utilization of ketone bodies are more efficient than adults. The serum concentration of ketone bodies is as high as 2–3 mM just after birth, and the neonatal brain uses ketone bodies as an important energy source.

Ketone bodies are produced by the liver and supplied to the brain, muscles, and kidneys during fasting, but the liver cannot utilize ketone bodies as an energy source because it does not express 3-keto acid CoA transferase (OXCT1/SCOT). β-Hydroxybutyrate is produced in the liver and released into the bloodstream via

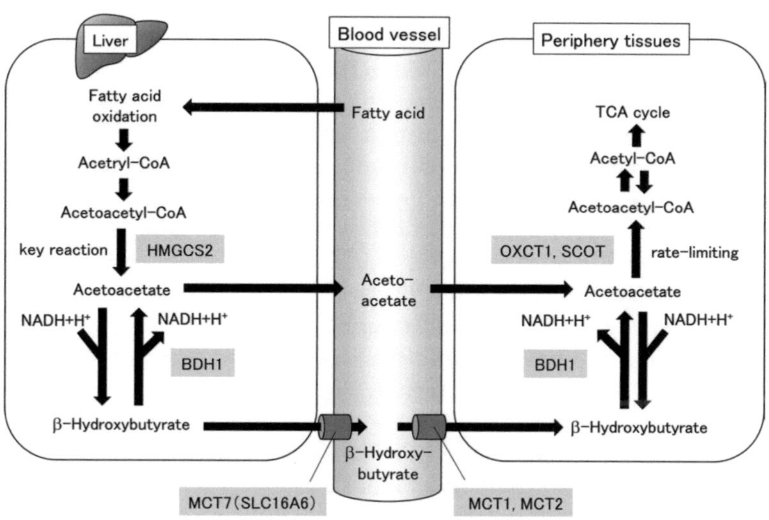


**Figure 5.**
*Production and utilization of ketone bodies.*

monocarboxylic acid transporter 7 (MCT7/SLC16A6) (**Figure 5**) [6]. During prolonged fasting, the high concentration of β-hydroxybutyrate in the blood is taken up by the brain through the blood–brain barrier via several monocarboxylic acid transporters, including MCT1 and MCT2 (**Figure 5**). Once taken up into neurons, β-hydroxybutyrate reverses the ketone body production pathway to produce acetoacetate by BDH1 and further converts to acetoacetyl-CoA by OXCT1/SCOT. The activity of BDH1 is promoted by NADH+$H^+$ produced during fatty acid oxidation (**Figures 3** and 5). In addition, the reaction of OXCT1/SCOT is the rate-limiting step to produce acetoacetyl-CoA, which is accompanied by the production of an intermediate metabolite of the TCA cycle, succinate, in a succinyl CoA-dependent manner (**Figure 5**).

In addition, acetate is also utilized as an energy source during prolonged fasting. In the liver, acetate is produced from acetyl-CoA by the action of acetyl-CoA hydroxylase during fasting, and is released from the liver to other organs. Acetate is utilized as an energy source for acetyl-CoA production via type 2 acetyl-CoA synthase (AceCS2), which is particularly abundant in mitochondria of the muscles [2].

## 5. Regulatory mechanisms of ketone body production

HMGCS2 is a key enzyme for the regulation of ketone body production. The expression of HMGCS2 is strongly regulated by forkhead box protein A2 (FOXA2), peroxisome proliferators-activated receptor α (PPARα), fibroblast growth factor 21 (FGF21), and mTOR, and its activity is enhanced through deacetylation by sirtuin 3 (SIRT3) [6]. FOXA2 binds directly to the promoter region of HMGCS2 and activates its transcription. The expression of FOXA2 is regulated by insulin and glucagon. Insulin-mediated phosphorylation inactivates FOXA2 by translocating it out of the nucleus, while glucagon activates FOXA2 through p300-mediated acetylation, thereby contributing to ketone body production. FOXA2 deacetylation is also regulated by class I and class II HDACs and SIRT1, a class III HDAC. In addition, mTORC1 complex is known to suppress PPARα, and rapamycin promotes ketone body production by inhibiting mTORC1 complex.

## 6. Regulation of metabolism under fasting conditions by PPARα and FGF21

PPARα is a nuclear receptor expressed in the liver, kidney, heart, and brown adipose tissue, which is activated by long-chain fatty acids and involved in fatty acid metabolism (**Figure 6**). PPARα forms a heterodimer with retinol X receptor (RXR) and regulates transcription by binding to the response sequence called PPAR response element (PPRE) in the gene regulatory regions. In the liver, PPARα promotes the expressions of a variety of genes related to β-oxidation, including FGF21, HMGCS2, CPT1a, and acyl-CoA oxidase (ACOX), which is the rate-limiting enzyme for peroxisomal β-oxidation (**Figure 6**).

FGF21, a target gene of PPARα, is a member of the FGF family, with 22 members in humans, and belongs to the same subfamily as FGF15/19 and FGF23 [7, 8]. FGFs in this subfamily characteristically function as hormones. FGF21 is expressed in the liver, adipose tissue, skeletal muscle, and pancreas, and the liver mainly secretes FGF21 as a hormone [9]. The expression of FGF21 is enhanced by fasting and ketogenic (or high-fat) diets [7, 10]. FGF21 levels in infants are higher than fasting FGF21 levels in adults, which is thought to be induced by milk-derived free fatty acids. In addition to PPARα, glucocorticoid receptors, activating transcription factor 4 (ATF4), cAMP response element binding protein

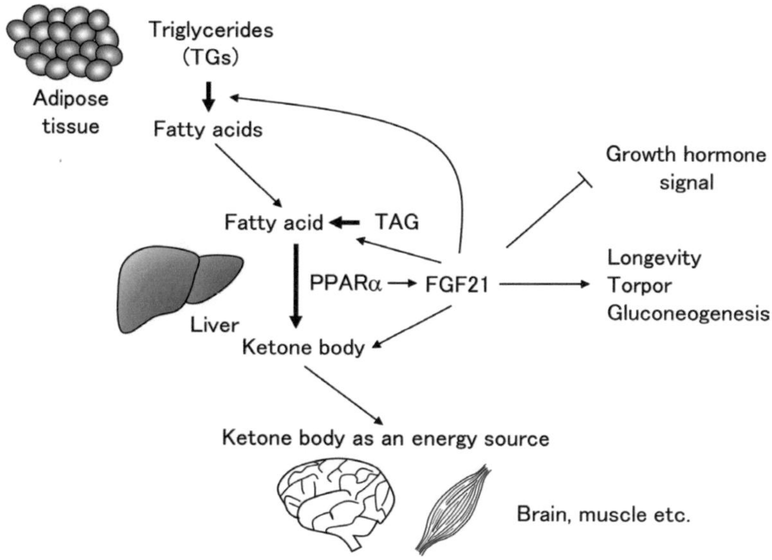


**Figure 6.**
*Regulation of energy metabolism by FGF21.*

H (CREBH), carbohydrate response element binding protein (ChREBP), PPARγ, farnesoid X receptor (FXR), and activin B induce the expression of FGF21 in the liver [11], while liver X receptor (LXR) inhibits the expression [12]. In the skeletal muscles, FGF21 is expressed through ATF4 under specific conditions such as metabolic stresses in mitochondria, and is also regulated by the phosphatidylinositol-3 kinase (PI3K) and Akt signals [12].

FGF21 plays an important role in the regulation of systemic energy metabolism during fasting. In the white adipose tissue, FGF21 induces lipolysis by enhancing the transcription of HSL and ATGL [7]. Free fatty acids produced by lipolysis promote fatty acid oxidation and the protein expression of HMGCS2, which induces the production of ketone bodies (**Figure 6**). FGF21 also enhances the expression of lipolytic enzymes in the liver, suppresses glycogenolysis, and promotes gluconeogenesis, but does not significantly affect glycolysis. FGF21 binds to the FGF receptor (FGFR) and its co-factor β-Klotho on the plasma membrane of target cells, and regulates transcription and translation of the target genes via phosphorylation cascades. FGF21 also regulates glucose metabolism in the liver partially via peroxisome proliferator-activated receptor γ coactivator 1-α (PGC-1α), which acts as a co-activator of transcriptional regulators and induces gene expression related to gluconeogenesis, fatty acid oxidation, and ketone body production during fasting [13]. In rodent models, pharmacological concentrations of FGF21 promote glucose uptake in adipocytes, increase insulin sensitivity, reduce blood triglyceride and hepatic fat, and suppress weight gain on a high-fat diet. In addition, it induces the expression of Glut1 in adipocytes [14], increases the number of pancreatic islets and the content of insulin per islet [15], and reduces blood glucagon levels by suppressing glucagon secretion [14]. In diabetic monkeys, FGF21 lowers blood glucose, serum insulin, triglyceride, and low density lipoprotein (LDL) cholesterol levels, increases high density lipoprotein (HDL) cholesterol levels in the blood, and induces weight loss without inducing hypoglycemia [16]. Human blood FGF21 levels were shown to be elevated in individuals with obesity, type 2 diabetes, and insulin resistance. It is also reported that blood FGF21 levels in hyperlipidemic patients are twice as high as in the normal group, and that administration of fibrate, a PPARα ligand, increases blood FGF21 levels.

In addition, FGF21 levels in humans are increased by prolonged fasting for 7 days [17]. Thus, even under feeding conditions, FGF21 induces a fasting-like metabolic states, such as gluconeogenesis, fatty acid oxidation, and ketone body production (**Figure 6**) [12].

Living organisms suppress GH and reproductive signals to reduce unnecessary energy consumption during fasting. Mice with excess FGF21 show reduced response to GH and suppressed reproductive signals (**Figure 6**) [18, 19]. In detail, FGF21 transgenic mice show reduced phosphorylation of signal transducer and activator of transcription 5 (STAT5) downstream of Janus kinase (JAK) 2 in response to GH in the liver and reduced blood IGF-1 levels [18]. In addition, FGF21 transgenic female mice have a suppressed luteinizing hormone (LH) surge due to inhibition of vasopressin signals in the hypothalamus [19]. The latest statistical analysis, which excluded the contribution of insulin resistance and body fat percentage, showed elevated blood FGF21 levels in human anorexia [20], suggesting that FGF21 may be involved in impaired GH signaling in anorexic patients. In addition, FGF21 plays a role in energy conservation by inducing a hibernation-like state (torpor) in mice [7]. During mouse torpor and squirrel hibernation, in addition to hypothermia and hypoactivity, it is known that pancreatic lipase is ectopically induced outside the pancreas and FGF21 induces the ectopic expression in the liver [7, 21]. The pancreatic lipase is capable of hydrolyzing TGs into glycerol and fatty acids over a wide temperature range, and thus may provide fatty acids as an energy source during torpor and hibernation.

Furthermore, FGF21 transgenic mice exhibit a long lifespan (**Figure 6**) [22]. It is reported that the median lifespan of wild-type mice was 28 months, while that of FGF21 transgenic mice was 38 months. Interestingly, the longevity of the FGF21 transgenic mice did not require restriction of food intake, and insulin sensitivity was maintained even when food intake was increased. This suggests that FGF21 increases lifespan by shifting systemic metabolism to a fasting-like state regardless of changes in food intake. These phenotypes are attributed to the suppression of GH/IGF-1 signaling accompanied by decreased IGF-1 production, but do not involve mTOR signaling, AMPK signaling, and $NAD^+$ metabolism. In the signaling of the endocrine FGF subfamily (FGF15/19, FGF21, and FGF23), β-Klotho on the plasma membrane is required for FGF15/19 and FGF21, and α-Klotho for FGF23. α-Klotho was originally reported as a longevity gene [23], and it inhibits insulin/IGF-1 signaling by its truncated extracellular region circulating in the bloodstream. Thus, it is possible that α-Klotho causes longevity through a similar mechanism to FGF21, but α-Klotho is different from FGF21 in that it causes insulin resistance [22]. FGF21 also decreases preference for sweetness and alcohol via the central nervous system [24–27], which may contribute to the regulation of eating behavior in response to the energy states.

## 7. Regulation of metabolism during fasting by insulin and glucagon

Low blood insulin levels play an important role in the regulation of energy metabolism during fasting. Insulin activates PI3K through phosphorylation of insulin receptor substrate (IRS), and subsequent activation of Akt leads to phosphorylation and translocation of FOXO1 out of the nucleus, resulting in the suppression of the expression of ATGL, the rate-limiting enzyme in lipolysis. In addition, insulin signaling phosphorylates FOXA2 and excludes it from the nucleus, thereby suppressing the expression of HMGCS2, the rate-limiting enzyme for ketone body production. Therefore, the decrease in insulin signaling during fasting is involved in the expression of ATGL, gluconeogenesis-related genes, and ketone body production-related genes. Fasting also regulates the expression of IRSs and the PI3K activity. The expression of IRS-2 and the PI3K activity are elevated during fasting and decrease immediately after food intake in the liver [28]. In this context, IRS-2 appears to act for a short time after food intake so that it can respond again to the next coming dietary stimuli, whereas the expression of IRS-1 is relatively constant regardless of feeding conditions [28]. Therefore, it is considered that while both IRS-1 and IRS-2 are involved in inhibition of gluconeogenesis immediately after food intake, IRS-1 is mainly involved in glycogen production that is initiated at an interval after that. IRS-1 and IRS-2 differ not only in their expression patterns but also in their functions. IRS-1 deficient mice do not show strong diabetic symptoms, because IRS-2 can compensate for glucose intolerance by promoting the proliferation of pancreatic β cells [29]. The increased transcription of the IRS-2 gene during fasting and its repression after refeeding are regulated by the glucagon receptor-PKA-CREB-regulated transcription coactivator 2 (CRTC2)-CREB pathway and the insulin receptor signaling in the liver, while the regulation mechanism in other tissues remains unclear [30]. Refeeding induces insulin binding to the insulin receptor and downstream PI3K activation, which represses IRS-2 transcription via FOXO1 phosphorylation by Akt.

During fasting, glucagon is secreted from pancreatic α cells in response to hypoglycemia and stimulates glucose production in the liver through gluconeogenesis and glycogenolysis. The glucagon receptor-cAMP-PKA pathway promotes gluconeogenesis by inducing the expression of the catalytic subunits of G6Pase and PEPCK in the liver. PKA-dependent phosphorylation of CREB and dephosphorylation of CRTC2 forms CREB-CRTC2 complex that recruits a histone acetyltransferase, CREB binding protein (CBP) and promotes transcription of the gene encoding PGC-1α. Furthermore, PGC-1α, which is activated by SIRT1-mediated deacetylation and inactivated by general control nonderepressible-5 (GCN5)-mediated acetylation, promotes gluconeogenesis together with FOXO1 and hepatocyte nuclear factor 4α (HNF4α) [30].

## 8. Caloric restriction and life span

Fasting and caloric restriction have received so much attention because of their relationship to longevity. Fasting and caloric restriction to the extent that they do not lead to malnutrition are associated with longevity from nematodes to vertebrates, and are effective against aging and age-related diseases. For example, it has already been known for 80 years that restricting food intake prolongs lifespan in rats and mice [31]. Studies in monkeys showed that feeding a calorie-restricted diet from a young age inhibits the development of obesity, type 2 diabetes, cardiovascular disease, and cancer, and delays the onset of sarcopenia, senile deafness, and brain atrophy [31]. Although the molecular mechanisms by which caloric restriction maintains health and extends lifespan are not yet fully understood, various factors have been identified to be involved, including FGF21, insulin and IGF-1 signaling, mTOR, AMPK, SIRTs, $NAD^+$, FOXO, heat shock factor (HSF), and nuclear factor-erythroid 2-related factor 2 (NRF2) [31].

FOXO is a DNA-binding transcriptional regulator, which promotes the expression of a group of genes involved in DNA repair, autophagy, antioxidant activity, stress tolerance, and cell proliferation [31]. NRF2 and HSF1 are thought to be involved in the maintenance of protein homeostasis and cell structure through induction of antioxidant and drug-metabolizing enzymes, thus extending lifespan [32].

mTOR, first found in bacteria collected from Easter Island soil, is a serine/threonine kinase that is activated by a variety of factors and regulates a wide range of biological processes. mTOR is activated by insulin and IGF-1 signaling, intracellular nutrients such as amino acids and glucose, and energy states as well as oxygen and stresses to regulate cell proliferation, metabolism, nutrition, and environmental stresses [33]. It was also shown that inhibition of mTOR signaling prolongs lifespan in yeast, *C. elegans*, Drosophila, and mouse, but the mechanism is not fully understood [32, 33]. mTOR forms two distinct protein complexes, mTORC1 and mTORC2, each of which phosphorylates different target substrates. While mTORC1 is strongly inhibited by rapamycin, mTORC2 is less affected [32]. Therefore, much remains to be learned about biological functions of mTORC2.

mTORC1 is activated by growth factors such as IGF-1, stresses, energy states, oxygen, and amino acids [33]. mTORC1 promotes ribosome biosynthesis and protein synthesis in the muscles, and inhibits ketone body production in the liver. In addition, it promotes adipocyte differentiation through activation of sterol regulatory element binding protein 1 (SREBP1) and PPARγ, and increases the number and the size of pancreatic β-cells. Furthermore, mTORC1 suppresses autophagy, enhances glycolytic gene expression, and regulates mitochondrial oxidative metabolism. Suppression of mTOR signaling by caloric restriction, methionine-restricted diet, and rapamycin is thought to be involved in longevity, presumably through the complex regulatory mechanisms described above [32].

mTORC2 is activated by insulin, IGF-1, and leptin through PI3K and other pathways, and then phosphorylates Akt, serum- and glucocorticoid-induced protein kinase 1 (SGK1), and protein kinase C (PKC) family members. Akt and SGK1 further phosphorylate FOXO1, which results in nuclear export of FOXO1 and repression of the expression of gluconeogenesis-related genes [32, 33]. Thus, mTORC2 is involved in the regulation of energy metabolism, but its role in longevity is still unclear.

SIRTs are known as "longevity genes," and forced expression of SIRTs extends lifespan in yeast, *C. elegans*, and Drosophila [34]. SIRTs are $NAD^+$-dependent deacetylases. Since $NAD^+$ and NADH levels are strongly related to fatty acid oxidation, ketone body production, and gluconeogenesis, SIRTs are thought to be involved in lifespan extension by fasting. Although the molecular mechanisms of longevity are not fully understood, it was reported that SIRT1 and AMPK activates PGC-1α, and that overexpression of SIRT1, SIRT3, and SIRT6 results in enhanced genomic stability, suppression of NF- κB signaling, and improvement of metabolic homeostasis via histone deacetylation [31]. In addition, Sir2.1 of *C. elegans* activates DAF-16, a FOXO-type transcription factor [34].

Insulin and IGF-1 signals function as a sensor of nutritional states, and are suppressed by fasting and caloric restriction. During fasting, IGF-1 signaling is repressed by FGF21 as described earlier. On the other hand, the mechanism of suppression of IGF-1 signaling by caloric restriction is complex and may differ among species. In humans, it was reported that protein intake is more important than total caloric intake for the suppression of IGF-1 signaling [31]. Insulin and IGF-1 signals have been shown to be involved in longevity, but its mechanism remains unclear. Genome-wide association studies (GWAS) showed an association between insulin and IGF-1 signaling and human lifespan, and also suggested that Akt, FOXO, PI3K, and SGK signaling pathways are involved in longevity [35]. Treatment of epithelial cells with serum from patients with Laron syndrome, which is characterized by refractoriness to GH, increases the expression of the superoxide dismutase 2 ($SOD_2$) and decreases the expression of mTOR [36]. In addition, FOXO transcription factors are upregulated in the absence of IGF-1 signaling [36]. These studies suggest that insulin and IGF-1 signaling suppresses stress resistance responses. In *C. elegans*, mutations of the daf-2 gene that suppresses the activity of DAF-2, a homolog of the insulin/IGF-1 receptor, increase lifespan through the inhibition of the PI3K-phosphoinositide-dependent kinase (PDK)-Akt pathway [34]. In Snell mice with mutations in pituitary-specific positive transcription factor-1 (PIT-1) and Ames mice with mutations in the gene encoding the regulator of PIT-1, their lifespan increased by up to 68% compared to control mice [36]. In these mice, in addition to GH, thyroid stimulating hormone (TSH) and prolactin levels were low. However, the observations that lifespan is extended in GH receptor-deficient mice and in mice lacking the gene encoding pregnancy-associated plasma protein A (PAPP-A), an activator of IGF-1 [36], support the idea that insulin and IGF-1 signaling contributes to longevity.

## 9. Energy states and epigenetics

The energy states of organisms, such as fasting and caloric restriction, are memorized in cells, and can lead to the development of future diseases. Recently, epigenetic mechanisms have received much attention in the field of metabolism. The epigenome is a mechanism for regulation of gene expression without changing the genome sequence. Due to its high plasticity, epigenetic regulation is suitable for the memory of metabolic states. Such epigenetic regulations include covalent modifications of DNA, histone, and RNA. More than 100 modifications have been identified, among which methylation, phosphorylation, ubiquitination, and acetylation are well studied, while glycosylation, crotonylation, and succinylation, although functional, are poorly understood [37]. These modifications influence spatial chromatin structure and recruitment of transcription factors and enzymes that are involved in chromatin remodeling. A number of studies have revealed that fasting and obesity-associated diseases that induce a fasting-like metabolic state have a functional link to the epigenome.

Accumulating evidence indicates that diet is one of the most important environmental factors that cause epigenetic changes in the growth process of organisms. One striking evidence of dietary effects on early development was found in honey bees [38]. Female honey bees have two distinct phenotypes, and female larvae that receive royal jelly exclusively develop into fertile queen bees while the other females develop into sterile workers. These phenotypic changes are accompanied by differential DNA methylation patterns and gene expressions between queens and workers through DNA methyltransferase 3 ($DNMT_3$). Such epigenetic alterations during development in response to nutritional states are also found in mammals. A well-known example is the nutritional effect on coat color of the mouse by DNA methylation of the Agouti viable yellow ($A^{vy}$) locus [38]. Insertion of an endogenous retrovirus (ERV) upstream of this gene locus causes constitutive expression of the Agouti gene as the ERV functions as an alternative promoter, resulting in yellow coat color and adult-onset of obesity. The DNA methylation level at the ERV locus increased in offspring but not in the mother in response to gestational intake of compounds related to the methionine cycle including folate. In rats, the locus-specific change in DNA methylation of the Ppara gene was also observed in offspring of the father or mother fed with a low protein diet [38]. It is also reported that feeding high-fat diet to pregnant Japanese macaques led to global hyperacetylation of histone H3 in their offspring [38]. In humans, epidemiological studies developed the important concept of 'Developmental Origins of Health and Disease' (DOHaD), which proposes that unfavorable adaptation to nutritional stress at the embryonic stage is a risk for abnormal growth and development and subsequent health disorders later in life [38]. Cohort studies on the Dutch Famine of 1944–1945 revealed that the severe maternal starvation during the peri-conceptional period induced mental and metabolic abnormalities such as obesity and type 2 diabetes along with changes in DNA methylation in the next generation.

Although epigenetic profiles are more prone to be altered by nutritional states during peri-conceptional, gestational, and early postnatal periods, dietary effects on the epigenetic state are also found in adult animals. Several lines of evidence have revealed that overnutrition induces epigenetic changes in adult organs. One study revealed 232 differentially methylated regions (DMRs) on the genomic DNA in the adipose tissue between mice fed a normal chow diet and those fed a high fat diet [39]. Importantly, the DMRs were also found in humans when comparing lean and obese subjects. Histone modifications are also influenced by diet. It is reported that mice fed a high-fat diet show the increased acetylation levels of histone H3K9 and H3K18 in the genomic regions encoding TNFα and CCL2 in the liver [40]. A mass spectrometry-based approach showed that high-fat diet increased the level of di-methylated histone H3K36 (H3K36me2) and other histone modifications in the mouse liver [41]. In human urine-derived podocyte-like cells, palmitate treatment induced sustained activation of FOXO1 even in the presence of insulin, which was accompanied by the increased H3K36me2 level in the promoter region of the FoxO1 gene [42]. The H3K27me3 in the FoxO1 promoter region decreased in the kidney of rat fed a high-fat diet. In addition to the DNA and histone modifications, RNA methylation is an emerging regulatory mechanism of epigenetics/epitranscriptomics. For example, there reported that a high-fat diet enhanced the expression of fat mass and obesity-associated protein (FTO)/alkB homolog 9 (ALKBH9), an RNA demethylase, and suppressed the N6-methyladenosine (m6A) levels in the mouse adipose tissue, which resulted in obesity [43]. The beneficial effects of fasting on health have also attracted attention in the field of epigenetics. Fasting is implicated in histone modifications via ketone body production as described below. In addition, a clinical human study showed that fasting stress increased methylated CpG sites of the Leptin and Adiponectin genes only in the group born with normal body weight but not in the group born with low body weight [44]. Collectively, epigenetic profiles reflect nutritional states not only in the fetus and infants but also in adults.

## 10. Metabolite and co-factor-mediated regulation of epigenetic enzymes

Although it is not well understood which component in the diets is responsible for epigenetic changes in organisms, it should be noted that the activity of epigenetic enzymes depends on metabolites and co-factors such as metals. These enzymes include acetyltransferases, deacetylases, methyltransferases, and demethylases for DNA, histone, and RNA. In reactions that add or remove epigenetic modifications, these enzymes utilize metabolites derived from metabolic pathways including glycolysis, fatty acid oxidation, the methionine cycle, and the TCA cycle. These metabolic pathways supply metabolites, such as acetyl-CoA, $NAD^+$, S-adenosylmethionine (SAM), and α-KG as substrates to the enzymes (**Figure 7**). Ferrous iron is also an essential co-factor for epigenetic demethylases. Considering that the kinetic and thermodynamic properties of the interaction between an epigenetic enzyme and a metabolite are in a similar range as the physiological concentrations of metabolites [37], it is possible that dynamic changes in the availability of metabolites and co-factors may affect epigenetic outcomes. Here, we discuss the potential for regulation of epigenetic modifications through metabolites and co-factors.

HATs, such as CBP/p300, are enzymes that transfer an acetyl group from acetyl-CoA to lysine residues on histone proteins (**Figure 7B**). Acetyl-CoA is supplied from various nutrients through metabolic pathways such as glycolysis, the TCA cycle, and fatty acid oxidation (**Figure 7A**). In a study examining which nutrient-derived acetyl-CoA alters histone acetylation, only lipids, among various nutrients, induced direct acetylation of histones via fatty acid oxidation in mammalian cells [45]. Another

A

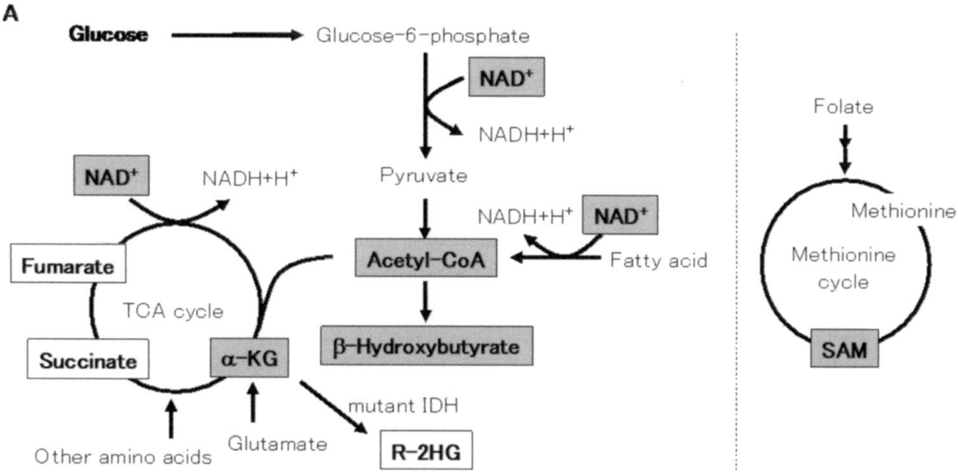


B

| Epigenetic enzymes | Substrates and co-factors | Inhibitory metabolites |
|---|---|---|
| **Histone acetyltransferase** | Acetyl-CoA | |
| **Histone deacetylase (SIRTs)** | $NAD^+$ | Butylate, **β**-hydroxybutyrate |
| **Methyltransferase** | SAM | |
| **Demethylase (2OGDDs)** | $O_2$, **α**-KG, $Fe^{2+}$ | R-2HG, succinate, fumarate |

**Figure 7.**
*Metabolite-mediated regulation of epigenetic enzymes. A. Production of substrates and co-factors of epigenetic enzymes in the metabolic process, B. Substrates, co-factors, and inhibitory metabolites of epigenetic enzymes.*

study showed that the treatment of pancreatic β cells with palmitate increased HAT activity and histone acetylation [44]. However, a mass spectrometry-based study demonstrated that a high-fat diet rather decreased acetyl-CoA levels in the mouse white adipose tissue, which correlated with histone acetylation [45], suggesting that the regulation of histone acetylation by metabolites is more complex in obesity.

Acetyl groups on histones are removed by the action of HDACs. SIRTs (SIRT1–7), a class III HDACs, are $NAD^+$-dependent deacetylases that sense the energy state in cells (**Figure 7**). They have been shown to be involved in longevity in a variety of species, including yeast, *C. elegans*, and Drosophila, although epigenetic mechanisms are not fully understood [32, 33]. Importantly, a decrease in $NAD^+$ levels due to activated glycolysis was sufficient to inhibit the activity of $NAD^+$-dependent deacetylases and promoted histone H4K16 acetylation during differentiation of murine muscle cells [37], suggesting that fasting can be involved in the regulation of epigenetic enzymes. Butylate, a short-chain fatty acid produced by intestinal fermentation, is known to inhibit histone deacetylases [45]. Butyrate and a class I HDAC inhibitor have been reported to suppress obesity-associated phenotype in a mouse model of high-fat diet induced obesity (**Figure 7B**) [45]. Similarly, β-hydroxybutyrate, one of the ketone bodies, inhibits class I HDACs (HDAC1, 2, 3, and 8) (**Figure 7B**) [6]. Considering that the inhibition potency (IC50) of β-hydroxybutyrate on these HDACs is around 2–5 mM in an in vitro assay, and that the concentration of β-hydroxybutyrate in humans during long-term fasting is 6–8 mM, β-hydroxybutyrate is a potential physiological inhibitor of HDACs [6]. In the mouse kidney, fasting induced hyperacetylation of histone H3K9 and H3K14, and the HDAC-mediated expression of FoxO3 enhanced the expression of oxidative stress resistance genes [46].

DNMTs, histone methyltransferases (e.g., enhancer of zeste homolog 2 (EZH2), SET domain-containing methyltransferases (SETs), and mixed-lineage leukemias

(MLLs)), and RNA methyltransferase (e.g., methyltransferase like 3 (METTL3) and METTL14) require SAM as a methyl donor for methylation of DNA, histone, and RNA, respectively (**Figure 7B**). SAM is provided by the methionine cycle from dietary components such as methionine and folate (**Figure 7A**). Decreased folate levels in the circulation was reported in patients with type 2 diabetes, and the folate levels were correlated with DNA methylation levels in the liver [44]. Additionally, administration of folate to mice fed a high-fat diet altered the DNA methylation patterns of genes in the adipose tissue and improved obesity-associated phenotype [44].

Among epigenetic demethylases, DNA demethylases (ten-eleven translocation methylcytosine dioxygenases (TETs)), histone lysine demethylases with a JmjC domain (e.g., KDMs), and RNA demethylases (ALKBH5 and FTO/ALKBH9 require oxygen and α-KG as substrates and ferrous iron as a cofactor (**Figure 7B**). α-KG is an intermediate metabolite of the TCA cycle and is also supplied by a flux of amino acids such as glutamate (**Figure 7A**), while ferrous iron is taken up from outside the cell via transferrin receptors or supplied internally by ferritin-selective autophagy [47]. Interestingly, these demethylases are classified into the 2-oxoglutarate-dependent dioxygenase (2OGD) family, and the structure of their catalytic domain is highly conserved among all the enzymes [48]. Notably, the iron-binding site of the enzymes is composed of a highly conserved amino acid sequence, that is, histidine, and aspartate or glutamate located two amino acids away from the histidine, followed by histidine located around a hundred amino acids away from the two amino acids (HXD/G...H). A ferrous iron molecule bound to these amino acids serve as a catalytic center of the demethylase, which oxidizes the methyl group of the substrates and removes the methyl group from DNA, histone, and RNA. Several studies suggested that both α-KG and iron are critical regulators of 2OGDs. α-KG has been shown to increase during adipocyte differentiation and to promote differentiation through demethylation of H3K9 at the Pparg locus [49]. Similarly, adipocyte differentiation in 3T3-L1 cells, which involves dynamic changes in the epigenome, is inhibited by iron depletion, although how the ferrous iron level is altered during differentiation has not been explored [50, 51]. It is also noteworthy that some types of cancer cells harboring mutations on IDH1 and IDH2 produce an inhibitor of 2OGDs, (R)-2-hydroxyglutarate (R-2HG) (**Figure** 7) and show characteristic DNA and histone hypermethylation [37]. Additionally, fumarate and succinate can inhibit 2OGDs (**Figure** 7), and deletion of fumarate dehydrogenase and succinate dehydrogenase induced histone and DNA hypermethylation [37]. Considering the recent findings that KDM5A/JARID1A and KDM6A/UTX function as oxygen sensors whose demethylase activity is inhibited under hypoxia [52, 53], it is possible that change in the concentrations of metabolites and cofactors may also affect the demethylase activity of 2OGDs, and thus control epigenetic consequences of cellular processes.

Therefore, it is conceivable that energy states could regulate epigenetic mechanisms and be memorized, subsequently influencing the onset of a variety of diseases. Thus, understanding the relationship between energy states and the epigenome is essential for establishment of an appropriate diet-based therapy. As future challenges, it is necessary to elucidate how concentrations of metabolites and cofactors change during biological processes, and which epigenetic enzymes are responsible for the metabolite- and/or cofactor-mediated epigenetic alterations. However, measuring local concentrations of metabolites and cofactors, especially in the nucleus, has been difficult due to technical barriers. We have recently developed a fluorescence resonance energy transfer (FRET)-based biosensor to measure nuclear α-KG concentrations and have found that nuclear α-KG concentrations increase with adipocyte differentiation [54]. The development of such tools will shed light on the regulatory mechanisms of the epigenome by biomolecules in the future.

## 11. Future perspectives

Now that the development of the internet and other factors have made it easy for non-medical professionals to obtain medical knowledge, the effects of caloric restriction, fasting, the order in which foods are eaten, and the nutritional composition of diets have become familiar topics of interest in the treatment of diabetes and obesity. Therefore, it is more and more important than ever for researchers to understand whole body metabolism based on accurate evidence. There is no doubt that diet plays an important role in the maintenance of health, and new molecular mechanisms including epigenetics have recently emerged in addition to the widely accepted concepts on metabolism. In addition, the involvement of unknown regulatory factors has been implicated. Extensive research will lead to a better understanding of energy metabolism in the body and contribute to the extension of healthy life.

## Conflict of interest

None.

## Author details

Tomohiro Suzuki, Tetsuro Komatsu, Hiroshi Shibata and Takeshi Inagaki*
Laboratory of Epigenetics and Metabolism, Institute for Molecular and Cellular Regulation, Gunma University, Gunma, Japan

*Address all correspondence to: inagaki@gunma-u.ac.jp

## References

[1] Cahill GF. Fuel metabolism in starvation. Annu Rev Nutr. 2006; 26:1-22.

[2] Sakakibara I, Fujino T, Ishii M, Tanaka T, Shimosawa T, Miura S, et al. Fasting-induced hypothermia and reduced energy production in mice lacking acetyl-CoA synthetase 2. Cell Metab. 2009;9(2):191-202.

[3] Owen OE. Ketone bodies as a fuel for the brain during starvation. Biochemistry and Molecular Biology Education. 2005;33(4):246-251.

[4] Liu N, Qiao K, Stephanopoulos G. 13C Metabolic Flux Analysis of acetate conversion to lipids by Yarrowia lipolytica. Metabolic Engineering. 2016;38:86-97.

[5] Owen OE, Felig P, Morgan AP, Wahren J, Cahill GF. Liver and kidney metabolism during prolonged starvation. Journal of Clinical Investigation. 1969;48(3):574-583.

[6] Newman JC, Verdin E. Ketone bodies as signaling metabolites. Trends in Endocrinology & Metabolism. 2014;25(1):42-52.

[7] Inagaki T, Dutchak P, Zhao G, Ding X, Gautron L, Parameswara V, et al. Endocrine Regulation of the Fasting Response by PPARα-Mediated Induction of Fibroblast Growth Factor 21. Cell Metabolism. 2007;5(6):415-425.

[8] Inagaki T, Choi M, Moschetta A, Peng L, Cummins CL, Mcdonald JG, et al. Fibroblast growth factor 15 functions as an enterohepatic signal to regulate bile acid homeostasis. Cell Metabolism. 2005;2(4):217-225.

[9] Markan KR, Naber MC, Ameka MK, Anderegg MD, Mangelsdorf DJ, Kliewer SA, et al. Circulating FGF21 Is Liver Derived and Enhances Glucose Uptake During Refeeding and Overfeeding. Diabetes. 2014;63(12): 4057-4063.

[10] Badman MK, Pissios P, Kennedy AR, Koukos G, Flier JS, Maratos-Flier E. Hepatic Fibroblast Growth Factor 21 Is Regulated by PPARα and Is a Key Mediator of Hepatic Lipid Metabolism in Ketotic States. Cell Metabolism. 2007;5(6):426-437.

[11] Ueki K. Role of Activin B/FSTL3 axis in the control of glucose homeostasis. Diabetes Research and Clinical Practice. 2016;120:S25-SS6.

[12] Inagaki T. Research Perspectives on the Regulation and Physiological Functions of FGF21 and its Association with NAFLD. Front Endocrinol (Lausanne). 2015;6:147.

[13] Potthoff MJ, Inagaki T, Satapati S, Ding X, He T, Goetz R, et al. FGF21 induces PGC-1 and regulates carbohydrate and fatty acid metabolism during the adaptive starvation response. Proceedings of the National Academy of Sciences. 2009;106(26):10853-10858.

[14] Kharitonenkov A, Shiyanova TL, Koester A, Ford AM, Micanovic R, Galbreath EJ, et al. FGF-21 as a novel metabolic regulator. Journal of Clinical Investigation. 2005;115(6): 1627-1635.

[15] Wente W, Efanov AM, Brenner M, Kharitonenkov A, Köster A, Sandusky GE, et al. Fibroblast Growth Factor-21 Improves Pancreatic β-Cell Function and Survival by Activation of Extracellular Signal–Regulated Kinase 1/2 and Akt Signaling Pathways. Diabetes. 2006;55(9):2470-2478.

[16] Kharitonenkov A, Wroblewski VJ, Koester A, Chen Y-F, Clutinger CK, Tigno XT, et al. The Metabolic State of Diabetic Monkeys Is Regulated by

Fibroblast Growth Factor-21. Endocrinology. 2007;148(2):774-781.

[17] Gälman C, Lundåsen T, Kharitonenkov A, Bina HA, Eriksson M, Hafström I, et al. The Circulating Metabolic Regulator FGF21 Is Induced by Prolonged Fasting and PPARα Activation in Man. Cell Metabolism. 2008;8(2):169-174.

[18] Inagaki T, Lin VY, Goetz R, Mohammadi M, Mangelsdorf DJ, Kliewer SA. Inhibition of Growth Hormone Signaling by the Fasting-Induced Hormone FGF21. Cell Metabolism. 2008;8(1):77-83.

[19] Owen BM, Bookout AL, Ding X, Lin VY, Atkin SD, Gautron L, et al. FGF21 contributes to neuroendocrine control of female reproduction. Nature Medicine. 2013;19(9):1153-1156.

[20] Fazeli PK, Misra M, Goldstein M, Miller KK, Klibanski A. Fibroblast Growth Factor-21 May Mediate Growth Hormone Resistance in Anorexia Nervosa. The Journal of Clinical Endocrinology & Metabolism. 2010;95(1):369-374.

[21] Zhang J, Kaasik K, Blackburn MR, Lee CC. Constant darkness is a circadian metabolic signal in mammals. Nature. 2006;439(7074):340-343.

[22] Zhang Y, Xie Y, Berglund ED, Coate KC, He TT, Katafuchi T, et al. The starvation hormone, fibroblast growth factor-21, extends lifespan in mice. eLife. 2012;1.

[23] Kuro-O M, Matsumura Y, Aizawa H, Kawaguchi H, Suga T, Utsugi T, et al. Mutation of the mouse klotho gene leads to a syndrome resembling ageing. Nature. 1997;390(6655):45-51.

[24] Talukdar S, Owen M, Bryn, Song P, Hernandez G, Zhang Y, Zhou Y, et al. FGF21 Regulates Sweet and Alcohol Preference. Cell Metabolism. 2016; 23(2):344-349.

[25] Søberg S, Sandholt CH, Jespersen NZ, Toft U, Madsen AL, Von Holstein-Rathlou S, et al. FGF21 Is a Sugar-Induced Hormone Associated with Sweet Intake and Preference in Humans. Cell Metabolism. 2017; 25(5):1045-53.e6.

[26] Holstein-Rathlou V, Stephanie, Bondurant D, Lucas, Peltekian L, Naber C, Meghan, Yin C, Terry, Claflin E, Kristin, et al. FGF21 Mediates Endocrine Control of Simple Sugar Intake and Sweet Taste Preference by the Liver. Cell Metabolism. 2016; 23(2):335-343.

[27] Matsui S, Sasaki T, Kohno D, Yaku K, Inutsuka A, Yokota-Hashimoto H, et al. Neuronal SIRT1 regulates macronutrient-based diet selection through FGF21 and oxytocin signalling in mice. Nature Communications. 2018;9(1).

[28] Kubota N, Kubota T, Itoh S, Kumagai H, Kozono H, Takamoto I, et al. Dynamic Functional Relay between Insulin Receptor Substrate 1 and 2 in Hepatic Insulin Signaling during Fasting and Feeding. Cell Metabolism. 2008;8(1):49-64.

[29] Kubota T, Kubota N, Kadowaki T. Imbalanced Insulin Actions in Obesity and Type 2 Diabetes: Key Mouse Models of Insulin Signaling Pathway. Cell Metabolism. 2017;25(4):797-810.

[30] Yano H, Sakai M, Matsukawa T, Yagi T, Naganuma T, Mitsushima M, et al. PHD3 regulates glucose metabolism by suppressing stress-induced signalling and optimising gluconeogenesis and insulin signalling in hepatocytes. Scientific Reports. 2018;8(1).

[31] Fontana L, Partridge L. Promoting Health and Longevity through Diet: From Model Organisms to Humans. Cell. 2015;161(1):106-118.

[32] Kennedy BK, Lamming DW. The Mechanistic Target of Rapamycin: The

Grand ConducTOR of Metabolism and Aging. Cell Metabolism. 2016;23(6):990-1003.

[33] Laplante M, Sabatini M, David. mTOR Signaling in Growth Control and Disease. Cell. 2012;149(2): 274-293.

[34] Kenyon CJ. The genetics of ageing. Nature. 2010;464(7288):504-512.

[35] Deelen J, Uh H-W, Monajemi R, Van Heemst D, Thijssen PE, Böhringer S, et al. Gene set analysis of GWAS data for human longevity highlights the relevance of the insulin/IGF-1 signaling and telomere maintenance pathways. AGE. 2013;35(1):235-249.

[36] Junnila RK, List EO, Berryman DE, Murrey JW, Kopchick JJ. The GH/IGF-1 axis in ageing and longevity. Nature Reviews Endocrinology. 2013;9(6):366-376.

[37] Reid MA, Dai Z, Locasale JW. The impact of cellular metabolism on chromatin dynamics and epigenetics. Nature Cell Biology. 2017;19(11): 1298-1306.

[38] Feil R, Fraga MF. Epigenetics and the environment: emerging patterns and implications. Nat Rev Genet. 2012;13(2):97-109.

[39] Multhaup L, Michael, Seldin M, Marcus, Jaffe E, Andrew, Lei X, Kirchner H, Mondal P, et al. Mouse-Human Experimental Epigenetic Analysis Unmasks Dietary Targets and Genetic Liability for Diabetic Phenotypes. Cell Metabolism. 2015;21(1):138-149.

[40] Mikula M, Majewska A, Ledwon JK, Dzwonek A, Ostrowski J. Obesity increases histone H3 lysine 9 and 18 acetylation at Tnfa and Ccl2 genes in mouse liver. International Journal of Molecular Medicine. 2014;34(6): 1647-1654.

[41] Nie L, Shuai L, Zhu M, Liu P, Xie Z-F, Jiang S, et al. The Landscape of Histone Modifications in a High-Fat Diet-Induced Obese (DIO) Mouse Model. Molecular & Cellular Proteomics. 2017;16(7):1324-1334.

[42] Kumar S, Pamulapati H, Tikoo K. Fatty acid induced metabolic memory involves alterations in renal histone H3K36me2 and H3K27me3. Molecular and Cellular Endocrinology. 2016;422:233-242.

[43] Zhou X, Chen J, Chen J, Wu W, Wang X, Wang Y. The beneficial effects of betaine on dysfunctional adipose tissue and N6-methyladenosine mRNA methylation requires the AMP-activated protein kinase α1 subunit. The Journal of Nutritional Biochemistry. 2015;26(12):1678-1684.

[44] Ling C, Rönn T. Epigenetics in Human Obesity and Type 2 Diabetes. Cell Metabolism. 2019;29(5):1028-1044.

[45] Xu L, Yeung MHY, Yau MYC, Lui PPY, Wong C-M. Role of Histone Acetylation and Methylation in Obesity. Current Pharmacology Reports. 2019;5(3):196-203.

[46] Shimazu T, Hirschey MD, Newman J, He W, Shirakawa K, Le Moan N, et al. Suppression of Oxidative Stress by -Hydroxybutyrate, an Endogenous Histone Deacetylase Inhibitor. Science. 2013;339 (6116):211-214.

[47] Santana-Codina N, Mancias J. The Role of NCOA4-Mediated Ferritinophagy in Health and Disease. Pharmaceuticals. 2018;11(4):114.

[48] Islam MS, Leissing TM, Chowdhury R, Hopkinson RJ, Schofield CJ. 2-Oxoglutarate-Dependent Oxygenases. Annu Rev Biochem. 2018;87:585-620.

[49] Okabe K, Nawaz A, Nishida Y, Yaku K, Usui I, Tobe K, et al. NAD+

Metabolism Regulates Preadipocyte Differentiation by Enhancing α-Ketoglutarate-Mediated Histone H3K9 Demethylation at the PPARγ Promoter. Front Cell Dev Biol. 2020;8:586179.

[50] Moreno-Navarrete JM, Ortega F, Moreno M, Ricart W, Fernández-Real JM. Fine-tuned iron availability is essential to achieve optimal adipocyte differentiation and mitochondrial biogenesis. Diabetologia. 2014;57(9):1957-1967.

[51] Lin Q, Lee Y-J, Yun Z. Differentiation Arrest by Hypoxia. Journal of Biological Chemistry. 2006;281(41):30678-30683.

[52] Chakraborty AA, Laukka T, Myllykoski M, Ringel AE, Booker MA, Tolstorukov MY, et al. Histone demethylase KDM6A directly senses oxygen to control chromatin and cell fate. Science. 2019;363(6432):1217-1222.

[53] Batie M, Frost J, Frost M, Wilson JW, Schofield P, Rocha S. Hypoxia induces rapid changes to histone methylation and reprograms chromatin. Science. 2019;363(6432):1222-1226.

[54] Suzuki T, Hayashi M, Komatsu T, Tanioka A, Nagasawa M, Tanimura-Inagaki K, et al. Measurement of the nuclear concentration of α-ketoglutarate during adipocyte differentiation by using a fluorescence resonance energy transfer-based biosensor with nuclear localization signals. Endocr J. 2021.

Chapter 8

# Role of Gut Microbiota in Bile-Acid Metabolism

*Yuji Naito, Tomohisa Takagi and Ryo Inoue*

## Abstract

The role of the gut microbiota in modifying the pathophysiology of various diseases, including neurodegenerative diseases, is increasingly becoming clear. Bile acids have been shown to be endogenous factors that affect gut microbiota, and bile-acid metabolites directly or indirectly affect host physiology and pathophysiology. The development of metagenomic analysis for gut microbiota and systematic bile-acid measurement using LC–MS/MS has triggered a breakthrough for research in this field. Clinically, an inhibitor of the ileal bile-acid transporter (Elobixibat) was used as a therapeutic agent for chronic constipation, which also paved the way for progress in bile-acid signal research. Additionally, this review emphasizes the importance of gut microbiota-bile acid-receptor signals when considering nutritional approaches to promote healthy longevity.

**Keywords:** *Akkermansia muciniphila*, bile acid, gut microbiota, ileal bile-acid transporter, TGR5

## 1. Introduction

Bile acids have been studied for more than 100 years, but recently, their interaction with intestinal flora has been drawing attention and is being increasingly clarified. Bile-acid research, which has been conducted mainly in the field of liver disease, has led to the development of ursodeoxycholic acid (UDCA), which is generally accepted to improve clinical and biochemical index values in patients with cholestatic liver disease. TGR5 (G protein-coupled bile-acid receptor 1, GPBAR-1), identified in 2002, is a G protein-coupled receptor with seven transmembrane domains and is widely distributed in various organs and tissues. TGR5 can be activated by primary and secondary bile acids, indicating the function of bile acids as signal transduction molecules and in regulating energy metabolism and glycolipid metabolism [1]. Bile acids undergo various metabolic processes such as deconjugation by intestinal bacteria; it has also been shown that the host response is regulated by the reaction between the metabolite and the receptor [2]. Under these circumstances, an inhibitor of the ileal bile-acid transporter (IBAT) localized at the terminal ileum has been shown to be effective in treating constipation [3, 4] and has become a topic of clinical research. This review focuses on the interaction between bile acids and gut microbiota.

## 2. Classification of bile acids and their metabolites

Bile acids are synthesized from cholesterol in the liver; in humans, cholic acid (CA) and chenodeoxycholic acid (CDCA) are typical primary bile acids [5]. In the rodent liver, chenodeoxycholic acid is further converted to muricolic acid (MCA). After biosynthesis, CA and CDCA undergo further glycine conjugation or taurine conjugation in the liver. Among human conjugated bile acids, taurine conjugates and glycine conjugates accumulate in the gallbladder at a concentration ratio of approximately 1:3 and are secreted from the bile duct into the duodenum in response to food intake. On secretion into the duodenum, taurine conjugates (tauro-CA, tauro-CDCA) and glycine conjugates (glyco-CA, glyco-CDCA) are deconjugated by the bile salt hydrolase (BSH) of the gut microbiota; these deconjugated bile acids are involved in the formation of micelles and the absorption of dietary fat (**Figure 1**).

*Lactobacillus plantarum*, *Lactobacillus johnsonii*, *Clostridium perfringens*, and *Bifidobacterium longum* have been reported to be specific bacteria carrying the BSH gene [6]. Because the BSH gene is expressed in many bacteria and the presence of BSH is favorable to the host, the presence of these bacteria can be interpreted to be a result of selection by the host. BSH has been suggested to play an important role in the colonization and survival of bacteria in the gut [7]. Jarocki et al. [8] first analyzed the occurrence of BSH in 14 strains belonging to the *Bifidobacterium* genus and purified and analyzed two BSHs from *B. pseudocatenulatum* and *B. longum* subsp. *suis* for their selected biochemical and molecular features. Deconjugation by BSH seems to be meaningful in human physiology and is involved in the lowering of cholesterol levels, maintenance of intestinal homeostasis, maintenance of the intestinal circadian rhythm, and supply of glycine and taurine to the surrounding bacteria [6]. In particular, free bile acids (CA, CDCA) have been reported to be directly involved in the expression of clock genes in intestinal epithelial cells that can control peripheral circadian rhythms in the intestinal tract and liver. Govindarajan et al. [9] demonstrated that unconjugated bile acids are potential chronobiological regulators of host circadian gene expression, especially in the intestine and liver. These data may indicate the potential role of microbiota-generated bile acids as chronological regulators of the peripheral circadian clock and

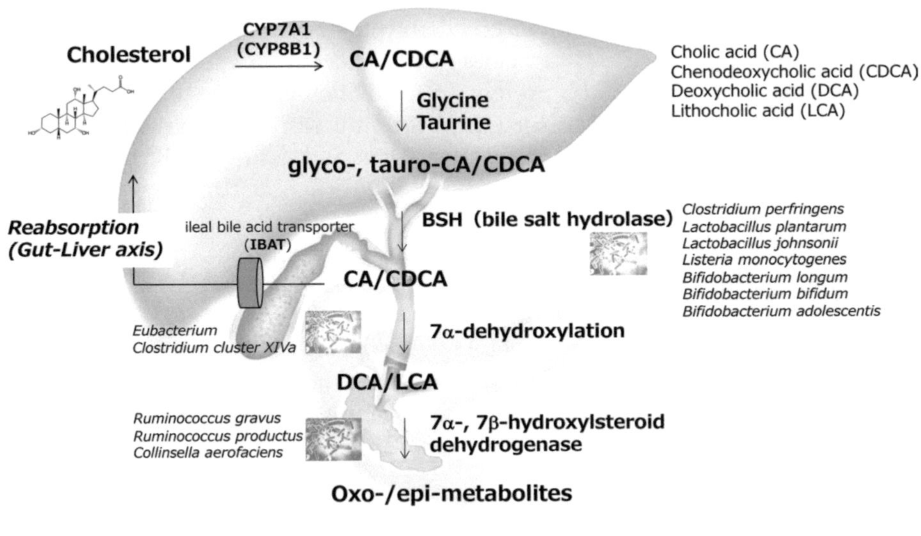


**Figure 1.**
*Synthesis, conjugation, and metabolism of bile acids by gut microbiota.*

suggest that intervention strategies that alter gut bile-acid profiles could influence the circadian clock. Joyce et al. [10] investigated the role bacterial BSH in the host physiology and have demonstrated that bacterial BSH activity significantly impacts the systemic metabolic processes and adiposity in the host and represents a key mechanistic target for the control of obesity and metabolic syndrome.

Primary bile acids are actively reabsorbed by the ileal bile-acid transporter (IBAT) present in the terminal ileum in addition to being passively absorbed. Consequently, bile acids secreted into the intestinal tract could return to the liver via the portal vein, 95% of which is reused. Bile acids are reported to be reused by enterohepatic circulation and circulated in the human body 4–12 times a day [11]. The details of the mechanism regulating IBAT expression have not yet been elucidated; however, IBAT expression appears to be affected by gut microbiota and is markedly enhanced in germ-free mice [12].

Bile acids that flow from the small intestine to the large intestine are further metabolized by abundant gut bacteria. First, multi-step reactions of specific bacteria result in the hydroxyl group at the C-7a position of the deconjugated bile acids (CA and CDCA) being dehydroxylated (7α-dehydroxylation) to form secondary bile acids, such as deoxycholic acid (DCA) and lithocholic acid (LCA). Specifically, CA is metabolized to deoxycholic acid (DCA), which in turn is metabolized to lithocholic acid (LCA). Specific *Eubacterium* and *Clostridium* cluster XIVa species, belonging to the Firmicutes phylum, are involved in this conversion in a complex manner, but the entire pathway has not yet been clarified. More than 90% of bile acids in feces are secondary bile acids, and in humans, DCA and LCA are the most abundant [13]. These bile acids affect host physiological function via the TGR5 receptor, which is a bile-acid receptor, and are involved in water secretion to the lumen of the large intestine and peristaltic movement of the tract. Therefore, secondary bile acids produced by the gut microbiota are essential for the physiological function of the host, and a decrease in their concentration could lead to a corresponding decrease in intestinal peristalsis. Thus, a decrease in bile-acid concentrations may not only induce constipation symptoms, but also adversely affect the gut-brain axis.

Furthermore, some amount of CDCA is further metabolized to UDCA by gut bacteria carrying the 7α- and 7β-hydroxylsteroid dehydrogenase (HSDH) genes. Bacteria such as *Ruminococcus gravus*, *Ruminococcus productus*, *Collinsella aerofaciens*, and *Clostridium absonum* have the HSDH gene but have not been studied in detail. Although the luminal concentrations of these bile-acid metabolites in the large intestine are low, recent reports have reported anti-inflammatory, anti-bacterial, and wound healing promoting effects of these metabolites [14]; thus, further studies are required.

As described above, primary bile acids secreted into the duodenum in a conjugated form are metabolized by various intestinal bacterial genes. This interaction is complex because bile acids also have a more direct effect on the survival of the gut microbiota. Islam et al. [15] have demonstrated that bile acid is a host factor that regulates the composition of the cecal microbiota in rats, and that CA feeding simplifies the composition of the microbiota, with outgrowth of several bacteria in the classes Clostridia and Erysipelotrichi. Furthermore, importantly, several bile-acid receptors have been discovered and each bile acid has differing binding ability to these receptors; these aspects should be considered to understand the bile acid-mediated host response. Metabolic disorders have an impact on longevity and the recent findings showed the relationship between bile acid metabolism and metabolic disorders [16–18]. Broeders et al. [16] have showed that CDCA promotes mitochondrial uncoupling via bile-acid receptor (TGR5) in human brown adipocytes and increases brown fat activity and energy expenditure in women.

Because it has been shown that TGR5 localizes in many cells and tissues, including enteroendocrine cells, neurons, macrophages, muscle and endothelial cells, the bile acid-mediated host response should be carefully analyzed.

## 3. Serum bile-acid profile as a biomarker

The profiles of various bile acids can be selectively measured using quantitative systematic liquid chromatography–tandem mass spectrometry (LC–MS/MS) for samples such as blood and stool. Furthermore, quantitative measurement using internal standard substances has made it possible to rapidly conduct research using a large number of clinical samples [19, 20]. Features of serum bile-acid profiles have been reported in patients with inflammatory bowel disease [19], colon cancer [21], irritable bowel syndrome [22], chronic constipation [23], liver diseases such as fatty liver and fatty hepatitis [24], and neurodegenerative diseases such as Alzheimer's disease and cognitive dysfunction [25, 26].

The relationship between colorectal cancer and the gut microbiota is a hot topic of research. *Fusobacterium nucreatum*, detected relatively specifically in colorectal cancer tissues, is a sulfate-reducing bacterium that can produce hydrogen sulfide, which is a gene mutagen. Taurine released from taurine-conjugated bile acids has been suggested to be a substrate for hydrogen sulfide production [27]; therefore, the carcinogenic-promoting effect of a high-fat diet may be partially explained by the increase in levels of taurine-conjugated bile acids caused by the diet. Bile-acid profile information for patients with colorectal cancer has also been reported. Uchiyama et al. [21] measured serum bile-acid profiles of healthy individuals, colorectal adenomatous polyps, and colorectal cancer at each clinical stage and analyzed the principal components of 30 types of bile acids. Free CA, 3epi-DCA, CDCA, 3-dehydro CA, glyco-CA, and tauro-CA were extracted as principal components (PC) 1 and free 3-dehydroDCA was extracted as PC 2 by canonical discriminant function coefficients. They concluded that the verification of discriminability using the cross-validation method revealed that the correct classification rate was 66.3% for the original data and 52.6% for the cross-validation data. Kuhn et al. [28] also demonstrated the association between serum concentrations of individual bile acids and colon cancer risk and was the first to show the importance of conjugated bile acids compared to that of unconjugated bile acids. They observed statistically significant positive associations between most conjugated primary bile acids (glyco-CA, tauro-CA, glyco-tauro-CDCA, tauro-CDCA, and glyco-hyocholic acid [GHCA]) and colon cancer risk.

The clinical usefulness of serum bile-acid profiles has also been analyzed in several diseases other than colorectal cancer. Recent reports have demonstrated that the concentration of conjugated secondary bile acids (glycol-DCA, glycol-LCA, tauro-DCA, and tauro-LCA), but not of the unconjugated forms, increases parallelly with the progression of the disease, especially in patients with Alzheimer's disease and dementia. Nho et al. [26] were the first to show that altered bile-acid profiles and increased ratios of glyco-DCA:CA, tauro-DCA:CA, and glyco-LCA:CDCA were significantly associated with structural and functional changes in the brain, as indicated by greater atrophy and reduced glucose metabolism. Higher levels of secondary conjugated bile acids (glyco-DCA, glycol-LCA, and tauro-LCA) were significantly associated with worse cognitive function in 1,464 subjects, including 370 cognitively normal older adults, 284 individuals with early mild cognitive impairment (MCI), 505 individuals with late MCI, and 305 patients with Alzheimer's disease [25]. The increase in the concentration of conjugated bile acids in the blood should be considered to be caused by the high-fat diet-stimulated increase in the bile-acid biosynthetic reactions in the liver and the decrease in the bile-acid deconjugation reactions in the intestinal tract, indicating a decrease in the gut microbiota carrying the deconjugation gene for BSH, as has been mentioned above.

We previously performed a correlation analysis between the bile-acid profile and gut microbiota in a fatty liver model and a colon cancer model in mice fed a high-fat diet and indicated that this correlation analysis is useful for assessing the functionality of dietary factors [29, 30]. High-fat dietary load increased serum levels of conjugated bile acids (tauro-CA, tauro-DCA) and decreased levels of unconjugated bile acids (such as CA), but the administration of epigallocatechin gallate (EGCG), a functional ingredient in tea, normalized bile-acid profiles. Furthermore, an analysis of gut microbiota revealed a positive correlation between an increase in the abundance of *Akkermansia* and their effects on bile acids [29]. Similarly, in the colon cancer model, we found that agarooligosaccharide suppressed the increase in levels of taurine-conjugated bile acids and suppressed the increase of bacteria classified into *Clostridium* subcluster XIVa that are involved in secondary bile-acid metabolism.

As described above, quantitative bile-acid profile measurement using the LC–MS/MS method has made it possible to obtain integrated bile-acid information that distinguishes between conjugated and unconjugated types; consequently, the roles of bile acids in physiology and pathophysiology are being elucidated. It is important to note that such analysis should be conducted with the understanding that the bile-acid profiles are influenced by dietary factors, including high-fat diet, liver function, lipid metabolism, cholesterol level, and gut microbiota.

## 4. An inhibitor of ileal bile-acid transporter (IBAT)

In a gnotobiotic experiment wherein feces of patients with chronic constipation, especially those with delayed intestinal transit time, were transplanted into germ-free mice, short chain fatty acids and secondary bile acids, which are metabolites of the gut microbiota, were identified to be factors that promote intestinal peristalsis, and the administration of butyric acid or DCA activated serotonin signals in the gut and restored the decreased intestinal peristalsis of these gnotobiotic mice [31]. In addition, the amount of bile acids in the feces of patients with chronic constipation and irritable bowel syndrome was found to be decreased, suggesting that improving this decrease in the bile-acid concentration in the large intestine may be a suitable therapeutic strategy.

Elobixibat, the first inhibitor of IBAT, expressed in epithelial cells in the terminal ileum and suppresses the reabsorption of bile acids, thereby causing bile acids to flow into the lumen of the large intestine (**Figure 2**). Elobixibat is effective as a therapeutic agent for chronic constipation as it induces a secondary bile-acid signal, causing water to be secreted into the lumen of the large intestine and thus promoting gastrointestinal peristalsis [3, 4]. These physiological effects of bile acids are thought to be mediated by the TGR5 receptor localized in intestinal cells. The analysis of bile acids in feces has indicated an increase in DCA levels after the administration of Elobixibat compared to those before administration [23]. Intestinal neuroendocrine cells (EC cells) are considered to be the main TGR5 receptor-expressing cells, and TGR5 receptor-deficient mice have been demonstrated to have decreased intestinal peristalsis [32]. The binding of bile acids to the TGR5 receptor expressed on the luminal side of EC cells is hypothesized to activate serotonin synthesis signals and enhance secretion, leading to the activation of peristalsis. The reactivity of the TGR5 receptor to different bile acids varies; the TGR5 receptor has high reactivity with LCA and DCA and low reactivity with CDCA and CA [33].

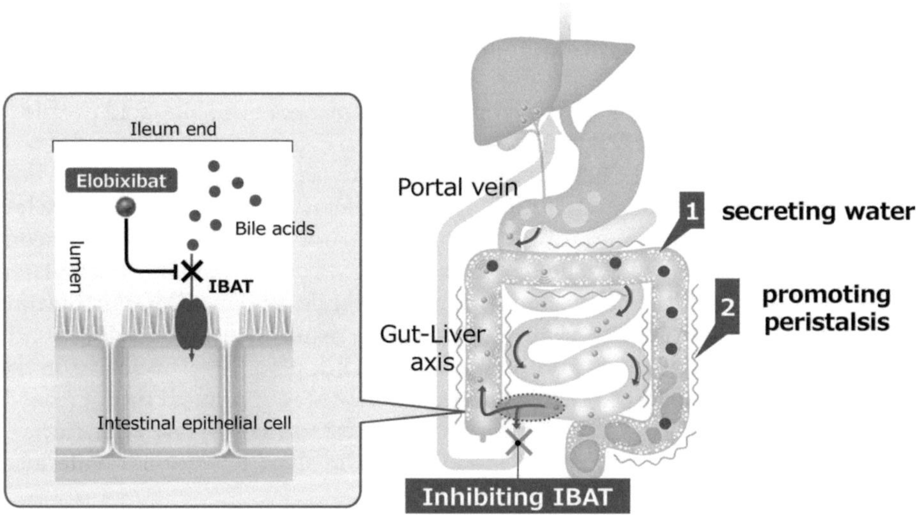


**Figure 2.**
*Ileal bile-acid transporter (IBAT) inhibitor (elobixibat) and its effect on the function of the large intestine. Elobixibat inhibits IBAT expressed in epithelial cells in the terminal ileum and partially suppresses bile-acid reabsorption. The flow of bile acids into the lumen of the large intestine activates TGR5 receptors, causing the secretion of water into the lumen of the large intestine and thus promoting gastrointestinal peristalsis.*

TGR5 receptor expression is also reported to be affected by gut microbiota [12]. In other words, the dose dependence of the efficacy of Elobixibat may be strongly influenced by the intestinal bile-acid profile and intestinal flora of each individual. In addition, Elobixibat activates bile-acid metabolism, and in future studies, it is necessary to consider the effects of Elobixibat on the whole body, including effects on cholesterol metabolism and fatty liver.

An observational study that used the Japanese version of the Patient Assessment of.

Constipation-Quality of Life (PAC-QOL) questionnaire has demonstrated that the scores of physical discomfort and psychosocial discomfort significantly decreased in patients with constipation after the treatment with Elobixibat for 4 weeks, indicating the possibility that Elobixibat could affect the gut-brain axis [34].

## 5. *Akkermansia muciniphila* and bile-acid signals for well-being

Well-being is a key word in the WHO's definition of health: a state of complete physical, mental, and social well-being and not merely the absence of disease or infirmity. Thus, medical care aimed at wellbeing is necessary. Recent reports have revealed the involvement of gut microbiota and bile-acid metabolism in extending healthspan and lifespan [35]. The gut microbiota of two different mouse models of progeria was characterized by intestinal dysbiosis with alterations including an increase in the abundance of Proteobacteria and Cyanobacteria and a decrease in the abundance of Verrucomicrobia compared to the gut microbiota of control mice. Fecal microbiota transplantation from wild-type mice enhanced healthspan and lifespan in both progeroid mouse models, and transplantation with the Verrucomicrobia *Akkermansia muciniphila* was sufficient to exert beneficial effects. Furthermore, an analysis of gut microbiota metabolites revealed that various bile acids were reduced in the progeroid mouse models, and this dysregulation in bile acids was improved by transplantation with *Akkermansia muciniphila* [35].

Morita et al. [36] reported that *Akkermansia* was more abundant in individuals from Ogimi and *Lachnospiraceae*, *Collinsella*, *Peptococcus*, and S24–7 were more abundant in individuals not from Ogimi. Ogimi is a village located in the northern region of Okinawa's main island and has a population of approximately 3,000; it is known as the village of longevity in Japan. Grajeda-Iglesias et al. [37] recently demonstrated that *Akkermansia muciniphila*, especially if it is pasteurized, causes major changes in metabolism, elevating the concentrations of several metabolites that have been previously associated with positive effects on health in mouse models. Pasteurized *Akkermansia muciniphila* was more efficient than live *Akkermansia muciniphila* in elevating the intestinal and circulatory concentrations of polyamines, short-chain fatty acids, 2-hydroxybutyrate, and multiple bile acids, all of which may have a positive impact on human health.

Bile-acid analysis by LC–MS/MS has enabled the identification of new metabolites related to health and longevity. Detailed metagenomic analysis and intestinal metabolite analysis of Japanese centenarians recently revealed a novel bile-acid metabolite, isoallo-lithocholic acid, which has a bactericidal effect on specific intestinal bacteria [38]. Although details of the effect of *Akkermansia muciniphila* on bile-acid metabolism are not fully understood, our previous analysis using a high-fat diet load mouse model suggests that the bacterium promotes the deconjugation of conjugated bile acids and suppresses the production of secondary bile acids [29]. A double-blind comparative study in obese individuals has already been conducted to investigate whether *Akkermansia muciniphila* improves the intestinal environment [39]. They demonstrated that Akkermansia muciniphila reduced the levels of the relevant blood markers for liver dysfunction and inflammation while the overall gut microbiome structure was unaffected after three months of supplementation [39].

The neuroprotective effect of tauroursodeoxycholic acid (TUDCA), a hydrophilic bile acid and naturally produced in the liver by conjugation of taurine to UDCA, has been recently elucidated [40]. Several studies have shown that TUDCA has neuroprotective action in several models of neurodegenerative disorders, including Alzheimer's disease, Parkinson's disease, and Huntington's disease [40]. Currently, there is one registered clinical trial with TUDCA in Alzheimer's disease, in the United States (Clinical Trials registration: NCT03533257).

Additionally, countermeasures against sarcopenia are important clinical issues in research aimed at improving well-being. Maintaining muscle strength with diet and exercise is important to prevent sarcopenia, and recent studies have shown that TGR5 present in the skeletal muscle plays an important role in muscle maintenance [41, 42]. Exercise-induced stimulation enhances TGR5 receptor expression in the skeletal muscle, and the increased after-meal levels of bile acids in the blood act as ligands for the TGR5 receptor, helping maintain muscle and prevent sarcopenia. Furthermore, TGR5 signaling in the muscle activates muscle metabolism and enhances glucose clearance, which also has a positive effect on glucose metabolism [41, 42]. Countermeasures against so-called frail complexes, such as sarcopenia, locomotive syndrome, and frailty, are extremely important clinical issues in supporting medical care aimed at improving well-being. It should be emphasized that the gut microbiota-bile acid-receptor signal is a novel therapeutic and prophylactic target molecule for improving frailty.

## Acknowledgements

This work was partly supported by the MAFF Commissioned Project Study on the "Project for the realization of foods and dietary habits to extend healthy life expectancy" (grant number JPJ009842).

## Author contributions

All authors were involved in the study design. This review was based on animal and human studies conducted by the group of YN and TT. RI performed metagenome analysis of gut microbiota. YN wrote the manuscript, and all authors reviewed and approved the paper.

## Competing interests

YN received scholarship funds from EA Pharma. Co. Ltd., a collaboration research fund from Taiyo Kagaku Co., Ltd., and received lecture fees from Mylan EPD Co., Takeda Pharma. Co. Ltd., Mochida Pharma. Co. Ltd., EA Pharma. Co. Ltd., Otsuka Pharma. Co. Ltd., and Miyarisan Pharma. Co. Ltd. TT received a collaboration research fund from Fujifilm Medical Co., Ltd., and received lecture fees by Mochida Pharma. Co. Ltd., and Yanssen Pharmaceutical K.K. This study was partly supported by these funds. Neither the funding agency nor any outside organization participated in the study design or had any competing interests. These companies approved the final version of the manuscript.

## Author details

Yuji Naito[1*], Tomohisa Takagi[2,3] and Ryo Inoue[4]

1 Department of Human Immunology and Nutrition Science, Graduate School of Medical Science, Kyoto Prefectural University of Medicine, Kyoto, Japan

2 Molecular Gastroenterology and Hepatology, Graduate School of Medical Science, Kyoto Prefectural University of Medicine, Kyoto, Japan

3 Department for Medical Innovation and Translational Medical Science, Graduate School of Medical Science, Kyoto Prefectural University of Medicine, Kyoto, Japan

4 Laboratory of Animal Science, Department of Applied Biological Sciences, Faculty of Agriculture, Setsunan University, Osaka, Japan

*Address all correspondence to: ynaito@koto.kpu-m.ac.jp

## References

[1] Ma K, Tang D, Yu C, Zhao L. Progress in research on the roles of TGR5 receptor in liver diseases. Scand J Gastroenterol 2021; 56(6): 717-726.

[2] Jia W, Xie G, Jia W. Bile acid-microbiota crosstalk in gastrointestinal inflammation and carcinogenesis. Nat Rev Gastroenterol Hepatol 2018; 15(2): 111-128.

[3] Nakajima A, Seki M, Taniguchi S. Determining an optimal clinical dose of elobixibat, a novel inhibitor of the ileal bile acid transporter, in Japanese patients with chronic constipation: a phase II, multicenter, double-blind, placebo-controlled randomized clinical trial. J Gastroenterol 2018; 53: 525-534.

[4] Nakajima A, Seki M, Taniguchi S, Ohta A, Gillberg P-G, Mattsson JP, Camilleri M. Safety and efficacy of elobixibat for chronic constipation: results from a randomised, double-blind, placebo-controlled, phase 3 trial and an open-label, single-arm, phase 3 trial. The Lancet Gastroenterology & Hepatology 2018; 3(8): 537-547.

[5] Camilleri M, Gores GJ. Therapeutic targeting of bile acids. Am J Physiol Gastrointest Liver Physiol 2015; 309(4): G209-G215.

[6] Long SL, Gahan CGM, Joyce SA. Interactions between gut bacteria and bile in health and disease. Mol Aspects Med 2017; 56: 54-65.

[7] Bustos AY, Font de Valdez G, Fadda S, Taranto MP. New insights into bacterial bile resistance mechanisms: the role of bile salt hydrolase and its impact on human health. Food Res Int 2018; 112: 250-262.

[8] Jarocki P, Podlesny M, Glibowski P, Targonski Z. A new insight into the physiological role of bile salt hydrolase among intestinal bacteria from the genus Bifidobacterium. PLoS One 2014; 9(12): e114379.

[9] Govindarajan K, MacSharry J, Casey PG, Shanahan F, Joyce SA, Gahan CG. Unconjugated Bile Acids Influence Expression of Circadian Genes: A Potential Mechanism for Microbe-Host Crosstalk. PLoS One 2016; 11(12): e0167319.

[10] Joyce SA, MacSharry J, Casey PG, Kinsella M, Murphy EF, Shanahan F, Hill C, Gahan CG. Regulation of host weight gain and lipid metabolism by bacterial bile acid modification in the gut. Proc Natl Acad Sci U S A 2014; 111(20): 7421-7426.

[11] Stellaard F, Lütjohann D. Dynamics of the enterohepatic circulation of bile acids in healthy humans. Am J Physiol Gastrointest Liver Physiol 2021; 321(1): G55-g66.

[12] Fu ZD, Selwyn FP, Cui JY, Klaassen CD. RNA-Seq Profiling of Intestinal Expression of Xenobiotic Processing Genes in Germ-Free Mice. Drug Metab Dispos 2017; 45(12): 1225-1238.

[13] Humbert L, Maubert MA, Wolf C, Duboc H, Mahé M, Farabos D, Seksik P, Mallet JM, Trugnan G, Masliah J, Rainteau D. Bile acid profiling in human biological samples: comparison of extraction procedures and application to normal and cholestatic patients. J Chromatogr B Analyt Technol Biomed Life Sci 2012; 899: 135-145.

[14] Doden HL, Ridlon JM. Microbial Hydroxysteroid Dehydrogenases: From Alpha to Omega. Microorganisms 2021; 9(3).

[15] Islam KB, Fukiya S, Hagio M, Fujii N, Ishizuka S, Ooka T, Ogura Y, Hayashi T, Yokota A. Bile acid is a host factor that regulates the composition of

the cecal microbiota in rats. Gastroenterology 2011; 141(5): 1773-1781.

[16] Broeders EP, Nascimento EB, Havekes B, Brans B, Roumans KH, Tailleux A, Schaart G, Kouach M, Charton J, Deprez B, Bouvy ND, Mottaghy F, Staels B, van Marken Lichtenbelt WD, Schrauwen P. The Bile Acid Chenodeoxycholic Acid Increases Human Brown Adipose Tissue Activity. Cell Metab 2015; 22(3): 418-426.

[17] Hansen M, Scheltema MJ, Sonne DP, Hansen JS, Sperling M, Rehfeld JF, Holst JJ, Vilsbøll T, Knop FK. Effect of chenodeoxycholic acid and the bile acid sequestrant colesevelam on glucagon-like peptide-1 secretion. Diabetes Obes Metab 2016; 18(6): 571-580.

[18] Kusumoto Y, Irie J, Iwabu K, Tagawa H, Itoh A, Kato M, Kobayashi N, Tanaka K, Kikuchi R, Fujita M, Nakajima Y, Morimoto K, Sugizaki T, Yamada S, Kawai T, Watanabe M, Oike Y, Itoh H. Bile acid binding resin prevents fat accumulation through intestinal microbiota in high-fat diet-induced obesity in mice. Metabolism 2017; 71: 1-6.

[19] Murakami M, Iwamoto J, Honda A, Tsuji T, Tamamushi M, Ueda H, Monma T, Konishi N, Yara S, Hirayama T, Miyazaki T, Saito Y, Ikegami T, Matsuzaki Y. Detection of Gut Dysbiosis due to Reduced Clostridium Subcluster XIVa Using the Fecal or Serum Bile Acid Profile. Inflamm Bowel Dis 2018; 24(5): 1035-1044.

[20] Honda A, Tanaka A, Kaneko T, Komori A, Abe M, Inao M, Namisaki T, Hashimoto N, Kawata K, Takahashi A, Ninomiya M, Kang JH, Arakawa M, Yamagiwa S, Joshita S, Umemura T, Sato K, Kaneko A, Kikuchi K, Itakura J, Nomura T, Kakisaka K, Fujii H, Kawada N, Takikawa Y, Masaki T, Ohira H, Mochida S, Yoshiji H, Iimuro S, Matsuzaki Y, Takikawa H. Bezafibrate Improves GLOBE and UK-PBC Scores and Long-Term Outcomes in Patients With Primary Biliary Cholangitis. Hepatology 2019; 70(6): 2035-2046.

[21] Uchiyama K, Naito Y, Yagi N, Mizushima K, Higashimura Y, Hirai Y, Dohi O, Okayama T, Yoshida N, Katada K, Kamada K, Ishikawa T, Takagi T, Konishi H, Kuriu Y, Nakanishi M, Otsuji E, Honda A, Itoh Y. Identification of colorectal cancer by using serum bile acid profile. Biomarker 2021; in press.

[22] Vijayvargiya P, Busciglio I, Burton D, Donato L, Lueke A, Camilleri M. Bile Acid Deficiency in a Subgroup of Patients With Irritable Bowel Syndrome With Constipation Based on Biomarkers in Serum and Fecal Samples. Clin Gastroenterol Hepatol 2018; 16(4): 522-527.

[23] Misawa N, Higurashi T, Takatsu T, Iwaki M, Kobayashi T, Yoshihara T, Ashikari K, Kessoku T, Fuyuki A, Matsuura T, Ohkubo H, Usuda H, Wada K, Naritaka N, Takei H, Nittono H, Matsumoto M, Honda A, Nakajima A, Camilleri M. The benefit of elobixibat in chronic constipation is associated with faecal deoxycholic acid but not effects of altered microbiota. Aliment Pharmacol Ther 2020; 52(5): 821-828.

[24] Caussy C, Hsu C, Singh S, Bassirian S, Kolar J, Faulkner C, Sinha N, Bettencourt R, Gara N, Valasek MA, Schnabl B, Richards L, Brenner DA, Hofmann AF, Loomba R. Serum bile acid patterns are associated with the presence of NAFLD in twins, and dose-dependent changes with increase in fibrosis stage in patients with biopsy-proven NAFLD. Aliment Pharmacol Ther 2019; 49(2): 183-193.

[25] MahmoudianDehkordi S, Arnold M, Nho K, Ahmad S, Jia W, Xie G, Louie G, Kueider-Paisley A, Moseley MA,

Thompson JW, St John Williams L, Tenenbaum JD, Blach C, Baillie R, Han X, Bhattacharyya S, Toledo JB, Schafferer S, Klein S, Koal T, Risacher SL, Kling MA, Motsinger-Reif A, Rotroff DM, Jack J, Hankemeier T, Bennett DA, De Jager PL, Trojanowski JQ, Shaw LM, Weiner MW, Doraiswamy PM, van Duijn CM, Saykin AJ, Kastenmuller G, Kaddurah-Daouk R, Alzheimer's Disease Neuroimaging Initiative the Alzheimer Disease Metabolomics Consortium. Altered bile acid profile associates with cognitive impairment in Alzheimer's disease-An emerging role for gut microbiome. Alzheimers Dement 2019; 15(1): 76-92.

[26] Nho K, Kueider-Paisley A, MahmoudianDehkordi S, Arnold M, Risacher SL, Louie G, Blach C, Baillie R, Han X, Kastenmuller G, Jia W, Xie G, Ahmad S, Hankemeier T, van Duijn CM, Trojanowski JQ, Shaw LM, Weiner MW, Doraiswamy PM, Saykin AJ, Kaddurah-Daouk R, Alzheimer's Disease Neuroimaging Initiative the Alzheimer Disease Metabolomics Consortium. Altered bile acid profile in mild cognitive impairment and Alzheimer's disease: Relationship to neuroimaging and CSF biomarkers. Alzheimers Dement 2019; 15(2): 232-244.

[27] Ridlon JM, Wolf PG, Gaskins HR. Taurocholic acid metabolism by gut microbes and colon cancer. Gut Microbes 2016; 7(3): 201-215.

[28] Kuhn T, Stepien M, Lopez-Nogueroles M, Machado AD, Sookthai D, Johnson T, Roca M, Husing A, Maldonado SG, Cross AJ, Murphy N, Freisling H, Rinaldi S, Scalbert A, Fedirco V, Severi G, Boutron-Ruault MC, Mancini FR, Sowah SA, Boeing H, Jakszyn P, Sanchez MJ, Merino S, Colorado-Yohar S, Barricarte A, Khaw KT, Schmidt JA, Perez-Cornago A, Trichopoulou A, Karakatsani A, Thriskos P, Palli D, Agnoli C, Tumino R, Sacerdote C, Panico S, Bueno-de-Mesquita B, van Gils CH, Heath A, Gunter MJ, Riboli E, Lahoz A, Jenab M, Kaaks R. Pre-diagnostic plasma bile acid levels and colon cancer risk: A prospective study. J Natl Cancer Inst 2020; 112(5): 516-524.

[29] Ushiroda C, Naito Y, Takagi T, Uchiyama K, Mizushima K, Higashimura Y, Yasukawa Z, Okubo T, Inoue R, Honda A, Matsuzaki Y, Itoh Y. Green tea polyphenol (epigallocatechin-3-gallate) improves gut dysbiosis and serum bile acids dysregulation in high-fat diet-fed mice. J Clin Biochem Nutr 2019; 65(1): 34-46.

[30] Higashimura Y, Naito Y, Takagi T, Uchiyama K, Mizushima K, Ushiroda C, Ohnogi H, Kudo Y, Yasui M, Inui S, Hisada T, Honda A, Matsuzaki Y, Yoshikawa T. Protective effect of agaro-oligosaccharides on gut dysbiosis and colon tumorigenesis in high-fat diet-fed mice. Am J Physiol Gastrointest Liver Physiol 2016; 310: G367-G375.

[31] Ge X, Zhao W, Ding C, Tian H, Xu L, Wang H, Ni L, Jiang J, Gong J, Zhu W, Zhu M, Li N. Potential role of fecal microbiota from patients with slow transit constipation in the regulation of gastrointestinal motility. Sci Rep 2017; 7(1): 441.

[32] Alemi F, Poole DP, Chiu J, Schoonjans K, Cattaruzza F, Grider JR, Bunnett NW, Corvera CU. The receptor TGR5 mediates the prokinetic actions of intestinal bile acids and is required for normal defecation in mice. Gastroenterology 2013; 144(1): 145-154.

[33] Kawamata Y, Fujii R, Hosoya M, Harada M, Yoshida H, Miwa M, Fukusumi S, Habata Y, Itoh T, Shintani Y, Hinuma S, Fujisawa Y, Fujino M. A G protein-coupled receptor responsive to bile acids. J Biol Chem 2003; 278(11): 9435-9440.

[34] Kamei D, Kamei Y, Nagano M, Mineshima M, Nitta K, Tsuchiya K. Elobixibat alleviates chronic constipation in hemodialysis patients: a questionnaire-based study. BMC Gastroenterol 2020; 20(1): 26.

[35] Bárcena C, Valdés-Mas R, Mayoral P, Garabaya C, Durand S, Rodríguez F, Fernández-García MT, Salazar N, Nogacka AM, Garatachea N, Bossut N, Aprahamian F, Lucia A, Kroemer G, Freije JMP, Quirós PM, López-Otín C. Healthspan and lifespan extension by fecal microbiota transplantation into progeroid mice. Nat Med 2019; 25(8): 1234-1242.

[36] Morita H, Ichishima M, Tada I, Shiroma H, Miyagi M, Nakamura T, Tanaka H, Ikematsu S. Gut microbial composition of elderly women born in the Japanese longevity village Ogimi. Biosci Microbiota Food Health 2021; 40(1): 75-79.

[37] Grajeda-Iglesias C, Durand S, Daillère R, Iribarren K, Lemaitre F, Derosa L, Aprahamian F, Bossut N, Nirmalathasan N, Madeo F, Zitvogel L, Kroemer G. Oral administration of Akkermansia muciniphila elevates systemic antiaging and anticancer metabolites. Aging (Albany NY) 2021; 13(5): 6375-6405.

[38] Sato Y, Atarashi K, Plichta DR, Arai Y, Sasajima S, Kearney SM, Suda W, Takeshita K, Sasaki T, Okamoto S, Skelly AN, Okamura Y, Vlamakis H, Li Y, Tanoue T, Takei H, Nittono H, Narushima S, Irie J, Itoh H, Moriya K, Sugiura Y, Suematsu M, Moritoki N, Shibata S, Littman DR, Fischbach MA, Uwamino Y, Inoue T, Honda A, Hattori M, Murai T, Xavier RJ, Hirose N, Honda K. Novel bile acid biosynthetic pathways are enriched in the microbiome of centenarians. Nature 2021.

[39] Depommier C, Everard A, Druart C, Plovier H, Van Hul M, Vieira-Silva S, Falony G, Raes J, Maiter D, Delzenne NM, de Barsy M, Loumaye A, Hermans MP, Thissen J-P, de Vos WM, Cani PD. Supplementation with Akkermansia muciniphila in overweight and obese human volunteers: a proof-of-concept exploratory study. Nature Medicine 2019; 25(7): 1096-1103.

[40] Zangerolamo L, Vettorazzi JF, Rosa LRO, Carneiro EM, Barbosa HCL. The bile acid TUDCA and neurodegenerative disorders: An overview. Life Sci 2021; 272: 119252.

[41] Sasaki T, Kuboyama A, Mita M, Murata S, Shimizu M, Inoue J, Mori K, Sato R. The exercise-inducible bile acid receptor Tgr5 improves skeletal muscle function in mice. J Biol Chem 2018; 293(26): 10322-10332.

[42] Sasaki T, Watanabe Y, Kuboyama A, Oikawa A, Shimizu M, Yamauchi Y, Sato R. Muscle-specific TGR5 overexpression improves glucose clearance in glucose-intolerant mice. J Biol Chem 2020; 296. Dec 1.

## Section 3

# Life Styles, Eating Disorders, and Psychology

Chapter 9

# Relations between Dietary Habits, Lifestyle and Leading Obesity

*Shradha Mistri*

## Abstract

Obesity, hypertension, depression currently in the rise are some of the many problems faced by a common person due to poor dietary and sleeping habits along with some genetic disorders. An extensive study has been done over two years with 205 subjects regarding their eating & sleeping habits and their mental & physical state on a day-to-day basis. The subjects include both males and females ranging from 15 years of age to 70 above. Altogether 12.68% of people suffer from obesity while just 51.21% of them have an appropriate weight. Women below the age of 25 have shown an overpowering presence of PCOS affecting their health and 38.53% of the population showcasing suffering from hypertension and 14.14% suffering from depression. Sleep has yet proven to be a defining factor in wellbeing. 17.07% of the population exhibit signs of sleep deprivation while just 63.9% of the population sleep over 7 hours daily. Like many other countries, in India, the shift from traditional healthy food to fast food & processed food is taking place, resulting in various health problems like obesity, heart problems, arthritis, weakness, diabetes, high blood pressure, difficulty in breathing, stroke & so on. The aim of this meta-analysis was to quantify the effects of nutrition, mental health and exercise on the various aspects of a person's well-being.

**Keywords:** Obesity, Hypertension, PCOS, Diet, Sleep, Depression

## 1. Introduction

Obesity is a chronic medical condition on the rise almost on the global epidemic level, which negatively impacts the health of people. The World Health Organization (WHO) defines it as the accumulation of excessive fat in the body creating risks for a healthy life [1]. In the year 2015, it was estimated that around 603.7 million adults were obese worldwide and then recently in 2018, it shows that the rate has increased and now 650 million adults suffer from obesity and 1.9 billion adults are overweight [2]. Studies have also shown that in the past 25 years, the prevalence of obesity has doubled in 73 countries globally [3]. In the last 30 years the rate of obesity has doubled amongst adults and children, and tripled amongst the adolescents [4]. In India, more than 135 million people are affected by obesity, prevalence rate of obesity and central obesity varies from 11.8% to 31.3% and 16.9% to 36.3% respectively according to the ICMR-INDIAB study conducted in 2015 [4].

Obesity is increasing globally in epidemic proportions over the past 50 years and has become a public burden with profound impacts on mortality, morbidity and cost of living, and thus has been recognised as a diseased state [4–6]. Therefore, to understand the general public's standing when it comes to health the commonly used metric is the Body Mass Index (BMI) for defining anthropometric height/weight characteristics in adults and for categorizing them into groups. BMI basically is the ratio between body weight and the square of body height which is commonly used to assess bodily mass in epidemiological studies, since it corrects for height [7]. BMI primarily represents an individual's fatness, along with the risk factors for the prevalence of various health issues. This survey uses BMI to categorize as well as decipher the prevalence of obesity amongst the 205 individuals who participated, due to its wide acceptance in defining specific categories of body mass as a health issue [3, 7]. Being overweight is defined as the BMI being equal to or higher than 25 $kg/m^2$. From the studies, it has been revealed that the mean BMI is increasing by the years and they are skewing towards the right, showcasing a hasty increase of obesity [8]. Multiple Factors create a chronic positive energy balance which leads to obesity. This excess energy gets converted to triglyceride that gets stored in the adipose tissue depots and increases body fat accumulation and weight gain [1].

Obesity rates are rapidly increasing, especially amongst those with low incomes and education levels, suggesting that the gap among socioeconomic strata for obesity rates may be closing [9]. Consequences of leading sedentary life and poor diet leads to obesity, which now is nothing short of a global health hazard. Studies have even shown from both cross-sectional and longitudinal ways that consuming more of Western or highly processed diet over Mediterranean-style diet leads one to develop depression, anxiety and obesity [10]. At same time, sometimes genetics can also play a role in gaining weight. It has been observed that one subjects show resistance towards adipocyte secreted hormone leptin; this hormone opposes fat accumulation [7].

Hypertension is closely associated with the prevalence, pathophysiology, and morbidity of obesity and bears a positive linear correlation with BMI [3]. Heightened inflammatory activity leads to vascular dysfunction, coronary and cardiovascular diseases, and development of hypertension in patients suffering from severe obesity. Therefore, Obesity has been identified as the most important determinant of hypertension [3]. High sodium intake causes increased renal sodium reabsorption along with the combination of amplified renin-angiotensin aldosterone and sympathetic nervous system activity in obesity. All these leads up to hypertension and extracellular volume expansion in obesity [3, 7]. It has been estimated that worldwide over 300 million people suffer from depression and over 650 million are affected by obesity (2019).

Mental health disorders, mood and anxiety disorders are frequently co-occurring with obesity. Studies suggest that exposure to childhood trauma generally contributes in developing obesity as one grows older, especially in women and that rates of obesity are much higher in people who suffer from problems. A recent cross-sectional study also found developing anxiety due to excess weight and vice versa are quite extensive [11, 12].

The relation of obesity and PCOS is intertwined, where obesity is taken under consideration for the pathophysiological cascade of PCOS through 2 major pathways- insulin resistance & hyperandrogenism at the same time the increase in visceral fat due to PCOS can lead to obesity [6]. PCOS is considered a multifactorial disorder with various genetic, endocrine, hormonal alterations like hyperandrogenaemia and environmental abnormalities [13]. During infancy and early childhood, a change in the pre- and postnatal weight gain leads to central obesity, which if not taken under control can develop into polycystic ovary syndrome (PCOS) after reaching adult height [14]. Women with PCOS have higher normal serum concentrations of androgen and show more clinically significant insomnia symptoms & daytime sleepiness in comparison to women without PCOS. Adolescents with PCOS and obesity have extremely poor actigraphy-estimated sleep, sleep efficiency and show longer sleep onset latency [15]. Thus, obese individuals are at a higher risk of developing sleep apnea, where the airway gets partially or completely obstructed while sleeping [6]. These obstructions in the night-time sleep leads to daytime somnolence, morning headache, systemic hypertension, which circles back and leads to hypertension and cardiac problems [9].

In this survey we also consider women above the age of 45 and women usually experience menopause during that time frame (42–50) which definitely alters the body composition, which usually is an increase in total and abdominal fat mass due to oestrogen deficiency. Usually, the average weight gain ranges between 2.2 kgs to 4.1 kgs during this period. Independent of weight modifications, the menopause has been shown to be associated with major changes in body composition and fat distribution [16].

## 2. Methods and materials

Interview surveys include questions on self-reported weight and height, which have been used to monitor trends over time. A total of 205 subjects participated in the study. Following convention, we defined prevalence of overweight and obesity (in adults (aged >18 years) overweight categorised as BMI $\geq$25 to <30 kg/m$^2$ and obesity as BMI $\geq$30 kg/m$^2$; in children, classification is based on the International Obesity Task Force [IOTF] definition; appendix). We did a systematic literature review with search criteria as those pertaining to our subjects under consideration. We identified all articles reporting prevalence of overweight and obesity based on BMI [5]. In totality data was collected from 120 female subjects and 85 male subjects with their consent. The age group ranged between 15 to 70 years of age. A few above 70-year-old subjects volunteered in this study as well. Data regarding their eating & sleeping habits and their mental & physical state on a day-to-day basis. A special interest was taken to understand the relation between mental and physical disorder, and their association with eating patterns as well as weight gain. The subjects hailed from Mumbai, Kolkata and Bangalore in India. The students were mostly high school and college going individuals, whilst the rest hailed from either corporate sectors (private companies) or government services. Few subjects were also hailing from impoverished backgrounds who have to work as labourers to earn a living. The height was recorded in either centimeters or foot whilst collecting data and converted into centimeters during tabulations. Although all the readings of height were converted into metre so that the BMI value could be calculated. On the other hand, the weight was collected, tabulated as well as implemented in the formula in the form of kilogram units. In our analysis, we recorded a systematic bias, but this bias is greater in some regions than in others. Self-reported weights for women in some countries tend to be under-reported and self-reported heights for men tend to be over-reported. However, self-reported weights and heights are a major source of information for studies of obesity [5]. The body mass index (BMI), calculated by dividing the body weight in kilograms by the square of height in meters, is a simple metric used to indicate overall body fatness [17]. WHO defines a normal BMI range as 18.5 to 24.9, whereas a BMI $\geq$25 kg/m2 is considered to be overweight, and a BMI $\geq$30 kg/m2 is classified as obese, with severe obesity defined as a BMI $\geq$40 kg/m2 [1, 2]. The daily diet of the subjects were segregated on the basis of them either being vegetarians or non-vegetarians, if they consumed dairy products, and if they had breakfast in the mornings. Breakfast is considered the important meal of the day and research findings have proven that skipping the most important meal of the day can lead to weight gain and a slew of other problems like elevated blood pressure, higher levels of total and low-density lipoprotein cholesterol, gastric problems etc. Another important factor which was considered and given importance was to sleep and the gap between the subject's last meal and going to sleep. A 7-to-8-hour continuous sleep in the night is an extremely crucial factor for a proper functioning of the human body. Studies have shown that when people don't get enough sleep, they have increased levels of a hunger hormone called ghrelin and decreased levels of the satiety/fullness hormone called leptin, which could lead to overeating and weight gain. Also, according to the experts it's crucial that we keep an interval of 3 hours between our dinner and sleep as it allows your body time to digest your food so you're not up at night with an upset stomach, indigestion or heartburn.

Most of the fast food contains a large amount of sugar, fats and carbs and less minerals and vitamins. They are energy dense food which means that one consumes large amounts of unhealthy calories in the shape of fast food which leads to weight gain and ultimately obesity. The frequency of fast food in a month is an important factor in deciding the reason behind rapid weight gain. The frequency has been recorded in terms of 1–2, 3–4, 5–6 and more than 6 (>6) times in a month. The cheapest foods are those containing high levels of fat and sugar. Thus, the way to get the most calories for the least money is to eat a diet that is high in fat and sugar [9].

Consuming water, at least 4 litres in a day is impertinent with mental and physical wellbeing. Drinking water helps in fighting infections all over your body by flushing out toxins, maintaining homeostasis and also flushing the wastes being generated by the body constantly. It's especially good for getting rid of and preventing urine infections and kidney stones. We have collected the data regarding consuming water in the form of cups as the standard measurement, where 4 cups of water are equivalent of a bottle of 1 litre water.

Studies have shown that whilst excessively working out to lose weight is not a beneficial method, as diets play more important role than exercise in maintaining body weight, still exercise is extremely important to build stamina, muscle mass, improve immunity, endurance, and keep the vital organs on high functionality. The burning of calories through physical activity, combined with reducing the number of calories you eat, creates a "calorie deficit" that results in weight loss. The record of exercise is more to understand if people devote even an hour of their day to properly exercise where most of today's work takes place by sitting in front of the computer monitor. The data on exercise was collected on 5 basis- Walking, Cardio regime, Weight's training, playing sports or none of the physical activities at all. Finally, the mental health disorders as well as hereditary syndromes were also recorded, as they play an important role in the overall wellbeing of a person. The leading disorders kept in mind were blood pressure, diabetes, asthma, thyroid, cholesterol and PCOS. There is a confirmed relationship between obesity and PCOS. Obesity is considered a factor in the pathophysiological cascade of PCOS through 2 major pathways: IR & hyperandrogenism. However, obesity can also be considered a complication of PCOS, considering the presence of increased visceral fat in PCOS [6]. The mental disorders considered in this study were Hypertension/stress, Depression, Anxiety and Sleep Apnea. We did not conduct an elaborate study on the eating patterns in individuals with Bulimia or Anorexia as it was a general public survey and provides scope for further research.

## 3. Result

The normal BMI defined by WHO ranges normal as 18.5 to 24.9, whereas a BMI $\geq 25$ kg/m$^2$ is considered to be overweight, and a BMI $\geq 30$ kg/m$^2$ is classified as obese, with severe obesity defined as a BMI ≥40 kg/m$^2$ [1, 2]. In the National Family Health Survey's report, it is revealed that the population of obese have doubled in the past decade.

**Figure 1** shows that from the information collected of the 205 individuals which were self-reported, we can deduce that around 48.78% individuals were harbouring abnormal weight, considering that BMI is directly linked to the body weight and not the fat content in the body. Being underweight also falls under the category of abnormal BMI. Under the abnormal BMI category of men and women, around 11.7% were underweight, 21.66% were overweight and 12.37% were Obese. Although the number of women were higher to men under the underweight and obese category, the populous of men under the overweight category was way higher, by almost a 7.5% hike.

Exercises were divided into four categories after determining that the subjects selected were practising these routines primarily. According to **Tables 1** and **2** the data collected shows that 53.65% of the populous exercised by walking for at least 30 minutes, around 20% of them took part in cardio exercises and 11.21% visited the gymnasium to be properly guided by a trainer, who helped them with weights and endurance training along with cardio exercises. Just about 3.9% of the populous practised Yoga, which was observed in individuals who were ageing between the 51 to 70 range. It was also revealed that just 63.9% of the populous were getting an adequate sleep of a minimum 7 hours. Only 58.33% of the women in this study got adequate sleep. Most of the women suffering from sleep apnea or who received inadequate sleep in the night usually were agonized by High blood pressure or Hypothyroidism if they were above 36 years old, whereas the women between the age range of 15 to 35 years couldn't sleep suffered from PCOS, hormonal disbalances and Hypertension.

In order, to understand the underlying relation between mental health and obesity. **Figure 2** shows that around 30.58% of male and 44.16% of female suffer from Hypertension, almost all the men and women who had developed high blood pressure and hypertension were either overweight or obese and the people having low pressures were mostly underweight. Thus, in the study around 10.73% of the populous were suffering from either high or low blood pressures. Just about 6.82%

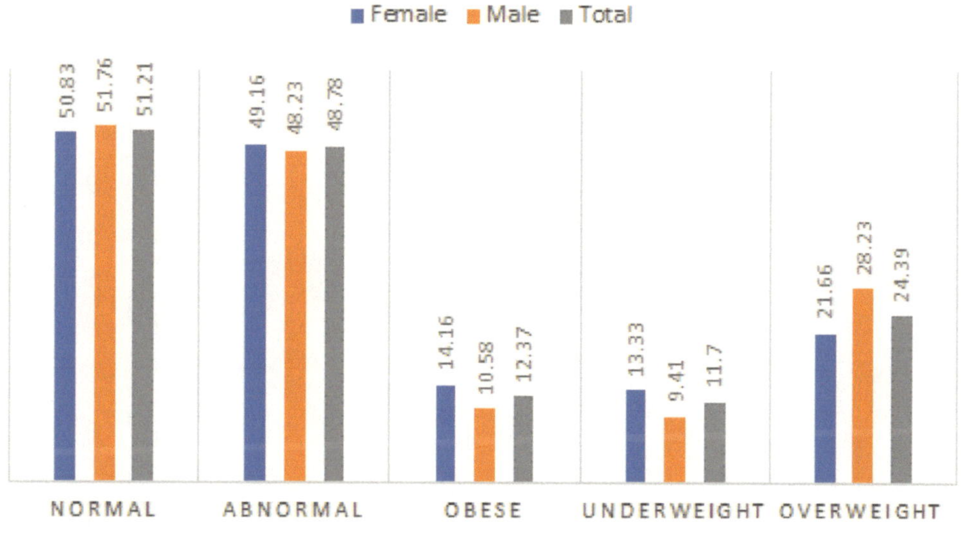


**Figure 1.**
*Graphical representation of the percentage of subjects having normal and abnormal BMI values. The abnormal BMI have been further divided into people who are underweight, overweight and obese (n = 205).*

| Sr. No. | Age | Occupation | Height (cm) | Weight (kg) | BMI | Status | Food | Milk | Breakfast | Sleep (hours) | Gap (hours) | Fast Food | Water (cups) | Exercise | Disease |
|---|---|---|---|---|---|---|---|---|---|---|---|---|---|---|---|
| 1 | 15–25 | Service | 154.94 | 52 | 21.7 | Normal | Non Veg | Yes | Yes | 7.5 | 1.5 | 3–4 | 10 | Walk + cardio | Hormonal |
| 2 | 15–25 | Student | 164.59 | 65 | 24 | Normal | Veg | Yes | 4 | 6 | 4 | 2 | 28 | Cardio | PCOS |
| 3 | 15–25 | Student | 167.64 | 63 | 23.1 | Normal | Veg | Yes | Yes | 6 | 3 | >6 | 8 | Walk | Stress |
| 4 | 15–25 | Student | 154.94 | 52 | 21.7 | Normal | Veg | Yes | Yes | 5 | 3 | >6 | 8 | Cardio | Sleep |
| 5 | 15–25 | Student | 164.59 | 69 | 26.3 | Over weight | Non Veg | No | Yes | 5 | 2 | >6 | 24 | Walk | — |
| 6 | 15–25 | Student | 167.67 | 70 | 28.4 | Over weight | Veg | No | 3–4 | 8 | 2 | >6 | 24 | Walk | Hypertension |
| 7 | 15–25 | Student | 161.54 | 75 | 29.3 | Over weight | Non Veg | No | 1–2 | 4 | 1 | >6 | 8 | Walk | None |
| 8 | 15–25 | Student | 146.30 | 80 | 39.5 | Obese class 2 | Non Veg | No | No | 6 | 2.5 | 5–6 | 6 | Walk | PCOS |
| 9 | 15–25 | Student | 158.49 | 43 | 17.3 | Under Weight | Non Veg | Yes | 1–2 | 6 | 2 | 5–6 | 12 | Walk | None |
| 10 | 15–25 | Student | 158.49 | 45 | 18.3 | Under Weight | Veg | Yes | 1–2 | 9 | 4 | >6 | 12 | Walk | None |
| 11 | 15–25 | Student | 158.49 | 54 | 21.9 | Normal | Veg | Yes | Yes | 8 | 1.5 | >6 | 4 | Walk | Stress |
| 12 | 15–25 | Student | 164.59 | 64 | 23.6 | Normal | Non Veg | Yes | 3–4 | 7 | 4 | 5–6 | 12 | GYM | PCOS+ Depression |
| 13 | 15–25 | Student | 161.54 | 48 | 18.7 | Normal | Veg | Yes | Yes | 8 | 2.5 | 5–6 | 13 | Cardio + Weight | Hypertension+Sleep+Anxiety |
| 14 | 15–25 | Corporate | 167.64 | 40 | 15.1 | Under Weight | Veg | Yes | Yes | 4 | 3 | >6 | 12 | Cardio | Hypertension+Sleep+Anxiety |
| 15 | 15–25 | Student | 161.54 | 48 | 18.5 | Under Weight | Non Veg | Yes | Yes | 8 | 1.5 | >6 | 8 | Walk | None |

DOI: http://dx.doi.org/10.5772/intechopen.98307

| Sr. No. | Age | Occupation | Height (cm) | Weight (kg) | BMI | Status | Food | Milk | Breakfast | Sleep (hours) | Gap (hours) | Fast Food | Water (cups) | Exercise | Disease |
|---|---|---|---|---|---|---|---|---|---|---|---|---|---|---|---|
| 16 | 15–25 | Student | 164.59 | 53 | 20.1 | Normal | Non Veg | Yes | Yes | 6 | 2 | >6 | 4 | Sports | None |
| 17 | 15–25 | Student | 164.59 | 56 | 21.3 | Normal | Non Veg | No | Yes | 5 | 1 | 1–2 | 7 | Walk | Depression |
| 18 | 15–25 | Student | 158 | 70 | 28 | Over weight | Non Veg | Yes | 3–4 | 5 | 3 | 1–2 | 17 | Walk | PCOS +Hypertension |
| 19 | 15–25 | Student | 173.73 | 48 | 16.6 | Under Weight | Non Veg | Yes | No | 7 | 2 | 5–6 | 10 | Walk | None |
| 20 | 15–25 | Corporate | 173.73 | 74 | 25.6 | Over weight | Non Veg | No | Yes | 7 | 1 | 1–2 | 5 | Walk | None |
| 21 | 15–25 | Student | 158.49 | 54 | 21.9 | Normal | Veg | Yes | Yes | 7 | 2 | 5–6 | 8 | Walk | None |
| 22 | 15–25 | Student | 155 | 60 | 25 | Normal | Non Veg | No | 3–4 | 7 | 3 | >6 | 4 | Walk | Anxiety |
| 23 | 15–25 | Student | 132 | 54 | 31 | Obese class 1 | Non Veg | Maybe | No | 5 | 3 | >6 | 5 | Walk | PCOS +Stress |
| 24 | 15–25 | Student | 164.59 | 50 | 19.1 | Normal | Non Veg | No | Yes | 6 | 2 | 5–6 | 10 | Walk | Diabetes |
| 25 | 15–25 | Student | 162 | 59 | 22.5 | Normal | Veg | No | 3–4 | 7 | 2 | 1–2 | 10 | Walk | None |
| 26 | 15–25 | Student | 170 | 55 | 19 | Normal | Non Veg | Maybe | Yes | 7 | 4 | >6 | 9 | GYM | None |
| 27 | 15–25 | Student | 160 | 74 | 28.9 | Over weight | Non Veg | Maybe | Yes | 6 | 3 | 5–6 | 20 | Walk | Depression |
| 28 | 15–25 | Service | 170 | 58 | 20.1 | Normal | Veg | No | 3–4 | 7 | 1.5 | 1–2 | 8 | Walk | Low BP |
| 29 | 15–25 | Student | 150 | 47 | 20.9 | Normal | Veg | Yes | 3–4 | 7 | 4 | 5–6 | 4 | Walk | Sleep |
| 30 | 15–25 | Corporate | 170 | 82 | 28.2 | Over weight | Non Veg | Yes | 1–2 | 8 | 4 | >6 | 4 | Walk | Thyroid |
| 31 | 15–25 | Student | 156 | 51 | 21 | Normal | Veg | Yes | 3–4 | 6 | 2 | 5–6 | 8 | Cyle + Walk | None |
| 32 | 15–25 | Student | 175 | 54 | 17.6 | Under Weight | Veg | Yes | Yes | 6 | 3 | >6 | 8 | Walk | None |

| Sr. No. | Age | Occupation | Height (cm) | Weight (kg) | BMI | Status | Food | Milk | Breakfast | Sleep (hours) | Gap (hours) | Fast Food | Water (cups) | Exercise | Disease |
|---|---|---|---|---|---|---|---|---|---|---|---|---|---|---|---|
| 33 | 15–25 | Corporate | 172 | 70 | 23.7 | Normal | Veg | No | 3–4 | 5 | 2 | 1–2 | 8 | None | Thyroid |
| 34 | 15–25 | Student | 165 | 60 | 22 | Normal | Non Veg | Maybe | 1–2 | 8 | 4 | >6 | 5 | Walk | Hypertension |
| 35 | 15–25 | Corporate | 155.44 | 75 | 31.6 | Obese class 1 | Veg | No | No | 6 | 5 | >6 | 2 | Dance | Hypertension |
| 36 | 15–25 | Student | 154 | 45 | 19 | Normal | Veg | Yes | Yes | 8 | 1 | >6 | 10 | Walk | None |
| 37 | 15–25 | Student | 160 | 88 | 34.4 | Obese class 1 | Non Veg | Yes | 1–2 | 5 | 4 | 1–2 | 24 | Cardio | PCOS+ Hypertension |
| 38 | 15–25 | Student | 160 | 54 | 21.1 | Normal | Non Veg | No | Yes | 6 | 1.5 | 5–6 | 14 | Walk | Hypertension |
| 39 | 15–25 | Student | 172 | 49 | 16.6 | Under Weight | Veg | Yes | Yes | 6 | 2 | 1–2 | 6 | Walk | PCOS+ Hypertension +Depression |
| 40 | 15–25 | Student | 157 | 45 | 18.3 | Under Weight | Veg | Yes | 3–4 | 7 | 1 | >6 | 8 | Walk | Hormones |
| 41 | 15–25 | Student | 160 | 47 | 18.4 | Under Weight | Veg | Yes | Yes | 7 | 3 | 5–6 | 10 | Walk | None |
| 42 | 15–25 | Student | 145 | 35 | 16.6 | Under Weight | Non Veg | No | 3–4 | 6 | 0.5 | >6 | 8 | None | None |
| 43 | 15–25 | Student | 162 | 45 | 17.1 | Under Weight | Veg | Yes | Yes | 6 | 1.5 | 5–6 | 3 | Walk | None |
| 44 | 15–25 | Student | 160 | 53 | 20.7 | Normal | Veg | Yes | Yes | 8 | 2 | 5–6 | 10 | Walk | None |
| 45 | 15–25 | Student | 183 | 78 | 23.3 | Normal | Non Veg | Yes | Yes | 8 | 2 | 5–6 | 10 | Walk | Depression |
| 46 | 15–25 | Student | 167.64 | 74 | 26.3 | Over weight | Non Veg | No | Yes | 8 | 2.5 | 1–2 | 15 | Walk | Sleep |
| 47 | 15–25 | Student | 161.54 | 52 | 19.9 | Normal | Veg | No | Yes | 7 | 3 | 1–2 | 10 | Cardio + Weights | None |

| Sr. No. | Age | Occupation | Height (cm) | Weight (kg) | BMI | Status | Food | Milk | Breakfast | Sleep (hours) | Gap (hours) | Fast Food | Water (cups) | Exercise | Disease |
|---|---|---|---|---|---|---|---|---|---|---|---|---|---|---|---|
| 48 | 15–25 | Student | 150 | 50 | 22.2 | Normal | Non Veg | Yes | Yes | 6 | 1 | 1–2 | 5 | Yoga + Dance | Hypertension+Depression +Anxiety |
| 49 | 15–25 | Student | 161 | 50 | 19.3 | Normal | Veg | Maybe | Yes | 8 | 4 | 1–2 | 6 | None | Hypertension |
| 50 | 15–25 | Corporate | 165 | 56 | 20.6 | Normal | Veg | Yes | Yes | 6 | 2 | 1–2 | 5 | Cardio + Gym | None |
| 51 | 15–25 | Corporate | 153 | 48 | 17 | Under Weight | Non Veg | Yes | Yes | 7 | 4 | 1–2 | 8 | Walk | None |
| 52 | 15–25 | Student | 161 | 44 | 20.5 | Normal | Veg | No | Yes | 8 | 3 | 1–2 | 6 | Walk | None |
| 53 | 15–25 | Student | 170.65 | 80 | 27.5 | Over weight | Non Veg | Yes | Yes | 7 | 2.5 | 5–6 | 4 | Walk | PCOS |
| 54 | 15–25 | Student | 164 | 60 | 22.3 | Normal | Non Veg | Yes | Yes | 7 | 4 | 5–6 | 7 | None | PCOS |
| 55 | 15–25 | Corporate | 161.54 | 59 | 22.6 | Normal | Non Veg | Yes | Yes | 8 | 3 | >6 | 5 | Walk + Sports + Weights | Hypertension |
| 56 | 15–25 | Student | 152.4 | 60 | 25.8 | Over weight | Veg | No | Yes | 8 | 2 | 1–2 | 5 | Walk | None |
| 57 | 15–25 | Student | 158 | 57 | 22.8 | Normal | Veg | Yes | Yes | 8 | 2 | 1–2 | 8 | Cardio | Anxiety |
| 58 | 15–25 | Student | 152.4 | 50 | 21.5 | Normal | Veg | Yes | Yes | 8 | 1 | 1–2 | 5 | Walk | Hypertension+Depression +Anxiety |
| 59 | 15–25 | Student | 152.4 | 50 | 21.5 | Normal | Non Veg | No | Yes | 8 | 2.5 | 1–2 | 20 | Walk + Cardio | Hypertension |
| 60 | 15–25 | Student | 162 | 49 | 18.7 | Normal | Non Veg | Yes | Yes | 8 | 2 | >6 | 10 | Walk | Anxiety |
| 61 | 15–25 | Student | 162 | 50 | 19.1 | Normal | Veg | Yes | Yes | 8 | 2 | 1–2 | 8 | Walk | Hypertension |
| 62 | 15–25 | Student | 170.6 | 66 | 22.7 | Normal | Non Veg | No | Yes | 8 | 3 | 5–6 | 12 | Walk | PCOS |
| 63 | 15–25 | Student | 167.64 | 50 | 17.8 | Under Weight | Non Veg | No | 3–4 | 8 | 2 | >6 | 6 | Walk | PCOS |
| 64 | 15–25 | Student | 170.6 | 60 | 20.6 | Normal | Non Veg | No | Yes | 7 | 2 | >6 | 28 | Walk + Weights | Hypertension + Depression + Anxiety |

| Sr. No. | Age | Occupation | Height (cm) | Weight (kg) | BMI | Status | Food | Milk | Breakfast | Sleep (hours) | Gap (hours) | Fast Food | Water (cups) | Exercise | Disease |
|---|---|---|---|---|---|---|---|---|---|---|---|---|---|---|---|
| 65 | 15–25 | Student | 152.4 | 61 | 26.2 | Over weight | Non Veg | No | Yes | 7 | 3 | 1–2 | 6 | Walk | PCOS |
| 66 | 15–25 | Student | 172 | 68 | 23 | Normal | Veg | Yes | Yes | 8 | 3 | 1–2 | 7 | Cardio | None |
| 67 | 15–25 | Corporate | 158.49 | 65 | 25.9 | Over weight | Veg | Yes | Yes | 9 | 3 | 5–6 | 8 | Walk | None |
| 68 | 15–25 | Corporate | 165 | 58 | 21.3 | Normal | Non Veg | Yes | 3–4 | 8 | 4 | 5–6 | 8 | Cardio | Anxiety |
| 69 | 15–25 | Student | 158 | 52 | 20.8 | Normal | Non Veg | Yes | No | 7 | 5 | 1–2 | 16 | Walk | Hypertension + Sleep + Anxiety + Depression |
| 70 | 15–25 | Student | 158.49 | 58 | 23.1 | Normal | Veg | Yes | Yes | 6 | 4 | >6 | 5 | Walk | None |
| 71 | 15–25 | Student | 165 | 50 | 18.4 | Under Weight | Veg | No | 3–4 | 8 | 5 | >6 | 6 | Walk | None |
| 72 | 15–25 | Student | 158 | 56 | 22.3 | Normal | Veg | Yes | Yes | 7 | 1 | 1–2 | 5 | Walk | Anxiety |
| 73 | 15–25 | Student | 149 | 40 | 18 | Under Weight | Veg | Yes | Yes | 7 | 2 | 5–6 | 6 | Yoga | Low BP |
| 74 | 15–25 | Student | 160 | 45 | 17.6 | Under Weight | Non Veg | Yes | 1–2 | 8 | 3 | >6 | 7 | Walk | None |
| 75 | 15–25 | Student | 164.59 | 70 | 25.8 | Over weight | Non Veg | No | 3–4 | 5 | 5 | 1–2 | 8 | Walk | Hypertension + Sleep + Anxiety |
| 76 | 15–25 | Student | 170.68 | 80 | 27.5 | Over weight | Veg | No | 3–4 | 7 | 2 | 1–2 | 8 | Cycle | Hypertension |
| 77 | 15–25 | Corporate | 161.54 | 51 | 19.5 | Normal | Veg | Yes | Yes | 7 | 5 | 5–6 | 6 | Sports | Asthma |
| 78 | 15–25 | Student | 159 | 53 | 21 | Normal | Veg | Yes | 3–4 | 8 | 5 | 5–6 | 8 | Walk | None |
| 79 | 15–25 | Corporate | 161.54 | 55 | 21.1 | Normal | Veg | Yes | Yes | 6 | 2 | >6 | 12 | None | PCOS+ Thyroid |
| 80 | 15–25 | Student | 173.73 | 102 | 33.8 | Obese class 1 | Veg | Yes | Yes | 6 | 2 | 5–6 | 8 | Walk + Cardio | Hypertension + Sleep + Depression + Anxiety |

| Sr. No. | Age | Occupation | Height (cm) | Weight (kg) | BMI | Status | Food | Milk | Breakfast | Sleep (hours) | Gap (hours) | Fast Food | Water (cups) | Exercise | Disease |
|---|---|---|---|---|---|---|---|---|---|---|---|---|---|---|---|
| 81 | 15–25 | Corporate | 164.59 | 75 | 27.7 | Over weight | Veg | No | 1–2 | 8 | 2 | 5–6 | 5 | Cardio + Cycle | PCOS |
| 82 | 15–25 | Student | 168 | 67 | 23.7 | Normal | Non Veg | Yes | Yes | 6 | 5 | 5–6 | 8 | Walk | Hypertension + Sleep + Depression + Anxiety |
| 83 | 15–25 | Student | 160 | 80 | 31.3 | Obese class 1 | Veg | Yes | Yes | 7 | 2.5 | 1–2 | 10 | Walk | Hypertension + Anxiety |
| 84 | 15–25 | Student | 167.64 | 40 | 14.2 | Under Weight | Veg | Yes | Yes | 8 | 4 | 1–2 | 15 | Cardio+ Dance | PCOS + Low BP |
| 85 | 15–25 | Student | 170.6 | 70 | 24 | Normal | Veg | Yes | 1–2 | 7 | 3.5 | 1–2 | 3 | Gym | PCOS + Sleep |
| 86 | 26–35 | Corporate | 162.56 | 60 | 25.3 | Normal | Veg | No | Yes | 7 | 3 | 5–6 | 4 | Walk | None |
| 87 | 26–35 | Student | 167.64 | 90 | 33.1 | Obese Class 1 | Non-Veg | No | 1–2 | 9 | 3 | >6 | 8 | Cardio | None |
| 88 | 26–35 | Corporate | 170.68 | 70 | 24 | Normal | Non-Veg | Yes | Yes | 7 | 3 | 1–2 | 10 | Cardio | PCOS + Thyroid |
| 89 | 26–35 | Corporate | 165 | 78 | 28.7 | Over weight | Non-Veg | Yes | Yes | 8 | 3 | 5–6 | 8 | None | None |
| 90 | 26–35 | Field Work | 173.73 | 60 | 19.9 | Normal | Veg | No | Yes | 7 | 2.5 | 5–6 | 10 | Walk + Cardio +Weights | Hormonal |
| 91 | 26–35 | Service | 152.4 | 50 | 21.5 | Normal | Veg | Yes | Yes | 5 | 2 | 1–2 | 12 | Walk | Low BP |
| 92 | 26–35 | Service | 162.56 | 58 | 21.9 | Normal | Veg | Yes | Yes | 6 | 2.5 | 5–6 | 16 | Walk | None |
| 93 | 26–35 | Corporate | 155.44 | 78 | 32.3 | Obese Class 1 | Veg | Maybe | Yes | 5 | 2 | 5–6 | 11 | Walk+ Cardio | Hypertension + Sleep + Depression + Anxiety + PCOS |
| 94 | 26–35 | Corporate | 158.75 | 78 | 31 | Obese Class 1 | Non-Veg | No | Yes | 7 | 4 | 5–6 | 4 | Walk | PCOS + Sleep |

| Sr. No. | Age | Occupation | Height (cm) | Weight (kg) | BMI | Status | Food | Milk | Breakfast | Sleep (hours) | Gap (hours) | Fast Food | Water (cups) | Exercise | Disease |
|---|---|---|---|---|---|---|---|---|---|---|---|---|---|---|---|
| 95 | 36–50 | Corporate | 154 | 58 | 24.5 | Normal | Non-Veg | Yes | 3–4 | 7 | 2.5 | 1–2 | 10 | Walk | Thyroid + Hypertension |
| 96 | 36–50 | Corporate | 165 | 74 | 27.2 | Obese Class 1 | Non-Veg | Yes | Yes | 8 | 1 | >6 | 7 | Walk | Sleep |
| 97 | 36–50 | Corporate | 162 | 69 | 26.3 | Obese Class 1 | Non-Veg | No | Yes | 5 | 1 | >6 | 10 | Cardio | None |
| 98 | 36–50 | Corporate | 170 | 80 | 27.7 | Obese Class 1 | Non-Veg | No | Yes | 7 | 0.5 | 5–6 | 10 | Yoga | Hypertension |
| 99 | 36–50 | Corporate | 160 | 72 | 28.1 | Obese Class 1 | Non-Veg | No | Yes | 6.5 | 2 | 5–6 | 14 | Walk + Yoga | None |
| 100 | 36–50 | Corporate | 165 | 70 | 25.7 | Over weight | Veg | Yes | Yes | 7 | 4 | 5–6 | 12 | Yoga | Hypertension |
| 101 | 36–50 | Home maker | 157 | 73 | 29.6 | Over weight | Veg | Yes | Yes | 7 | 1 | >6 | 10 | Walk | Fatty Liver |
| 102 | 36–50 | Service | 157 | 58 | 23.5 | Normal | Non-Veg | No | Yes | 7 | 3 | 5–6 | 8 | Gym | Stress |
| 103 | 36–50 | Home maker | 152 | 59 | 25.5 | Over weight | Veg | No | 3–4 | 8 | 1 | 5–6 | 8 | Walk | Asthma |
| 104 | 36–50 | Service | 158.49 | 69 | 27.5 | Over weight | Non-Veg | Yes | Yes | 6 | 2 | 5–6 | 10 | Walk | High BP and Hormones |
| 105 | 36–50 | Home maker | 164.59 | 78 | 28.8 | Over weight | Non-Veg | Yes | Yes | 7 | 2 | 5–6 | 10 | Walk + Dance | Hypertension |
| 106 | 36–50 | Service | 157.48 | 60 | 24.3 | Normal | Veg | Yes | No | 6 | 2 | 1–2 | 9 | None | Anxiety |
| 107 | 36–50 | Service | 152.4 | 59 | 25.4 | Over weight | Veg | No | Yes | 7 | 1 | 1–2 | 9 | Walk | Hypertension + Sleep |
| 108 | 36–50 | Service | 172.72 | 80 | 26.8 | Over weight | Veg | Yes | Yes | 5 | 2 | 5–6 | 6 | Walk | Hypothyroidism |
| 109 | 36–50 | Home maker | 158.49 | 65 | 25.9 | Over weight | Non-Veg | Yes | Yes | 5 | 3 | 5–6 | 8 | None | High BP |

| Sr. No. | Age | Occupation | Height (cm) | Weight (kg) | BMI | Status | Food | Milk | Breakfast | Sleep (hours) | Gap (hours) | Fast Food | Water (cups) | Exercise | Disease |
|---|---|---|---|---|---|---|---|---|---|---|---|---|---|---|---|
| 110 | 36–50 | Home maker | 160 | 58 | 22.7 | Normal | Veg | Yes | Yes | 9 | 3 | 1–2 | 12 | Walk | Hypertension + Sleep + Depression + Anxiety |
| 111 | 36–50 | Service | 157.48 | 78 | 31.6 | Obese Class 1 | Veg | Yes | Yes | 8 | 2.5 | 1–2 | 10 | Weights | Thyroid |
| 112 | 36–50 | Home maker | 154.94 | 82 | 34.2 | Obese Class 1 | Non-Veg | No | Yes | 5 | 1 | 1–2 | 10 | Walk | High BP + Sleep |
| 113 | 51–70 | Home maker | 155.44 | 60 | 24.8 | Normal | Non-Veg | Yes | Yes | 6 | 2 | None | 7 | Walk | None |
| 114 | 51–70 | Field Work | 152.4 | 45 | 21.5 | Normal | Non-Veg | Yes | Yes | 7 | 1.5 | 1–2 | 9 | Walk | Acidity |
| 115 | 51–70 | Service | 152.4 | 64 | 27.7 | Over weight | Veg | Maybe | Yes | 7 | 4 | 1–2 | 10 | Walk + Cardio | Diabetes |
| 116 | 51–70 | Home maker | 157.48 | 75 | 30.2 | Obese Class 1 | Veg | No | Yes | 5 | 2 | 1–2 | 8 | Walk | High BP + Thyroid |
| 117 | 51–70 | Home maker | 161.54 | 61 | 23.4 | Normal | Non-Veg | Yes | Yes | 8 | 2 | 1–2 | 10 | Walk | High BP + Asthma |
| 118 | 51–70 | Service | 152 | 60 | 26 | Obese Class 1 | Non-Veg | Yes | Yes | 7 | 1 | 1–2 | 15 | Walk | None |
| 119 | 51–70 | Service | 146.3 | 55 | 25.7 | Over weight | Non-Veg | Yes | Yes | 6 | 1 | 1–2 | 16 | Walk | None |
| 120 | 51–70 | Service | 164 | 64 | 23.6 | Normal | Veg | Yes | Yes | 7 | 2 | 1–2 | 20 | Yoga | High BP |

**Table 1.**
*Compilation of all the information collected by Females in the study* ($n = 120$).

| Sr. No. | Age (years) | Occupation | Height (cm) | Weight (kg) | BMI | Status | Food | Milk | Break fast | Sleep (hrs) | Gap (hrs) | Fast Food | Water (cups) | Exercise | Disease |
|---|---|---|---|---|---|---|---|---|---|---|---|---|---|---|---|
| 1 | 15–25 | Student | 157 | 64 | 26 | Over weight | Veg | Yes | 1–2 | 7 | 1 | >6 | 12 | Walk | None |
| 2 | 15–25 | Student | 177 | 105 | 33.5 | Obese Class 1 | Non-Veg | Yes | Yes | 7 | 3 | 5–6 | 8 | Walk | High BP |
| 3 | 15–25 | Student | 168 | 64 | 22.7 | Normal | Veg | Yes | Yes | 7.5 | 1.5 | 5–6 | 8 | Weight | None |
| 4 | 15–25 | Student | 175 | 74 | 24.2 | Normal | Non-Veg | No | Yes | 5 | 1 | >6 | 15 | Walk | Hormonal + Stress |
| 5 | 15–25 | Student | 182 | 84 | 25.4 | Over weight | Non-Veg | Yes | Yes | 7 | 1 | 5–6 | 15 | Sports | Hypertension |
| 6 | 15–25 | Student | 172 | 65 | 22 | Normal | Non-Veg | Yes | Yes | 6 | 4 | >6 | 6 | Walk | None |
| 7 | 15–25 | Student | 180 | 78 | 24.1 | Normal | Non-Veg | No | Yes | 8 | 4 | 5–6 | 20 | Walk | Hypertension |
| 8 | 15–25 | Student | 185 | 73 | 21.3 | Normal | Veg | Yes | Yes | 6 | 2 | 1–2 | 15 | Sports | None |
| 9 | 15–25 | Student | 170 | 70 | 24.2 | Normal | Veg | Yes | Yes | 6 | 2.5 | >6 | 10 | Sports | None |
| 10 | 15–25 | Student | 180 | 94 | 29 | Over weight | Non-Veg | Yes | Yes | 6 | 3 | >6 | 15 | Walk | Hormonal + Stress + Depression + Anxiety |
| 11 | 15–25 | Student | 170 | 61 | 21.1 | Normal | Non-Veg | Yes | Yes | 7 | 2.5 | >6 | 7 | Weight | Anxiety |
| 12 | 15–25 | Student | 172 | 56 | 18.9 | Normal | Veg | Yes | No | 7 | 4 | >6 | 10 | Walk | None |
| 13 | 15–25 | Student | 190 | 73 | 20.2 | Normal | Veg | Yes | Yes | 7 | 1 | 1–2 | 25 | Sports | None |
| 14 | 15–25 | Student | 172 | 59 | 19.9 | Normal | Veg | Yes | No | 7 | 2 | >6 | 12 | Sports | Hypertension |
| 15 | 15–25 | Student | 182 | 80 | 24.2 | Normal | Veg | Yes | Yes | 6 | 3 | >6 | 20 | Weight | Hormonal + Stress + Depression + Anxiety |
| 16 | 15–25 | Student | 183 | 90 | 26.9 | Over weight | Veg | Yes | Yes | 8 | 2 | 5–6 | 15 | Cardio | Hypertension + Anxiety |
| 17 | 15–25 | Student | 168 | 85 | 30.1 | Obese Class 1 | Non-Veg | Yes | Yes | 8 | 0.5 | 5–6 | 18 | Weight | None |

DOI: http://dx.doi.org/10.5772/intechopen.98307

| Sr. No. | Age (years) | Occupation | Height (cm) | Weight (kg) | BMI | Status | Food | Milk | Break fast | Sleep (hrs) | Gap (hrs) | Fast Food | Water (cups) | Exercise | Disease |
|---|---|---|---|---|---|---|---|---|---|---|---|---|---|---|---|
| 18 | 15–25 | Student | 172 | 71 | 24 | Normal | Non-Veg | Yes | Yes | 6 | 2 | 5–6 | 7 | Weight | None |
| 19 | 15–25 | Student | 175 | 75 | 26 | Over weight | Non-Veg | Yes | Yes | 7 | 0.5 | >6 | 10 | Walk + Cardio + Weights Sports | None |
| 20 | 15–25 | Student | 180 | 65 | 20.1 | Normal | Veg | Yes | Yes | 7 | 1 | 5–6 | 15 | None | None |
| 21 | 15–25 | Student | 182 | 49 | 14.8 | Under weight | Veg | Yes | Yes | 6 | 2 | >6 | 10 | None | None |
| 22 | 15–25 | Student | 180.34 | 70 | 21.5 | Normal | Veg | No | Yes | 8 | 1 | 1–2 | 5 | Walk | Hypertension + Depression |
| 23 | 15–25 | Student | 172 | 83 | 28.1 | Over weight | Non-Veg | No | Yes | 8 | 2 | >6 | 4 | Walk | Hormonal + Stress + Depression + Anxiety |
| 24 | 15–25 | Field Work | 181 | 109 | 33.3 | Obese Class 1 | Non-Veg | Yes | Yes | 6 | 4 | 1–2 | 20 | Walk + Cardio | Hypertension |
| 25 | 15–25 | Student | 182.88 | 85 | 25.4 | Over weight | Non-Veg | No | Yes | 9 | 2 | 1–2 | 20 | Walk + Cardio + Weights | None |
| 26 | 15–25 | Student | 167.64 | 60 | 21.3 | Normal | Non-Veg | Yes | Yes | 10 | 1 | >6 | 8 | Walk + Sports | Asthma |
| 27 | 15–25 | Corporate | 172 | 62 | 21 | Normal | Veg | Yes | Yes | 8 | 3 | 1–2 | 6 | Weight | None |
| 28 | 15–25 | Student | 182.88 | 65 | 19.4 | Normal | Veg | Yes | Yes | 7 | 3 | 1–2 | 5 | Weight | None |
| 29 | 15–25 | Student | 175 | 80 | 26.1 | Over weight | Veg | Yes | Yes | 7 | 4 | 5–6 | 6 | Walk | None |
| 30 | 15–25 | Student | 183 | 100 | 29.9 | Over weight | Non-Veg | Yes | Yes | 7 | 3 | 5–6 | 12 | None | None |
| 31 | 15–25 | Student | 182.88 | 81 | 24.2 | Normal | Non-Veg | Yes | Yes | 8 | 3 | 5–6 | 6 | Walk + Sports | None |
| 32 | 15–25 | Student | 172.72 | 50 | 16.8 | Under weight | Veg | Yes | Yes | 10 | 3.5 | 5–6 | 8 | Walk | None |

| Sr. No. | Age (years) | Occupation | Height (cm) | Weight (kg) | BMI | Status | Food | Milk | Break fast | Sleep (hrs) | Gap (hrs) | Fast Food | Water (cups) | Exercise | Disease |
|---|---|---|---|---|---|---|---|---|---|---|---|---|---|---|---|
| 33 | 15–25 | Field Work | 182.88 | 50 | 14.9 | Under weight | Non-Veg | No | Yes | 9 | 0.5 | 3–4 | 10 | Labour | None |
| 34 | 15–25 | Field Work | 144.78 | 50 | 23.9 | Normal | Non-Veg | No | Yes | 9 | 1.5 | 1–2 | 8 | Labour | None |
| 35 | 15–25 | Field Work | 167.64 | 65 | 23.1 | Normal | Non-Veg | Yes | Yes | 10 | 1 | 1–2 | 9 | Labour | None |
| 36 | 15–25 | Field Work | 152.4 | 51 | 22 | Normal | Non-Veg | Yes | Yes | 9 | 1 | 1–2 | 8 | Labour | None |
| 37 | 15–25 | Field Work | 170.18 | 45 | 15.5 | Under weight | Non-Veg | Yes | Yes | 9 | 1 | 1–2 | 10 | Labour | None |
| 38 | 15–25 | Student | 172.72 | 65 | 21.8 | Normal | Veg | Yes | Yes | 5 | 0.5 | 5–6 | 24 | Walk + Sports | Hormonal |
| 39 | 15–25 | Student | 177.8 | 60 | 19.2 | Normal | Non-Veg | Yes | No | 4 | 5 | >6 | 8 | Walk | Sleep |
| 40 | 15–25 | Student | 170 | 63 | 21.8 | Normal | Veg | Yes | Yes | 7 | 0.5 | >6 | 4 | Walk | Sleep |
| 41 | 15–25 | Student | 162.56 | 60 | 22.7 | Normal | Non-Veg | Yes | Yes | 8 | 1 | 5–6 | 20 | Walk + cardio Weights + sports | None |
| 42 | 15–25 | Student | 172.72 | 95 | 31.8 | Obese Class 1 | Non-Veg | Yes | No | 10 | 2 | >6 | 20 | Cardio + Weights | None |
| 43 | 15–25 | Corporate | 172.72 | 66 | 22.1 | Normal | Veg | Yes | Yes | 8 | 3 | 5–6 | 20 | Walk | Hormonal |
| 44 | 15–25 | Student | 187.96 | 64 | 18.1 | Under weight | Non-Veg | Yes | Yes | 6 | 1.5 | 1–2 | 4 | None | Stress + Depression |
| 45 | 15–25 | Student | 172.72 | 95 | 31.8 | Obese Class 1 | Veg | Yes | Yes | 6 | 2 | >6 | 16 | Weight | None |
| 46 | 15–25 | Student | 177.8 | 71 | 22.5 | Normal | Veg | Yes | Yes | 8 | 3 | >6 | 12 | Sports | None |
| 47 | 26–35 | Corporate | 173 | 75 | 25.1 | Over weight | Non-Veg | No | Yes | 7 | 3 | >6 | 10 | Walk | Diabetes |
| 48 | 26–35 | Service | 170 | 75 | 26 | Over weight | Non-Veg | No | Yes | 6 | 1 | 5–6 | 5 | Walk + cardio | None |

DOI: http://dx.doi.org/10.5772/intechopen.98307

| Sr. No. | Age (years) | Occupation | Height (cm) | Weight (kg) | BMI | Status | Food | Milk | Break fast | Sleep (hrs) | Gap (hrs) | Fast Food | Water (cups) | Exercise | Disease |
|---|---|---|---|---|---|---|---|---|---|---|---|---|---|---|---|
| 49 | 26–35 | Corporate | 177.8 | 80 | 25.3 | Over weight | Veg | Yes | Yes | 8 | 2 | 5–6 | 5 | Walk | None |
| 50 | 26–35 | Field Work | 160.02 | 57 | 22.3 | Normal | Non-Veg | Yes | Yes | 10 | 2 | 1–2 | 12 | Labour | Stress |
| 51 | 26–35 | Field Work | 172.72 | 67 | 22.5 | Normal | Non-Veg | Yes | Yes | 10 | 2 | 1–2 | 15 | Labour | None |
| 52 | 26–35 | Field Work | 182.88 | 50 | 14.9 | Under weight | Non-Veg | No | Yes | 10 | 2 | 3–4 | 12 | Labour | None |
| 53 | 26–35 | Field Work | 165 | 50 | 18.4 | Under weight | Non-Veg | No | Yes | 9 | 2 | None | 12 | Labour | None |
| 54 | 26–35 | Service | 182.88 | 100 | 30.2 | Obese Class 1 | Non-Veg | No | Yes | 8 | 2 | >6 | 12 | Walk | High BP |
| 55 | 26–35 | Service | 67 | 68 | 24.4 | Normal | Veg | Yes | Yes | 6 | 2 | 1–2 | 8 | Walk | None |
| 56 | 26–35 | Service | 177.8 | 63 | 19.9 | Normal | Veg | No | Yes | 6 | 1 | >6 | 6 | Walk | None |
| 57 | 26–35 | Service | 182.88 | 93 | 28.1 | Over weight | Non-Veg | No | Yes | 7 | 2 | 1–2 | 12 | Walk | None |
| 58 | 26–35 | Field Work | 172 | 60 | 20.3 | Normal | Veg | Yes | Yes | 10 | 2 | 1–2 | 12 | Labour | None |
| 59 | 36–50 | Corporate | 167.64 | 69 | 24.6 | Normal | Non-Veg | No | Yes | 7 | 1.5 | 5–6 | 20 | Walk | Diabetes |
| 60 | 36–50 | Corporate | 177.8 | 89 | 28.2 | Over weight | Non-Veg | No | Yes | 7 | 2 | 5–6 | 12 | Walk | None |
| 61 | 36–50 | Corporate | 174 | 90 | 29.7 | Over weight | Veg | No | Yes | 6 | 2.5 | >6 | 10 | Cardio | High BP |
| 62 | 36–50 | Corporate | 185.4 | 125 | 36.4 | Obese Class 2 | Non-Veg | Yes | Yes | 8 | 1.5 | 5–6 | 8 | Walk | High BP |
| 63 | 36–50 | Service | 170 | 65 | 22.5 | Normal | Veg | Yes | Yes | 8 | 3.5 | 1–2 | 10 | Walk | None |
| 64 | 36–50 | Service | 172.72 | 51 | 17.1 | Under weight | Veg | Yes | Yes | 6 | 1.5 | 5–6 | 5 | Walk | Hypertension |

| Sr. No. | Age (years) | Occupation | Height (cm) | Weight (kg) | BMI | Status | Food | Milk | Break fast | Sleep (hrs) | Gap (hrs) | Fast Food | Water (cups) | Exercise | Disease |
|---|---|---|---|---|---|---|---|---|---|---|---|---|---|---|---|
| 65 | 36–50 | Service | 165.1 | 67 | 24.6 | Normal | Non-Veg | Yes | Yes | 8 | 1 | 5–6 | 16 | Walk | Diabetes |
| 66 | 36–50 | Service | 165.1 | 68 | 24.9 | Normal | Non-Veg | No | Yes | 7 | 1 | 5–6 | 4 | Walk | Diabetes + High BP |
| 67 | 36–50 | Corporate | 165.1 | 65 | 23.9 | Normal | Veg | No | No | 7 | 2 | 5–6 | 4 | Walk | Sleep |
| 68 | 36–50 | Service | 193.04 | 88 | 23.6 | Normal | Non-Veg | Yes | Yes | 8 | 2 | 1–2 | 16 | Walk | Diabetes + Stress + Depression |
| 69 | 36–50 | Corporate | 177.8 | 94 | 30 | Obese class 1 | Non-Veg | No | No | 7 | 2 | >6 | 8 | Walk + Weights | High BP + Depression |
| 70 | 36–50 | Service | 157 | 72 | 29.2 | Over weight | Non-Veg | No | Yes | 5 | 2 | >6 | 8 | Walk | None |
| 71 | 36–50 | Service | 162.56 | 75 | 28.6 | Over weight | Veg | Yes | Yes | 7 | 2 | 1–2 | 16 | Walk | Sleep + Depression80 |
| 72 | 36–50 | Service | 182.88 | 93 | 27.8 | Normal | Veg | Yes | Yes | 8 | 3 | 5–6 | 12 | Walk + Cardio | None |
| 73 | 36–50 | Field Work | 170 | 80 | 27.7 | Overweight | Veg | Yes | Yes | 8 | 2 | 1–2 | 12 | Labour | None |
| 74 | 51–70 | Field Work | 165.1 | 70 | 25.7 | Over weight | Non-Veg | No | Yes | 6 | 1 | None | 12 | Labour | None |
| 75 | 51–70 | Service | 176 | 78 | 25.2 | Over weight | Non-Veg | No | Yes | 7 | 1.5 | 1–2 | 20 | Walk | High BP |
| 76 | 51–70 | Service | 158 | 65 | 26 | Over weight | Veg | Yes | Yes | 7 | 2 | 1–2 | 8 | Walk | High BP |
| 77 | 51–70 | Corporate | 160 | 57 | 22.3 | Normal | Veg | Yes | Yes | 6 | 0.5 | 1–2 | 8 | Yoga + Walk | Diabetes |
| 78 | 51–70 | Service | 172.72 | 99 | 33.2 | Obese class 1 | Non-Veg | No | Yes | 7 | 1.5 | 5–6 | 6 | Walk | High BP |
| 79 | 51–70 | Service | 177 | 70 | 22.3 | Normal | Non-Veg | No | Yes | 7 | 0.5 | 1–2 | 20 | Walk | None |
| 80 | 51–70 | Service | 175 | 70 | 22.9 | Normal | Veg | No | Yes | 7 | 1 | 5–6 | 20 | Walk | Diabetes + High BP |

| Sr. No. | Age (years) | Occupation | Height (cm) | Weight (kg) | BMI | Status | Food | Milk | Break fast | Sleep (hrs) | Gap (hrs) | Fast Food | Water (cups) | Exercise | Disease |
|---|---|---|---|---|---|---|---|---|---|---|---|---|---|---|---|
| 81 | 51–70 | Service | 180.33 | 78 | 24 | Normal | Non-Veg | Yes | Yes | 7 | 0.5 | 1–2 | 12 | Walk | Cholesterol |
| 82 | 51–70 | Corporate | 180.34 | 70 | 21.5 | Normal | Veg | No | Yes | 7 | 5 | 1–2 | 16 | Walk + cardio | High BP |
| 83 | 51–70 | Service | 172 | 80 | 27 | Over weight | Non-Veg | No | Yes | 6 | 1 | 5–6 | 20 | Walk | Diabetes + High BP + Sleep |
| 84 | 51–70 | Service | 167.64 | 74 | 26.4 | Over weight | Non-Veg | Yes | Yes | 7 | 1.5 | 5–6 | 16 | Walk + cardio | None |
| 85 | >70 | Retired | 172.72 | 78 | 26.1 | Over weight | Non-Veg | No | Yes | 4 | 3 | None | 10 | Yoga + Walk | Kidney, Thyroid, High BP |

**Table 2.**
*Compilation of all the information collected by Males in the study ($n$ = 85).*

of the entire populous under observation were diabetic, where the men suffered from this metabolic disorder far more than the women. Around 10.58% out of the 85 men in this study were diabetic. 8.51% of the overweight and obese women gained weight due to metabolic and hormonal imbalance of the blood-sugar; whereas 8.57% of the overweight/obese men gained weight due to the very same reason. One of the major reasons for weight gain in women of the age range of 15 to 50 was due to PCOS and Hyperthyroidism. Around 15% of the women involved in this study were suffering from PCOS and around 19.14% females who were either overweight or obese had this syndrome as a contributing factor for the weight gain. People who abnormally put on a lot of weight or by lineage, have a high chance of developing polycystic ovaries and that inherently causes hormonal disbalance, fat accumulation, hair loss, facial hair growth and weight gain amongst other things. Women above the age of 50 showed a hike in weight either due to diabetes or menopause. Although there is no proof that menopause is the sole reason for weight gain. These women gained weight despite sleeping properly, eating well, having a proper gap between supper and bedtime, and exercising; thus, further research is required to understand the weight gain in elderly women.

Amongst the overweight/obese women, around 48.93% of the females did not suffer from any sort of major health problems, and still gained weights due to amalgam of reasons, like lesser sleep time, less water intake, lesser gap time between the last meal and bedtime, no exercises. On the other hand, 57.14% of the obese or overweight men who did not have any major health issues, were following a very healthy lifestyle in all aspects. The extra weight could be muscle mass or heavier bones rather than fat accumulation, a factor which is not transparent with a BMI reading.

**Figure 2** shows that 16.66% of the women and 10.58% of the men suffered from Depression and 21.66% of women and 11.76% of the men were plagued by anxiety. Lack of sound sleep of at least 7 hours was observed mainly in the youth (15–35) with a 24.39% and 34.14% overall. Although, 17.07% of the study populous

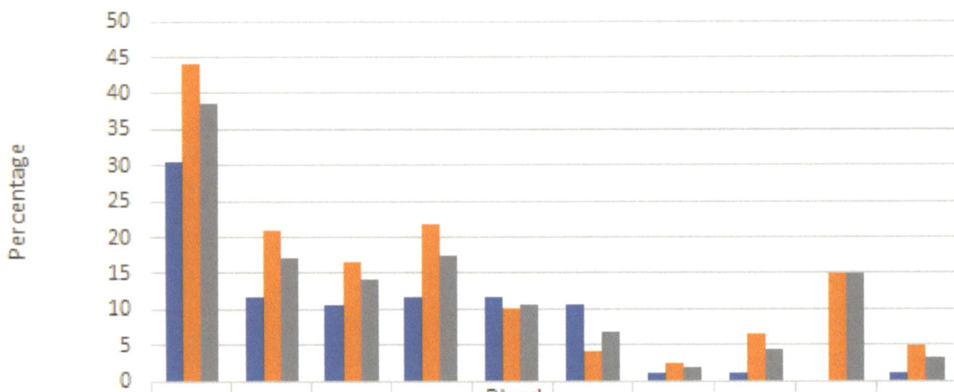


| | Hypertension | Sleep | Depression | Anxiety | Blood Pressure | Diabetes | Asthma | Thyroid | PCOS | Others |
|---|---|---|---|---|---|---|---|---|---|---|
| Male | 30.58 | 11.76 | 10.58 | 11.76 | 11.76 | 10.58 | 1.17 | 1.17 | 0 | 1.17 |
| Female | 44.16 | 20.83 | 16.66 | 21.66 | 10 | 4.16 | 2.5 | 6.66 | 15 | 5 |
| Percentage | 38.53 | 17.07 | 14.14 | 17.56 | 10.73 | 6.82 | 1.95 | 4.39 | 15 | 3.41 |

**Figure 2.**
*Graphical representation of women and men, who suffer from mental disorders such as Anxiety, Sleep apnea, Depression and other disorders such as Hypertension, Blood pressure dysregulation, Diabetes, Asthma, Thyroid and others (n = 120 for females and n = 85 for males).*

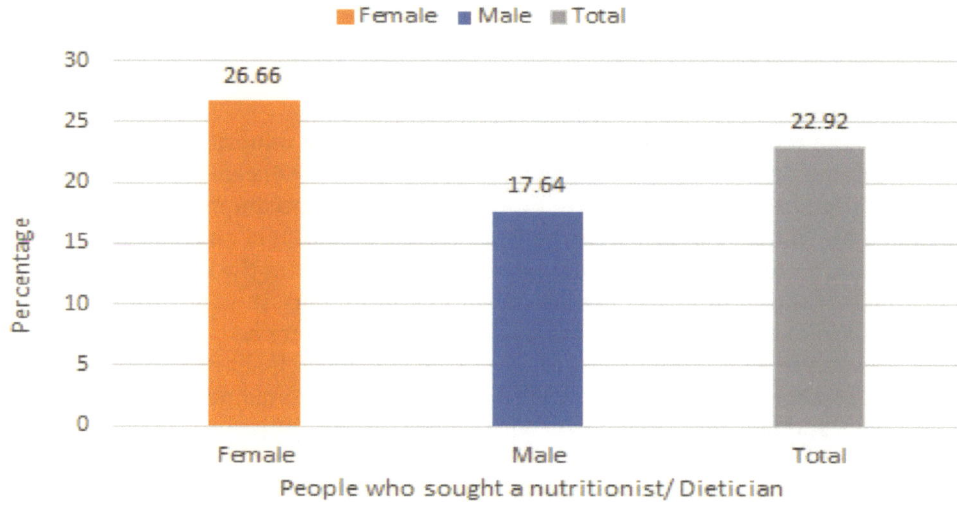


**Figure 3.**
*Graphical representation of women and men, who sought the help of health and nutrition specialists like dietician or a nutritionist (n = 120 for females and n = 85 for males).*

complained of suffering from Sleep Apnea. Amongst all the subjects 43.95% of the individuals suffering from mental disorders of anxiety and depression showed irregular BMI. The study was conducted in the city, while few subjects hailed from the underprivileged part of the city who earned their keep by manual labour, most of them belonged to the upper middle-class part of the society. Despite this from **Figure 3** we can see that only 22.92% of these people sought the professional guidance of a dietician or nutritionist, out of which 26.66% were women and 17.64% were men.

From **Tables 1** and **2**, another interesting fact is pointed out was 80% of the labourers involved in this study were either in the normal or underweight BMI range despite having a high carbohydrate diet. The working class consume high energy dense food, a lot of vegetables all freshly prepared. On the other hand, 62.5% of the homemakers were overweight and obese despite following all the healthy habits considered to maintain a healthy BMI.

## 4. Discussion

The prevalence of obesity has vigorously increased in the past three decades speculating the composition of current diet, decreasing levels of physical activities, changes in energy intake versus the expenditure to be the cause. Tackling this problem has to be the main priority as the rate of obesity refuses to settle down. Therefore, conducting field physical examination surveys that provide robust measurements as well as routine surveys which collect self-reported heights and weights is necessary. A combination of both these methods shall reveal a better periodic assessment of self-report bias and strengthen surveillance over the general public. Member States of WHO in 2013 made a resolution of stopping the rise in obesity by 2025, although noble this target is overambitious considering no countries showed downwards trend in the past 3 decades [5].

In this survey as mentioned earlier, BMI index has been used as the determining factor to understand overall wellbeing of an individual. Body mass index (BMI) is the ratio between body weight and the square of body height, and is commonly used to assess bodily mass in epidemiological studies [7]. This entire survey was conducted to understand the rise in obesity, especially in the youth and thus was conducted in colleges primarily to observe the physical activities of students as well as their eating habits. Overweight is defined by a BMI equal to or higher than 25 kg/m2 and obese is 30 kg/m2 or higher [7, 18].

Due to the socio-economic strata, it is observed that the minority and low-income individuals are disproportionately affected by obesity as the cheapest and accessible food is high in fats and sugar. Due to rapid changes in socioeconomic status and demographic in a developing country like India, the adoption of an energy- and fat-rich diet and a sedentary lifestyle has become the norm [1]. In the study itself, it was observed that the youth especially the college going students, indulged in junk food possibly for two reasons, as they are not earning, they prefer cheaper food on a daily basis, also due to 'Westernization' of lifestyles [4]. People who have more financial resources combat these circumstances more easily and, consequently, are more physically active and less obese than those with fewer resources [9].

From these results, it's evident that the rise in mental disorders like depression, anxiety and hypertension is quite prevalent. Mood disorders and anxiety, and weight gain are closely related and recognized as common conditions among adolescents and young adults [19]. The weight gain after diagnosing depression, lower HRQOL and anxiety is just as common as developing depression and other mental issues due to obesity [20–22]. There is a common factor between obesity and depression, i.e., the lower availability of rewarding dopamine D2 receptors. This leads them towards emotional eating as means of feeling better in response to negative emotions, which intake is proven as one behavioural mechanism between depression and subsequent development of obesity [20]. The brain treats high palatable foods that are energy-dense, especially high sugar and fat food as rewards. People under stress usually are attracted towards sugar and fat concentrated food to cope with negative emotions or confusing internal states of hunger and satiety with physiological changes associated with emotions, also called as the 'comfort food hypothesis' [6, 23]. Obstructive sleep apnea (OSA) accompanied with elevated blood pressure is extremely common in patients with obesity, due to fat deposition around the upper respiratory airways, chest wall, and truncal fat, which leads to a decrease in the functional residual capacity [3, 6]. Mechanistically, partial sleep modulates with hormones leading to increased serum ghrelin and reduced serum leptin, both of which result in elevated appetite [23].

From this survey, many girls were seen suffering from PCOS, which now has been declared as a rising epidemic among young girls. Usually children, before hitting puberty do not have gonadotropic and/or ovarian disorder, but have an excess of central that triggers an adaptive mode of accelerated growth and adaptive mode of subfertility (PCOS) [14]. PCOS shows clinical features of insulin resistance (IR), hyperandrogenism. The presence of IR appears as impaired insulin-mediated suppression of lipolysis and lipid oxidation, resulting in increased serum free fatty acids, which is associated with obesity [24, 25].

Weight gain after achieving menopause is a very common occurrence, although studies conducted on these aspects are quite contradictory. Women have been shown to gain weight the most between the ages of 25–34, rather than postmenopausal. Menopause does influence the body composition due to ageing but not any distinct increase in weight gain [16] From this survey, we do observe that women are extremely health conscious in their 30s and on the other hand men especially take major steps of looking after their health in comparison to the women in their 50s. From the study we can also deduce that both men and women prefer to walk for at least half an hour (Females - 59.16% and Males- 45.88%) over exercising in the gyms (Females- 8.33% and Males - 15.29%).

One interesting observation noticed in this survey study was that men and women doing labour work in the field, by default follow a high carbohydrate diet and stay healthy. The labourers do not have the privilege of consuming four whole meals a day, due to shortage of time and workload. Therefore, they were seen consuming high carbohydrate foods like rice, beets, potatoes etc. twice a day to endure the entire day's labour. The high carbohydrate food acts as a fuel for their sane functioning. The key is naturally occurring high carbohydrates to keep them full, provide energy, improve insulin function and heavy labour to create calorie deficit. Another interesting hypothesis is that the dramatic decrease in smoking could also likely be a cause of global increase in BMI. Smoking impairs appetite as well as causes chronic obstructive pulmonary disease, which itself results in a lower body mass [8].

## 5. Conclusion

In Summary, the prevalence of obesity is greater in women than men which increases with age. Overweight and obesity rates have increased considerably during the past 35 years to the extent that more than one-third of the world's population is now classified as overweight or obese [1]. Though a mammoth task, it's imperative that obesity epidemic is reversed through prevention. Countries need to get involved and effectively intervene against major determinants such as excessive caloric intake, physical inactivity, active promotion of food consumption by industry and stopping the gradual weight gain in children [5, 9]. These interventions could help resolve the increase in BMI associated with mood disorders especially in females [19]. According to WHO measures to prevent obesity by individual's choice of healthy foods and regular physical activity are the easiest, most accessible and affordable ones [4]. At the same time sleep also should be incorporated into management plans for obesity [26].

This study has few limitations which provide a scope for further investigation. BMI was considered as a classification source of the populous under scrutiny which is a rather poor indicator of percent of body fat and deposition [1, 8]. There is a known subset of the obese population devoid, of cardiometabolic complications such as diabetes mellitus, IR, and cardiovascular disease who show normal BMI yet have excess visceral adiposity, and are known as metabolically healthy obese (MHO) which is particularly observed in Asian men [6]. Also, in this survey we observed men leading a rather healthy life in all aspects yet having a higher BMI, as BMI doesn't differentiate between muscle or fat mass. Also in this study, we have considered mental health disorders such as depression, anxiety, sleep apnea along with lifestyle habits. As the survey was done to understand the all-round behaviour of the public to maintain a healthy lifestyle, we could not delve further into eating disorders such anorexia and bulimia, which has a wide scope of understanding the increase in the rate of obesity especially amongst the youth [17].

Apart from the country taking rigorous surveys and collaborating with the industries to balance the socio-economic situation to steadily bring down the growth curve of obesity, individuals too can lead and maintain a healthy life and BMI. Grains should be consumed in a minimally refined, high-fibre form, and intakes of refined starches and sugars should be minimized. Non hydrogenated dietary fats must be consumed. Vegetables and fruits must be eating in abundance while red meat should be considerably reduced. Daily exercise of any sort is always recommended [27].

## Acknowledgements

This work is supported by Thakur College of Science & Commerce, Mumbai-400101 and Jain University School of Sciences Centre of postgraduate studies, Bangalore- 560011 for allowing me to conduct my research in their premises. I am thankful to the Dr. Shirley Agwuocha and Dr. Salamun DE for the encouragement and support.

## Author details

Shradha Mistri[1,2]

1 Thakur College of Science and Commerce, Mumbai, India

2 Jain University School of Sciences Centre for Postgraduate Studies, Bangalore, India

*Address all correspondence to: shradhamistri@gmail.com

## References

[1] Yu Chung Chooi, Cherlyn Ding, Faidon Magkos, The epidemiology of obesity, Metabolism, Volume 92, 2019, Pages 6-10, ISSN 0026-0495, https://doi.org/10.1016/j.metabol.2018.09.005.

[2] Ahirwar, R., & Mondal, P. R. (2019). *Prevalence of obesity in India: A systematic review. Diabetes & Metabolic Syndrome: Clinical Research & Reviews, 13(1), 318–321.* doi:10.1016/j.dsx.2018.08.032

[3] Cohen, J.B. Hypertension in Obesity and the Impact of Weight Loss. *Curr Cardiol Rep* 19, 98 (2017). https://doi.org/10.1007/s11886-017-0912-4

[4] Blüher, M. Obesity: global epidemiology and pathogenesis. *Nat Rev Endocrinol* 15, 288–298 (2019). https://doi.org/10.1038/s41574-019-0176-8

[5] Ng, M., Fleming, T., Robinson, M., Thomson, B., Graetz, N., Margono, C., ... Abera, S. F. (2014). *Global, regional, and national prevalence of overweight and obesity in children and adults during 1980–2013: a systematic analysis for the Global Burden of Disease Study 2013. The Lancet, 384(9945), 766–781.* doi:10.1016/s0140-6736(14)60460-8

[6] Jagriti Upadhyay, Olivia Farr, Nikolaos Perakakis, Wael Ghaly, Christos Mantzoros, Obesity as a Disease, Medical Clinics of North America, Volume 102, Issue 1, 2018, Pages 13-33, ISSN 0025-7125, ISBN 9780323566438, https://doi.org/10.1016/j.mcna.2017.08.004.

[7] Díaz, M. Hypertension and obesity. J Hum Hypertens 16, S18–S22 (2002). https://doi.org/10.1038/sj.jhh.1001335

[8] Nuttall, F. Q. (2015). *Body Mass Index. Nutrition Today, 50(3), 117–128.* doi:10.1097/nt.0000000000000092

[9] Mitchell, N. S., Catenacci, V. A., Wyatt, H. R., & Hill, J. O. (2011). Obesity: overview of an epidemic. *The Psychiatric clinics of North America*, *34* (4), 717–732. https://doi.org/10.1016/j.psc.2011.08.005

[10] Owen, L., & Corfe, B. (2017). The role of diet and nutrition on mental health and wellbeing. *Proceedings of the Nutrition Society, 76*(4), 425-426. doi: 10.1017/S0029665117001057

[11] Health Organization. Depression [fact sheet]. 2018; Available at: http://www.who.int/en/news-room/fact-sheets/detail/depression. Accessed 8 July 2018.

[12] Tronieri, J. S., Wurst, C. M., Pearl, R. L., & Allison, K. C. (2017). Sex Differences in Obesity and Mental Health. Current Psychiatry Reports, 19 (6). doi:10.1007/s11920-017-0784-8

[13] De Leo, V., Musacchio, M.C., Cappelli, V. *et al.* Genetic, hormonal and metabolic aspects of PCOS: an update. *Reprod Biol Endocrinol* 14, 38 (2016). https://doi.org/10.1186/s12958-016-0173-x

[14] De Zegher, F., López-Bermejo, A., & Ibáñez, L. (2018). Central Obesity, Faster Maturation, and "PCOS" in Girls. Trends in Endocrinology & Metabolism. doi:10.1016/j.tem.2018.09.005

[15] Simon, S., Rahat, H., Carreau, A.-M., Garcia-Reyes, Y., Halbower, A., Pyle, L., ... Cree-Green, M. (2020). *Poor Sleep is Related to Metabolic Syndrome Severity in Adolescents with PCOS and Obesity. The Journal of Clinical Endocrinology & Metabolism.* doi:10.1210/clinem/dgz285

[16] G. Panotopoulos, J. Raison, J.C. Ruiz, B. Guy-Grand, A. Basdevant, Weight gain at the time of menopause, *Human Reproduction*, Volume 12, Issue suppl_1, October 1997, Pages 126–133, https://doi.org/10.1093/humrep/12.suppl_1.126

[17] Tatjana van Strien, Hanna Konttinen, Judith R. Homberg, Rutger C.M.E. Engels, Laura H.H. Winkens, Emotional eating as a mediator between depression and weight gain, Appetite, Volume 100, 2016, Pages 216-224, ISSN 0195-6663, https://doi.org/10.1016/j.appet.2016.02.034.

[18] World Health Organization. Obesity and overweight [fact sheet]. 2017; Available at:http://www.who.int/en/news-room/fact-sheets/detail/obesity-and-overweight. Accessed 8 July 2018.

[19] Sahle, B.W., Breslin, M., Sanderson, K. *et al.* Association between depression, anxiety and weight change in young adults. *BMC Psychiatry* 19, 398 (2019). https://doi.org/10.1186/s12888-019-2385-z

[20] Konttinen, H., van Strien, T., Männistö, S. *et al.* Depression, emotional eating and long-term weight changes: a population-based prospective study. *Int J Behav Nutr Phys Act* 16, 28 (2019). https://doi.org/10.1186/s12966-019-0791-8

[21] M. Morrison, Sabina Shin, Mark Tarnopolsky, Valerie H. Taylor, Association of depression & health related quality of life with body composition in children and youth with obesity, Journal of Affective Disorders, Volume 172, 2015, Pages 18-23, ISSN 0165-0327, https://doi.org/10.1016/j.jad.2014.09.014.

[22] Ma J, Rosas LG, Lv N, et al. Effect of Integrated Behavioral Weight Loss Treatment and Problem-Solving Therapy on Body Mass Index and Depressive Symptoms Among Patients With Obesity and Depression: The RAINBOW Randomized Clinical Trial. *JAMA.* 2019;321(9):869–879. doi: 10.1001/jama.2019.0557

[23] Maddahi, N.S., Yarizadeh, H., Setayesh, L. *et al.* Association between dietary energy density with mental health and sleep quality in women with overweight/obesity. *BMC Res Notes* 13, 189 (2020). https://doi.org/10.1186/s13104-020-05025-1

[24] N S Kakoly, M B Khomami, A E Joham, S D Cooray, M L Misso, R J Norman, C L Harrison, S Ranasinha, H J Teede, L J Moran, Ethnicity, obesity and the prevalence of impaired glucose tolerance and type 2 diabetes in PCOS: a systematic review and meta-regression, *Human Reproduction Update*, Volume 24, Issue 4, July-August 2018, Pages 455–467, https://doi.org/10.1093/humupd/dmy007

[25] Shengxian Li, Qianqian Chu, Jing Ma, Yun Sun, Tao Tao, Rong Huang, Yu Liao, Jiang Yue, Jun Zheng, Lihua Wang, Xinli Xue, Mingjiang Zhu, Xiaonan Kang, Huiyong Yin, Wei Liu, Discovery of Novel Lipid Profiles in PCOS: Do Insulin and Androgen Oppositely Regulate Bioactive Lipid Production?, *The Journal of Clinical Endocrinology & Metabolism*, Volume 102, Issue 3, 1 March 2017, Pages 810–821, https://doi.org/10.1210/jc.2016-2692

[26] Li, Y., Xie, J., Chen, B., Basta, M., & Vgontzas, A. (2020). *1035 Sleep Duration and Metabolic Syndrome: An Updated Systematic Review and Meta-Analysis. Sleep, 43(Supplement_1), A393–A393.* doi:10.1093/sleep/zsaa056.1031

[27] Walter C. Willett and Meir J. Stampfer Current Evidence on Healthy Eating Annual Review of Public Health 2013 34:1, 77-95

Chapter 10

# Hypertension as Three Systematic Dysregulations of $Na^+$ Homeostasis in Terrestrial Mammal, and Salt in Gut Might Cause Brain Inflammation

*Mizuo Mifune and Yoshihiko Kanno*


## Abstract

Although $Na^+$ homeostasis in vivo is essential for mammals, it is known that excessive salt (NaCl) intake has played a major role in the development of hypertension. In vivo, there is a hormonal system, the renin-angiotensin-aldosterone system (RAAS), that specializes in regulating $Na^+$ retention, especially the amount of $Na^+$ in plasma. $Na^+$ homeostasis in vivo has been achieved mainly by the RAAS, through regulation of vascular tonus (blood pressure) and $Na^+$ handling in the kidney ($Na^+$ diuresis). Recent studies have revealed a third mechanism of $Na^+$ homeostasis in vivo: regulation of interstitial $Na^+$ levels in tissues, such as subcutaneous tissues, by tissue macrophage immunity. In the pathogenesis of salt-sensitive hypertension, Recent research have been revealed that three molecular axes (Ang II - Rho/NOX-eNOS system, Aldosterone-rac1 -ENaC system, and tissue $Na^+$ – TonEBP in macrophage -VEGF-c) are significantly involved in maintaining $Na^+$ homeostasis in salt induced hypertension. Furthermore, the mechanism by which salt causes hypertension via the immune system (intestinal, local mucosal, and tissue immunity) has also been reported. In this article, we would like to propose that three molecular dysfunctions are involved in the development of salt-sensitive hypertension through three immunological mechanisms in the maintenance of $Na^+$ homeostasis. Next, I would like to explain the importance of gut-RAAS and abnormality of intestinal microflora (dysbiosis) in salt-sensitive hypertension. It has been known that the metabolites (e.g., short-chain fatty acid neural amino) produced by microflora are deeply involved in central (CNS) and sympathetic nervous system (SNS) activity. In addition, we would like to explain of the importance of brain-RAAS and cerebral inflammation in salt-sensitive hypertension. Moreover, recent research have revealed that the detection-mechanism in the brain for $Na^+$ concentration($[Na^+]$) in vivo and in the tongue for $[Na^+]$ in diet. These finding suggests that excessive salt intake may cause brain dysfunction, most delicate organ, before the onset of salt sensitive hypertension, and may also destroy brain structure after the onset of salt sensitive hypertension. Thus, we would like to insist that excessive salt intake might not only induce hypertension, but also be toxic especially for brain. Finally, we would like to explain that The DASH diet (Dietary Approaches to Stop Hypertension) is one of the universal diets for adult human, not only by reducing salt, but also by reducing metabolic stress and improving of dysbiosis.




IntechOpen

**Keywords:** homeostasis, multisystem, immunity, dysbiosis, taste

## 1. Introduction

For terrestrial mammals, dehydration is fatal. Because, dehydration cause lowering circulating plasma volume (plasma $Na^+$), lowering blood pressure, and decrease of organ blood flow, leading to death. To prevent dehydration, terrestrial mammals have been developed the mechanisms to maintain BP and Na in the body. This defense mechanism against dehydration is the renin–angiotensin–aldosterone system (RAAS) which is a hormone system that regulates blood pressure, systemic vascular resistance and maintain [$Na^+$]in the body [1, 2]. To prevent tissue hypo-reflux due to hypotension during dehydration and to maintain the effective circulating plasma volume, Ang-II caused vascular contraction and re-absorption of $Na^+$ (**Figure 1**).

In the detailed description, when renal blood flow is reduced, juxtaglomerular cells in the kidneys secrete renin into circulation. Plasma renin then carries out the conversion of angiotensinogen, released from the liver to angiotensin I. Angiotensin I is subsequently converted to angiotensin II(Ang-II) by the angiotensin-converting enzyme (ACE) found on the surface of capillary endothelial cells, predominantly those of the lungs. Ang -II is octapeptide described as Ang- [1-8]. There are two receptors for Ang-II, type 1 receptor (AT1R) and type II receptor (AT2) [3]. Ang-II is a biologically active peptide that mediates its effects via the angiotensin-II type 1 receptor (AT1R). On the other side, AT2R exerts mainly anti-AT1R [4]. Ang-II stimulation via AT1R was originally known as a circulating hormone that regulates blood pressure and electrolyte balance by acting on vascular contraction, renal sodium handling, sympathetic activity, and vasopressin release. As detailed description, Moreover, Ang II stimulates the secretion of aldosterone also via AT1R in the adrenal cortex [5].

Aldosterone increases the reabsorption of $Na^+$ via epithelial sodium channels (ENaC) in the renal tubules (collecting ducts), at the same time causing the excretion of potassium [6]. In this way, systematic RAAS was defined as an endocrine system involved in blood pressure regulation and body electrolyte balance. This pathway (renin – Ang-II-aldosterone axis) is called as "classical and systematic RA(A)S".

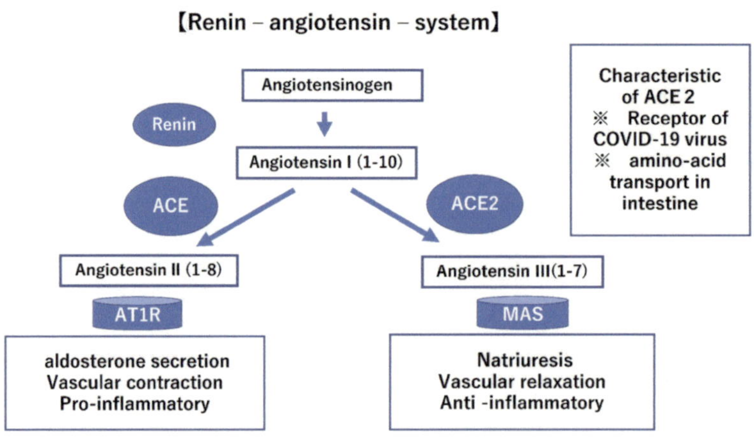


**Figure 1.**
*Bipolarity of pathophysiological effects in renin – angiotensin- system.*

Moreover, RAAS is now considered a "ubiquitous" system that expressed locally in various tissue and exerts multiple paracrine/autocrine effects involved in tissue physiology and homeostasis. This concept is considered as "tissue RAAS". Local angiotensin pathway and their physiological importance were elucidated in different tissues including the heart, blood vessels, kidney, brain, adipose tissue, liver, lymphatic tissue, reproductive system, and eye. In these tissues, local RAAS acts independently from systematic RAAS in a paracrine and paracrine manner but may still interact with systematic RAAS to exert endocrine effects [7].

If the RAS is abnormally active, blood pressure will be too high. There are several types of drugs which includes ACE inhibitors, Angiotensin-II type I receptor blocker (ARBs), and renin inhibitors that interrupt different steps in this system to improve blood pressure. These drugs are one of the primary ways to control high blood pressure, heart failure, kidney failure, and harmful effects of diabetes [8].

On the other side, a novel axis of the renin-angiotensin system (RAS) was unveiled by the discovery of angiotensin- (1-7) [Ang- (1-7)]. Angiotensin-converting enzyme 2 (ACE2), not ACE, was shown to be the main mediator of this reaction (Ang-I (1-10) to Ang (1-7), not Ang-II (1-8)), and Mas was found to be the receptor for the heptapeptide. Compared to classical RAS axis (ACE-AngII-AT1R), novel RAS axis (ACE2-Ang(1–7))-MAS act anti-hypertensive and anti-inflammatory effect [9].

In this chapter, we explained that the RAAS system is most pivotal hormonal mechanism for sodium retention in vivo. Apart from the systemic RAAS system, organ-specific effects have been recognized in various organs (kidney, cardiovascular, and brain) involved in sodium retention and blood pressure formation (renal RAAS, cardiovascular RAAS, and brain RAAS). Ang-II and aldosterone have been found to have pro-inflammatory effects via AT1R and MR. Originally, the balance between Na and aldosterone should be a seesaw-relationship, but it has been found that this relationship is broken in the development of salt-sensitive hypertension. Thus, a boost and runway of RAAS, the most important mechanism to maintain of Na homeostasis for terrestrial mammals, has been recognized as the basis for the development of hypertension.

## 2. Vascular tonus dysfunction by AngII-RhoA/NADPH-eNOS axis

Ang-II has three physiological effects to elevate blood pressure via AT1R, vascular contraction, renal absorption, and aldosterone secretion. As detailed description, Ang II is a potent vasoconstrictive peptide that causes blood vessels to construct via AT1R in vascular smooth muscle cell, resulting in increased blood pressure. Ang II also activate sodium reabsorption through NHE3 via AT1R in the renal tubules (proximal duct). Moreover, Ang II stimulates the secretion of aldosterone also via AT1R in the adrenal cortex.

Ang-II also exerts three pathological effect, oxidative stress production, induction of inflammation and fibrosis [10]. Ang II stimulation can activate NAD(P)H oxidase to produce ROS, resulting in oxidative stress damage [11]. ROS production in VSMC by Ang II caused also mitochondrial dysfunction and cellular injury [12].

In vascular smooth muscle cells, RhoA/ROCK determine sensitivity to vasoconstrictors by Ang II in salt-sensitive hypertension [13, 14]. The Rho family small GTP binding protein, what is called Rho GTPase (consist of Rho (RhoA, C), Rac (Rac1,2) and Cdc42), is part of the Ras superfamily and has important functions in regulating intracellular signaling and cell morphology. The Rho family has various cellular functions such as cell migration, phagocytosis, endocytosis, morphogenesis, and cytokinesis. The Rho family is also involved in cell cycle progression and gene expression, cell polarity, hematopoiesis, and Wnt signaling [15].

In endothelial cells, the RhoA/ROCK activation and ROS production via Ang-II stimulation in VSMC pathway negatively regulates NO production through eNOS dysfunction [16]. Endothelial dysfunction is caused by reducing NO bioavailability, leading to peroxynitrite (ONOO-) formation which is reactant superoxide with NO. Endogenous NO is critical for regulating renal hemodynamics and sodium homeostasis, including renal vasodilation and natriuresis [17], and is also control cerebral blood flow and Cerebrospinal fluid Na concentration [18].

The importance of NO in vivo cannot be overestimated. To maintain of homeostasis, the cellular action of nitric oxide, which is second messenger is as important as oxygen [19]. At first, vascular smooth muscle is dilated by NO produced by endothelial Nitric Oxide Synthase (eNOS), which is present in vascular endothelial cells. NO is a molecule with a simple chemical structure that exists in a gaseous state at room temperature. NOS is an enzyme involved in the metabolic reaction that synthesizes L-citrulline from the amino acid L-arginine to form L-citrulline and NO. There are three types of NOS: eNOS, which is found in the vascular endothelium; neural NOS (nNOS), which is found in nerve cells; and inducible NOS (NOS), which is induced by stress. It has been reported that excessive salt overload reduces the vascular dilation response, and arginine administration is known to restore this function. In the development of essential hypertension, oxidative stress (superoxide (O2-), hydrogen peroxide (H2O2)) produced by NADPH oxidase and xanthine oxidase in blood vessels reduces the production of NO by eNOS, which is thought to be one of the mechanisms of essential hypertension [20].

In addition, the activation of eNOS in the export and import arteries increases the renal medullary blood flow. Activation of nNOS in the macula dense decreases the regulatory capacity of TGF. In addition, iNOS decreases the renal Na reabsorption capacity. Thus, impaired endothelial function via dysfunction of eNOS due to increased oxidative stress is the cause of the development of hypertension from resistance vascular dysfunction. Furthermore, dysfunction of other NOS (nNOS and iNOS) is also involved in impaired medullary blood flow and tubular function in the kidney [20]. Thus, NOS in vascular endothelial cells is the most important molecule for the regulation of total peripheral vascular resistance, and other NOS also function in specific roles in the kidney and brain, and under specific conditions such as during inflammation. This suggests that dysfunction of these three NOSs may be the cause of the development of hypertension. In addition, the dysfunction of NOS is thought to be caused by increased oxidative stress, both systemic and local. Therefore, the activation of RhoA and the production of ROS by Ang II in VSMC caused NO production system in eNOS in endothelial cell might be pivotal mechanism of contractile augmentation and reducing renal blood flow, resulting Na retention in salt induced hypertension [21].

We would like to propose that the dysfunction of AngII-RhoA/NADPH-eNOS axis found in salt-sensitive hypertension cause vascular dysfunction by tissue local oxidative stress formation [22].

## 3. $Na^+$ retention by aldosterone-rac1-ENaC axis cause in vivo

Ang II is a typical hormone that contracts the vascular smooth muscle of resistance vessels, but Ang II also has two other effects, such as sodium reabsorption in the proximal tubule and aldosterone secretion from the adrenal gland [23]. The action of aldosterone is mediated by serum and glucocorticoid-regulated kinase 1 (SGK1) as a transcription factor, which is involved in the synthesis of ENaC protein in the luminal membrane, the synthesis of $Na^+$ pump ($Na^+/K$ + - ATPase) in the lateral basement membrane, and the inhibition of endogenous sodium pump, and activation of endogenous sodium pump inhibitory factor (digitalis-like substance) [24].

Essentially, the kidneys promote sodium diuresis by increasing blood pressure, increasing renal medullary blood flow, leading to increasing intraglomerular pressure. This is called baroreflex diuresis, which was firstly pointed out by Guyton. In other words, the kidneys regulate the amount of sodium in the body through the excretion of $Na^+$, which is called the sodium handling action of the kidneys [25]. This is called renal sodium handling. Renal handling consists of the production of primary urine by maintaining renal medullary blood flow with Ang II and NO, and the reabsorption of sodium in the tubules. To maintain renal medullary blood flow, there is tonus regulation of the two resistance vessels, glomerular export and import arteries, and a tubular feedback mechanism (TGF). $Na^+$ reabsorption by the tubules is mediated by NHE ($Na^+/K^+$ exchanger in the proximal tubules [26], NKCC ($Na^+/K^+/2Cl$- co-transporter) in the ascending Henle loop, NCC ($Na^+$/ Cl- co-transporter) in the distal tubules, and mineralocorticoid receptors in the collecting ducts. The epithelial sodium channel (ENaC) by the mineral corticoid receptor (MR) in the collecting duct, and four main $Na^+$ reabsorption transporters [27]. At the onset of hypertension, functional changes in renal sodium handling are observed due to changes in renal medullary blood flow and renal tubular $Na^+$ reabsorption. First, in the proximal tubule NHE, stimulation of tubular AT1 receptors by systemic circulating Ang II enhances Na reabsorption by NHE. Secondly, NCCs in the distal tubule promote Na reabsorption from NCCs with increased metabolic stress (hyperinsulinemia, hypokalemia, glucocorticoids, acidosis) (WNK-NCC system) [28] and activation of the sympathetic nervous system (β3-adrenalegic NCC system) [29]. The final effector of $Na^+$ reabsorption is the activation of MR by aldosterone stimulation, which results in $Na^+$ reabsorption from ENaC. Notably, homeostatic activation of rac1 was observed in the abnormal increase in $Na^+$ reabsorption by MR-ENaC, and it has been reported that MR-ENaC is activated and $Na^+$ reabsorption is enhanced independently of aldosterone stimulation [30]. In addition, aldosterone is known to promote pathological cardiovascular remodeling by inducing inflammation [31]. Therefore, eplerenone, an anti-aldosterone drug, has been reported to have a predominant inhibitory effect on cardiovascular events in large clinical studies. In addition, eplerenone, an anti-MR drug, has been reported to have a significant inhibitory effect on cardiovascular events in large clinical studies [32].

Aldosterone-activated ENaC is most pivotal in the mechanism of $Na^+$ retention in kidney was observed. Interestingly, the activation of ENaC was not dependent on the elevation of aldosterone concentration itself, but on the constitutive activation of rac1, a small G protein family with RhoA. We would like to propose that this increased renal sodium reabsorption observed in salt-sensitive hypertension is an abnormality of the aldosterone-rac1-ENaC axis.

## 4. Three immune mechanisms are involved in the development of salt-sensitive hypertension

Recent studies have revealed that three immune mechanisms are involved in the development of salt-sensitive hypertension [33]. First, excess salt from the diet is involved in blood pressure dysregulation through cytokine production by intestinal immunity [34]. $Na^+$ in the intestine activates T lymphocytes (TH17 cells) that produce interleukin-17 (IL-17), a strong pro-inflammatory cytokine, in the intestine, where 70% of the systemic immune cells are located. The increased oxidative stress produced by NADPH oxidase in neutrophils activated by circulating IL-17 was found to be a mechanism that greatly reduced the function of eNOS in the vascular endothelium [35]. It has also been reported that the activation of TH17 cells simultaneously causes a decrease in the function of regulatory T cells (Treg), which control the allergic reaction, a runaway immune response [36]. In other words, excessive salt induces systemic vascular endothelial dysfunction and immunodeficiency through systemic activation of IL-17 by dysbiosis. Therefore, excessive salt is also involved in cognitive dysfunction by decreasing blood flow to the brain [37], and in the development of multiple sclerosis, an autoimmune disease of the brain [38]. We hypothesize that dietary salt impairs the function of the Ang II-RhoA/NADPH-eNOS axis, a blood pressure regulating system, by impairing eNOS function (vascular endothelial dilatation) associated with hyper-cytokine induced oxidative stress via intestinal immunity abnormality.

Second, it has been reported that the acquired immune system, mainly T lymphocytes, may be involved in the function of renal tubules in the regulation of renal $Na^+$ handling [39, 40]. T-lymphocytes may be involved in the regulation of renal tubular function via stimulation from sympathetic nerve activation (via β3-adrenal receptors) and glucocorticoids (via SGK1 (serum glucocorticoid - regulated kinase 1)) in the renal medulla through activation of mTOR (mammalian target of receptor) [41, 42]. We would like to propose that abnormal activation of T lymphocytes of the acquired immune system reduces the regulatory function of renal $Na^+$ handling mechanisms manipulated by the aldosterone-rac1-ENaC axis.

Third, tissue immunity, which is controlled by macrophages [43] has been found to regulate the amount of interstitial $Na^+$ in skin by regulating tissue lymphatic reflux, and it has been reported that dysfunction of this mechanism contributes to the development of hypertension [44]. Excess interstitial $Na^+$ was found to accumulate in skin and muscle before increasing the amount of circulating plasma $Na^+$, which might cause salt-sensitive hypertension, by imaging the concentration of 23 $Na^+$ in tissues using sodium-magnetic resonance imaging (23Na-MRI) [45]. Although the amount of plasma $Na^+$ is regulated by the RAAS system, high concentrations of $Na^+$ in the interstitial fluid in subcutaneous tissues activate the mononuclear phagocytic cell lineage (macrophages and monocytes) and induce the transcription of their own osmotic-responsive enhancer binding protein (TonEBP). The increased expression of this transcription factor, TonEBP (tonicity-responsive enhancer binding protein), activate mononuclear phagocytic action. The TonEBP activation increases the expression and secretion of vascular endothelial growth factor (VEGF)-C, induces hyperplasia of lymphatic vessels in the subcutaneous tissue, and removes excess $Na^+$ via lymphatic vessels [46]. However, the drainage of interstitial $Na^+$ by increased lymphatic vessels, which is activated by TonEBP-VEGF-C in tissue-macrophage, may not be effective in condition of the loss of intercellular matrix, such as proteoglycans, for some reason, and the buffering and retention effect of $Na^+$ as interstitial $Na^+$ is lost, resulting in increased plasma $Na^+$. In this way, it is assumed that an increase in the amount of $Na^+$ in the plasma leads to the development of salt-sensitive hypertension. In practice, it has been reported that the amount of $Na^+$ in the skin and muscles of patients with hypertension is higher than that of normal subjects [47], and that the accumulation of $Na^+$ in the skin of patients with chronic kidney disease is associated with left ventricular hypertrophy [48]. Therefore, it has been proposed that dysfunction of lymphatic vessels regulated by tissue macrophage in the skin may cause excessive interstitial $Na^+$ accumulation and associated salt-sensitive hypertension. This mechanism may also be involved in local immunity against bacterial infections, as activation of TonEBP in the skin leads to bactericidal NO production by activating iNOS [49].

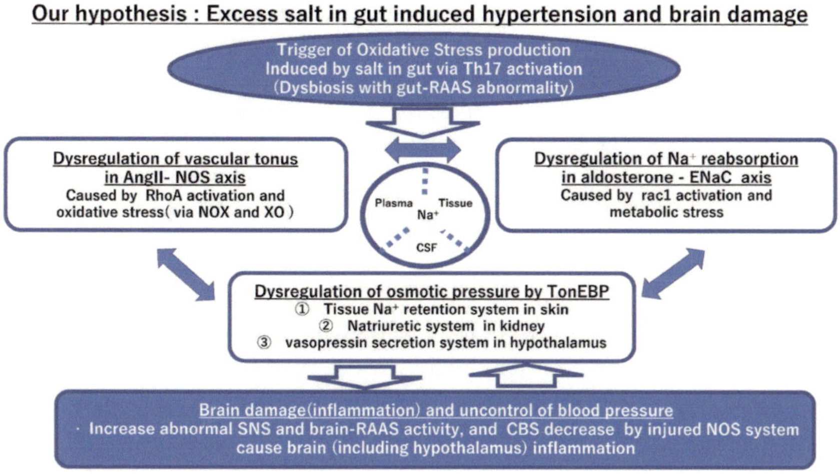


**Figure 2.**
*$Na^+$ homeostasis in terrestrial mammal body is architected by three axes, $Na^+$ circulation in side, $Na^+$ absorption from outside, and $Na^+$ concentration maintenance in tissue and body fluid.*

Surprisingly, TonEBP is also reported to be expressed in the renal medulla and hypothalamus and is involved in the urine concentration mechanism in the renal medulla [50] and the secretion of arginine vasopressin in the hypothalamus [51].

In other words, salt-sensitive hypertension, which is a dis-regulation of $Na^+$ homeostasis in the body, is caused not only by abnormalities in the regulation of plasma $Na^+$ by RAAS, but also by the dysregulation of interstitial $Na^+$ through the tissue immune system (tissue macrophage-TonEBP (macrophage)-VEGF-C/NO). VEGF-C/NO axis) (**Figure 2**).

## 5. Salt in gut, mediating through microbiome and gut-RAAS, cause hypertension

As mentioned earlier in this chapter, excessive salt in the intestine is assumed to be trigger of onset of hypertension via dysbiosis of the gut microbiome (GM) [52]. In an animal study, it was reported that a decrease in lactobacillus murinus caused by salt intake altered the intestinal microbiome and contributed to the development of hypertension [53]. The effects of dietary content on the intestinal microflora are not limited to salt, but also include due to excessive sugar and carbohydrate, causing abnormalities in glucose metabolism, and to dietary fiber deficiency in the development of hypertension, causing constipation. Single-chain fatty acids such as acetic acid and butyric acid produced by the intestinal microflora have been reported to play a favorable role in the regulation of blood pressure [54]. On the other hand, trimethylamine N-oxide (TMAO), a gut-microbiota of choline and L-carnitine, has been reported to exert vascular injury effects. Thus, the gut and hypertension are closely related, based on the metabolic and immune effects of the intestinal microbiota [55].

Furthermore, the GM is also thought to be involved in sympathetic nerve dysregulation by abnormal metabolism of tyrosine, which is a neurogenic amino acid, synthetized to sympathetic neurotransmitters (dopamine, norepinephrine, and epinephrine) [56]. Among these, tryptophan is the most important neurogenic amino acid [57]. Tryptophan is converted to serotonin, which has various effects on the nervous system, including the central nervous system, peripheral nervous system, and enteric nervous system [57]. Tryptophan is also involved in the function of T-lymphocytes and has been found to have effects on the immune system [58].

Thus, monoamine metabolism in the intestine is very important, and the intestinal microbiota is greatly involved in the control of blood pressure through regulation of the sympathetic nervous system and immunity.

In addition, the intestine has a local RAAS to regulate water uptake of sodium in colon. This is called gut RASS. In this mechanism, Ang-II - AT1R - aldosterone axis is responsible for bowel movement and sodium absorption via ENaC. On the other hand, this Ang-II - AT1 - aldosterone axis influences intestinal inflammation. On the other hand, the Ang-(1–7)- ACE2- MASR axis has been reported to have anti-hypertensive and anti-inflammatory effects [59]. Recent studies have shown that ACE2 is involved in the regulation of amino acid transport in the intestine [60]. In addition, ACE2 is a receptor for the COVID-19 virus, and cytokine storm caused by this viral infection has been found to be due to attenuation of the anti-inflammatory and anticoagulant effects of ACE2. Therefore, this property of ACE2 has led to the development of therapeutic agents for coronaviruses [61].

## 6. $Na^+$ sensor in brain cause Na appetite

The brain controls systemic blood pressure and maintains homeostasis of $Na^+$ in the body through the HPA (hypothalamus - pituitary – adrenal grand) system and the sympathetic nervous system (SNS). In addition, it has been reported that oxidative stress is involved in the pathogenesis of salt-sensitive hypertension by abnormal enhancement of the brain RAAS and SNS [62].

Recent studies have shown that $Na^+$ homeostasis in the body is maintained by $Na^+$ sensors (Nax) in the brain that detect cerebrospinal fluid $Na^+$ (CSF $Na^+$) [63], and that the brain detects $Na^+$ in the diet by ENaC in the taste cells on the tongue [64]. Recent studies have shown that the $Na^+$ concentration in the cerebrospinal fluid (CSF) of salt-sensitive hypertensive rodents is significantly higher than that of the control group, even though the blood $Na^+$ concentration is the same. Nax exist at the subfornical organ (SFO) and the vasculosum of the lamia terminalis (OVLT) in circumventricular organ (CVO) belonging to the of the third ventricle, which is exceptionally lacking a blood–brain barrier (BBB) [65]. Nax senses changes in cerebrospinal sodium (CSF $Na^+$) in the SFO and OVLT, and its signals regulate fluid and salt intake behavior in response to dehydrate condition [66]. The signal of increased CSF $Na^+$ concentration activates the peripheral sympathetic nervous system through activation of the paraventricular nucleus (PVN) and the rostral ventrolateral medulla (RVLM), which are both sympathetic control centers. In addition, this signal is transmitted to the hypothalamus to regulate the vasopressin (antidiuretic hormone) secretion [51]. Thus, the homeostasis of $Na^+$ in the body is controlled by the activation of SNS and RAAS functions in the brain via CSF [$Na^+$] signals.

Humans perceive five basic tastes: sweet, sour, bitter, umami, and salty. ENaC, which is present in taste cells in the taste buds of the tongue, detects salty taste. This ENaC, as mentioned earlier section, is in the renal collecting ducts and is also the final regulator of natriuresis. In vertebrates, ENaC is found in the colon, lungs, and sweat glands, in addition to the kidney and tongue, and regulates sodium reabsorption. In addition, ENaC and MR have been found to coexist in the brain choroid plexus, where SFO and OVLT, those which sense CSF $Na^+$, are located. In other words, humans sense $Na^+$ in the ENaC of the tongue and regulate the excretion of $Na^+$ out of the body through urine (kidneys), sweat (sweat glands), and stool (colon). This $Na^+$ balance for $Na^+$ homeostasis is controlled by the brain, which senses $Na^+$ in the CSF and controls the $Na^+$ input via the tongue and $Na^+$ output via kidneys [67, 68].

In addition, it is known that excessive salt intake and emotional stress can cause a significant increase in blood pressure. Emotional stress increases blood pressure by activating SNS and RAAS, and the blood pressure elevation caused by this stress is greater in salt-sensitive patients than in salt-resistant patients [69]. As a reason why salt preference, in concert with emotional stress, exacerbates salt-sensitive hypertension, it has been shown that Ang-II activation of AT1R occurs in various brain regions (amygdala, anterior hypothalamic area, PVN) related to stress response [70]. In salt-sensitive hypertension, abnormalities of the RAAS and SNS are observed also in the brain, and this is mediated by increased oxidative stress and inflammation in the brain, which in turn leads to dysfunction of salt-tasting taste cells in the tongue and increased $Na^+$ concentration in the CSF [71]. Furthermore, as mentioned above, it has been found that excessive salt causes inflammation in the brain by decreasing cerebral blood flow due to dysfunction of NOS in systemic blood vessels caused by salt-induced dysbiosis.

Thus, in salt-sensitive hypertension, excessive salt causes brain RAAS and SNS abnormal activity through increased intracerebral inflammation and oxidative stress, when the mechanism of the regulation of $Na^+$ homeostasis in the bran is disrupted, leading to systemic circulatory failure, neurological dysfunction, and chronic inflammation.

## 7. Epigenetics in salt-sensitive hypertension

In addition to genetic predisposition, environmental factors experienced during fetal life and childhood have been found to influence brain and nervous system functions through epigenetic changes. For example, the DOHaD theory (developmental origins of health and disease) has been proposed that inadequate nutrition during fetal life may lead to the risk of chronic diseases such as hypertension in adulthood [72]. It has also been pointed out that excess salt also may induce epigenetic salt-sensitive hypertension [73]. For example, it has been reported that salt-sensitive hypertension is caused by abnormalities of the glucocorticoid system in uterine environment. In addition, transcriptional changes in genetic activity due to DNA methylation and histone modifications in ENaC and NCC, which regulate sodium reabsorption in the kidney, have also been reported [74]. These finding suggests that excessive salt intake may lead to the development of salt-sensitive hypertension through acquired genetic changes, and the importance of salt reduction education from an early age [75].

## 8. Preventive diet for hypertension

The INTERSALT study, which is an international study that compared blood pressure in populations in the world with different amount of salt intakes, has revealed the relationship between salt intake and blood pressure. There was a strong positive correlation between daily urinary sodium excretion and the degree of increase in blood pressure with age [76]. This suggests the importance of reducing $Na^+$ intake. The antagonistic effect of $K^+$ on $Na^+$ has been recognized [77], and it has an antihypertensive effect on the kidneys by promoting the excretion of $Na^+$. According to Eaton et al.'s estimate, $K^+$ intake in the Paleolithic period was 6070 mg/day, but in modern society, it has dropped to 2500 mg/day, about 1/3 [78]. In fact, in a meta-analysis on the antihypertensive effect of $K^+$ loading, it has been pointed out that the higher the NaCl intake, the more marked the antihypertensive effect of $K^+$ in salt sensitive hypertension [79].

In the United States, the DASH diet (Dietary Approaches to Stop Hypertension) has been proposed as a hypertensive diet. This diet was recommended by the National Heart, Lung, and Blood Institute (NHLBI) of the National Institutes of Health (NIH) in the United States to improve hypertension. The DASH diet recommends fruits, vegetables, whole grains, and low-fat dairy products, and has been established as evidence in large-scale studies [80, 81]. The DASH-diet is based on $Na^+$ restriction and $K^+$ supplementation, suppression of intestinal inflammation by limiting fat, and intake of prebiotics such as dietary fiber. Among these, the production of short-chain fatty acids such as butyric acid, lactic acid, and acetic acid from dietary fiber by microbiota is said to contribute significantly to anti-inflammatory effects and improvement of energy metabolism. From this point of view, it is no exaggeration to say that the DASH diet is an all-round health food formula because of its low $Na^+$ content, proper intake of $K^+$ that excretes sodium, low fat content that suppresses inflammation in the intestines, and high fiber content. However, a risk of salt restriction in daily diet is attended in the special but often patients in Japan. They are elderly patient with hypertension, and patients receiving hemodialysis. As both have a risk of malnutrition by carrying out the salt restriction, the Japanese Society of Hypertension Guidelines for the Management of Hypertension (JSH 2019) allowed them to take salt over 6 gram per day [82]. We also emphasize that decreasing salt intake from 20 gram to 15 gram per day has enough meaning as salt restriction [83].

## 9. Finally, low-salt diet may protect our brain

As vertebrates evolved from the sea to the land, they developed the RAAS system and came to have a $Na^+$ retention system that could withstand desiccation and dehydration.

Furthermore, humans began to develop a taste for salt, finding it delicious in their meals. With the increase in industrial production of cheap NaCl, excessive

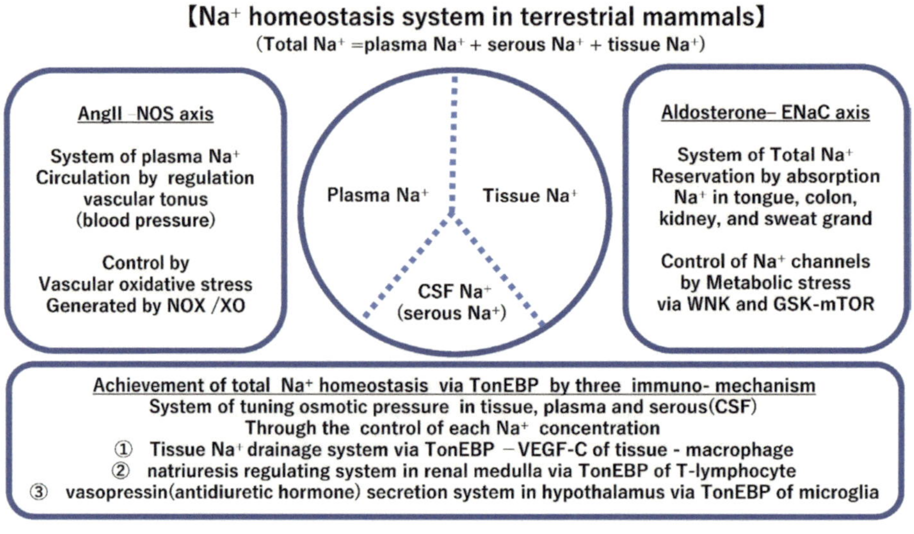


**Figure 3.**
*Our hypothesis: Excess salt in gut induced hypertension and brain damage in a deterioration spiral manner among three systematic dysregulation of $Na^+$ homeostasis.*

salt intake first became possible, causing hypertension and hypertensive diseases such as stroke. Furthermore, it has very recently been pointed out that excess salt can trigger dysbiosis of the intestinal microflora, which can lead to autoimmune brain diseases. In this study, we clarified that three mechanisms that maintain $Na^+$ homeostasis (the circulating plasma $Na^+$ system (AngII-eNOS axis), the total $Na^+$ retention system in body (Aldosterone-ENaC axis), and the tissue $Na^+$ sensing system (TonEBP (in macrophage)-VEGF-C axis) are impaired in salt-sensitive hypertension (**Figure 3**).

In the brain, which is the command center of $Na^+$ homeostasis in vivo, excessive salt causes cerebral blood flow (CBF) decrease because of NOS dysfunction. Secondly, ENaC dysfunction in taste cells causes taste disorder, which leads to a preference for strong salt tastes. In addition, the increase in CSF $Na^+$ leads to the activation of tissue macrophages in the brain (microglia) via TonEBP activation, which causes inflammation in the brain. Thus, we pointed out that the same molecular biological mechanism that leads to the development of salt-sensitive hypertension may also lead to brain toxicity in the form of exacerbation of salt preference (toxicity), emotional instability (CBF decrease), and pathological brain remodeling (structural damage in the brain such as atrophy). Excess salt may also lead to further development of acquired salt-sensitive organ damage through epigenetics. Therefore, we would like to emphasize that it is extremely important to be aware of salt reduction in our daily diet.

## Author details

Mizuo Mifune[1] and Yoshihiko Kanno[2]*

1 Shinozaki HD Clinic, Tokyo, Japan

2 Department of Nephrology, Tokyo Medical University, Tokyo, Japan

*Address all correspondence to: kannoyh@tokyo-med.ac.jp

## References

[1] Fountain JH, Lappin SL. Physiology, Renin Angiotensin System. StatPearls. Treasure Island (FL): StatPearls Publishing Copyright © 2021, StatPearls Publishing LLC.; 2021.

[2] Paul M, Poyan Mehr A, Kreutz R. Physiology of local renin-angiotensin systems. Physiol Rev. 2006;86(3): 747-803.

[3] Mifune M, Sasamura H, Nakazato Y, Yamaji Y, Oshima N, Saruta T. Examination of angiotensin II type 1 and type 2 receptor expression in human kidneys by immunohisto chemistry. Clin Exp Hypertens. 2001;23(3):257-266.

[4] Mifune M, Sasamura H, Shimizu-Hirota R, Miyazaki H, Saruta T. Angiotensin II type 2 receptors stimulate collagen synthesis in cultured vascular smooth muscle cells. Hypertension. 2000;36(5):845-850.

[5] Brewster UC, Perazella MA. The renin-angiotensin-aldosterone system and the kidney: effects on kidney disease. Am J Med. 2004;116(4): 263-272.

[6] Sztechman D, Czarzasta K, Cudnoch-Jedrzejewska A, Szczepanska-Sadowska E, Zera T. Aldosterone and mineralocorticoid receptors in regulation of the cardiovascular system and pathological remodelling of the heart and arteries. J Physiol Pharmacol. 2018;69(6).

[7] Nehme A, Zouein FA, Zayeri ZD, Zibara K. An Update on the Tissue Renin Angiotensin System and Its Role in Physiology and Pathology. J Cardiovasc Dev Dis. 2019;6(2).

[8] Ferrario CM, Mullick AE. Renin angiotensin aldosterone inhibition in the treatment of cardiovascular disease. Pharmacol Res. 2017;125(Pt A):57-71.

[9] Santos RAS, Oudit GY, Verano-Braga T, Canta G, Steckelings UM, Bader M. The renin-angiotensin system: going beyond the classical paradigms. Am J Physiol Heart Circ Physiol. 2019;316(5):H958-Hh70.

[10] Benigni A, Cassis P, Remuzzi G. Angiotensin II revisited: new roles in inflammation, immunology and aging. EMBO Mol Med. 2010;2(7):247-257.

[11] Griendling KK, Minieri CA, Ollerenshaw JD, Alexander RW. Angiotensin II stimulates NADH and NADPH oxidase activity in cultured vascular smooth muscle cells. Circ Res. 1994;74(6):1141-1148.

[12] de Cavanagh EM, Inserra F, Ferder M, Ferder L. From mitochondria to disease: role of the renin-angiotensin system. Am J Nephrol. 2007;27(6): 545-553.

[13] Guilluy C, Brégeon J, Toumaniantz G, Rolli-Derkinderen M, Retailleau K, Loufrani L, et al. The Rho exchange factor Arhgef1 mediates the effects of angiotensin II on vascular tone and blood pressure. Nat Med. 2010;16(2):183-190.

[14] Wirth A, Benyó Z, Lukasova M, Leutgeb B, Wettschureck N, Gorbey S, et al. G12-G13-LARG-mediated signaling in vascular smooth muscle is required for salt-induced hypertension. Nat Med. 2008;14(1):64-68.

[15] Heasman SJ, Ridley AJ. Mammalian Rho GTPases: new insights into their functions from in vivo studies. Nat Rev Mol Cell Biol. 2008;9(9):690-701.

[16] Loirand G, Pacaud P. The role of Rho protein signaling in hypertension. Nat Rev Cardiol. 2010;7(11):637-647.

[17] Bragulat E, de la Sierra A. Salt intake, endothelial dysfunction, and

salt-sensitive hypertension. J Clin Hypertens (Greenwich). 2002;4(1): 41-46.

[18] Hiyama TY, Noda M. Sodium sensing in the subfornical organ and body-fluid homeostasis. Neurosci Res. 2016;113:1-11.

[19] Thomas DD. Breathing new life into nitric oxide signaling: A brief overview of the interplay between oxygen and nitric oxide. Redox Biol. 2015;5:225-233.

[20] Hsu CN, Tain YL. Regulation of Nitric Oxide Production in the Developmental Programming of Hypertension and Kidney Disease. Int J Mol Sci. 2019;20(3).

[21] Kawarazaki W, Fujita T. Role of Rho in Salt-Sensitive Hypertension. Int J Mol Sci. 2021;22(6).

[22] Boegehold MA. The effect of high salt intake on endothelial function: reduced vascular nitric oxide in the absence of hypertension. J Vasc Res. 2013;50(6):458-467.

[23] Valinsky WC, Touyz RM, Shrier A. Aldosterone, SGK1, and ion channels in the kidney. Clin Sci (Lond). 2018; 132(2):173-183.

[24] Satoh N, Nakamura M, Suzuki M, Suzuki A, Seki G, Horita S. Roles of Akt and SGK1 in the Regulation of Renal Tubular Transport. Biomed Res Int. 2015;2015:971697.

[25] Lifton RP, Gharavi AG, Geller DS. Molecular mechanisms of human hypertension. Cell. 2001;104(4): 545-556.

[26] Li J, He Q, Li Q, Huang R, Wei X, Pan X, et al. Decreased expression of Na(+)-H(+) exchanger isoforms 1 and 3 in denervated spontaneously hypertensive rat kidney. Clin Exp Hypertens. 2019;41(3):235-243.

[27] Garty H, Palmer LG. Epithelial sodium channels: function, structure, and regulation. Physiol Rev. 1997;77(2):359-396.

[28] Mu S, Shimosawa T, Ogura S, Wang H, Uetake Y, Kawakami-Mori F, et al. Epigenetic modulation of the renal β-adrenergic-WNK4 pathway in salt-sensitive hypertension. Nat Med. 2011;17(5):573-580.

[29] Furusho T, Uchida S, Sohara E. The WNK signaling pathway and salt-sensitive hypertension. Hypertens Res. 2020;43(8):733-743.

[30] Shibata S, Mu S, Kawarazaki H, Muraoka K, Ishizawa K, Yoshida S, et al. Rac1 GTPase in rodent kidneys is essential for salt-sensitive hypertension via a mineralocorticoid receptor-dependent pathway. J Clin Invest. 2011;121(8):3233-3243.

[31] Blasi ER, Rocha R, Rudolph AE, Blomme EA, Polly ML, McMahon EG. Aldosterone/salt induces renal inflammation and fibrosis in hypertensive rats. Kidney Int. 2003;63(5):1791-1800.

[32] Pitt B, White H, Nicolau J, Martinez F, Gheorghiade M, Aschermann M, et al. Eplerenone reduces mortality 30 days after randomization following acute myocardial infarction in patients with left ventricular systolic dysfunction and heart failure. J Am Coll Cardiol. 2005;46(3):425-431.

[33] Rucker AJ, Rudemiller NP, Crowley SD. Salt, Hypertension, and Immunity. Annu Rev Physiol. 2018;80:283-307.

[34] Wenzel UO, Bode M, Kurts C, Ehmke H. Salt, inflammation, IL-17 and hypertension. Br J Pharmacol. 2019;176(12):1853-1863.

[35] Wilck N, Matus MG, Kearney SM, Olesen SW, Forslund K, Barto

lomaeus H, et al. Salt-responsive gut commensal modulates T(H)17 axis and disease. Nature. 2017;551(7682):585-589.

[36] Hernandez AL, Kitz A, Wu C, Lowther DE, Rodriguez DM, Vudattu N, et al. Sodium chloride inhibits the suppressive function of FOXP3+ regulatory T cells. J Clin Invest. 2015;125(11):4212-4222.

[37] Faraco G, Brea D, Garcia-Bonilla L, Wang G, Racchumi G, Chang H, et al. Dietary salt promotes neurovascular and cognitive dysfunction through a gut-initiated TH17 response. Nat Neurosci. 2018;21(2):240-249.

[38] Kleinewietfeld M, Manzel A, Titze J, Kvakan H, Yosef N, Linker RA, et al. Sodium chloride drives autoimmune disease by the induction of pathogenic TH17 cells. Nature. 2013;496(7446): 518-522.

[39] Mikolajczyk TP, Guzik TJ. Adaptive Immunity in Hypertension. Curr Hypertens Rep. 2019;21(9):68.

[40] Ren J, Crowley SD. Role of T-cell activation in salt-sensitive hypertension. Am J Physiol Heart Circ Physiol. 2019;316(6):H1345-H1h53.

[41] Gleason CE, Frindt G, Cheng CJ, Ng M, Kidwai A, Rashmi P, et al. mTORC2 regulates renal tubule sodium uptake by promoting ENaC activity. J Clin Invest. 2015;125(1):117-128.

[42] Sørensen MV, Saha B, Jensen IS, Wu P, Ayasse N, Gleason CE, et al. Potassium acts through mTOR to regulate its own secretion. JCI Insight. 2019;5(11).

[43] Wynn TA, Chawla A, Pollard JW. Macrophage biology in development, homeostasis and disease. Nature. 2013;496(7446):445-455.

[44] Machnik A, Neuhofer W, Jantsch J, Dahlmann A, Tammela T, Machura K, et al. Macrophages regulate salt-dependent volume and blood pressure by a vascular endothelial growth factor-C-dependent buffering mechanism. Nat Med. 2009;15(5):545-552.

[45] Titze J, Lang R, Ilies C, Schwind KH, Kirsch KA, Dietsch P, et al. Osmotically inactive skin $Na^+$ storage in rats. Am J Physiol Renal Physiol. 2003;285(6):F1108-F1117.

[46] Wiig H, Schröder A, Neuhofer W, Jantsch J, Kopp C, Karlsen TV, et al. Immune cells control skin lymphatic electrolyte homeostasis and blood pressure. J Clin Invest. 2013;123(7): 2803-2815.

[47] Kopp C, Linz P, Dahlmann A, Hammon M, Jantsch J, Müller DN, et al. 23Na magnetic resonance imaging-determined tissue sodium in healthy subjects and hypertensive patients. Hypertension. 2013;61(3):635-640.

[48] Schneider MP, Raff U, Kopp C, Scheppach JB, Toncar S, Wanner C, et al. Skin Sodium Concentration Correlates with Left Ventricular Hypertrophy in CKD. J Am Soc Nephrol. 2017;28(6):1867-1876.

[49] Jantsch J, Schatz V, Friedrich D, Schröder A, Kopp C, Siegert I, et al. Cutaneous $Na^+$ storage strengthens the antimicrobial barrier function of the skin and boosts macrophage-driven host defense. Cell Metab. 2015;21(3):493-501.

[50] Kitada K, Daub S, Zhang Y, Klein JD, Nakano D, Pedchenko T, et al. High salt intake reprioritizes osmolyte and energy metabolism for body fluid conservation. J Clin Invest. 2017;127(5): 1944-1959.

[51] Kim DH, Kim KK, Lee TH, Eom H, Kim JW, Park JW, et al. Transcription Factor TonEBP Stimulates Hyperosmolality-Dependent Arginine Vasopressin Gene Expression in the

Mouse Hypothalamus. Front Endocrinol (Lausanne). 2021;12:627343.

[52] Elijovich F, Laffer CL, Sahinoz M, Pitzer A, Ferguson JF, Kirabo A. The Gut Microbiome, Inflammation, and Salt-Sensitive Hypertension. Curr Hypertens Rep. 2020;22(10):79.

[53] Miranda PM, De Palma G, Serkis V, Lu J, Louis-Auguste MP, McCarville JL, et al. High salt diet exacerbates colitis in mice by decreasing Lactobacillus levels and butyrate production. Microbiome. 2018;6(1):57.

[54] Miyamoto J, Kasubuchi M, Nakajima A, Irie J, Itoh H, Kimura I. The role of short-chain fatty acid on blood pressure regulation. Curr Opin Nephrol Hypertens. 2016;25(5):379-383.

[55] Tang WH, Wang Z, Kennedy DJ, Wu Y, Buffa JA, Agatisa-Boyle B, et al. Gut microbiota-dependent trimethylamine N-oxide (TMAO) pathway contributes to both development of renal insufficiency and mortality risk in chronic kidney disease. Circ Res. 2015;116(3):448-455.

[56] Ge X, Ding C, Zhao W, Xu L, Tian H, Gong J, et al. Antibiotics-induced depletion of mice microbiota induces changes in host serotonin biosynthesis and intestinal motility. J Transl Med. 2017;15(1):13.

[57] Morris G, Berk M, Carvalho A, Caso JR, Sanz Y, Walder K, et al. The Role of the Microbial Metabolites Including Tryptophan Catabolites and Short Chain Fatty Acids in the Pathophysiology of Immune-Inflammatory and Neuroimmune Disease. Mol Neurobiol. 2017;54(6):4432-4451.

[58] O'Mahony SM, Clarke G, Borre YE, Dinan TG, Cryan JF. Serotonin, tryptophan metabolism and the brain-gut-microbiome axis. Behav Brain Res. 2015;277:32-48.

[59] Cole-Jeffrey CT, Liu M, Katovich MJ, Raizada MK, Shenoy V. ACE2 and Microbiota: Emerging Targets for Cardiopulmonary Disease Therapy. J Cardiovasc Pharmacol. 2015;66(6):540-550.

[60] Perlot T, Penninger JM. ACE2 - from the renin-angiotensin system to gut microbiota and malnutrition. Microbes Infect. 2013;15(13): 866-873.

[61] Gheblawi M, Wang K, Viveiros A, Nguyen Q, Zhong JC, Turner AJ, et al. Angiotensin-Converting Enzyme 2: SARS-CoV-2 Receptor and Regulator of the Renin-Angiotensin System: Celebrating the 20th Anniversary of the Discovery of ACE2. Circ Res. 2020;126(10):1456-1474.

[62] Kishi T, Hirooka Y. Oxidative stress in the brain causes hypertension via sympathoexcitation. Front Physiol. 2012;3:335.

[63] Noda M, Hiyama TY. Sodium sensing in the brain. Pflugers Arch. 2015;467(3):465-474.

[64] Nomura K, Nakanishi M, Ishidate F, Iwata K, Taruno A. All-Electrical Ca(2+)-Independent Signal Transduction Mediates Attractive Sodium Taste in Taste Buds. Neuron. 2020;106(5):816-29.e6.

[65] Huang BS, Van Vliet BN, Leenen FH. Increases in CSF [Na$^+$] precede the increases in blood pressure in Dahl S rats and SHR on a high-salt diet. Am J Physiol Heart Circ Physiol. 2004;287(3):H1160-H1166.

[66] Watanabe U, Shimura T, Sako N, Kitagawa J, Shingai T, Watanabe E, et al. A comparison of voluntary salt-intake behavior in Nax-gene deficient and wild-type mice with reference to peripheral taste inputs. Brain Res. 2003;967(1-2):247-256.

[67] Fu Y, Vallon V. Mineralocorticoid-induced sodium appetite and renal salt retention: evidence for common signaling and effector mechanisms. Nephron Physiol. 2014;128(1-2):8-16.

[68] Sakamoto T, Fujii A, Saito N, Kondo H, Ohuchi A. Alteration of amiloride-sensitive salt taste nerve responses in aldosterone/NaCl-induced hypertensive rats. Neurosci Res. 2016;108:60-66.

[69] Esler M, Eikelis N, Schlaich M, Lambert G, Alvarenga M, Dawood T, et al. Chronic mental stress is a cause of essential hypertension: presence of biological markers of stress. Clin Exp Pharmacol Physiol. 2008;35(4):498-502.

[70] Chen D, Jancovski N, Bassi JK, Nguyen-Huu TP, Choong YT, Palma-Rigo K, et al. Angiotensin type 1A receptors in C1 neurons of the rostral ventrolateral medulla modulate the pressor response to aversive stress. J Neurosci. 2012;32(6):2051-2061.

[71] Shigemura N, Iwata S, Yasumatsu K, Ohkuri T, Horio N, Sanematsu K, et al. Angiotensin II modulates salty and sweet taste sensitivities. J Neurosci. 2013;33(15):6267-6277.

[72] Lacagnina S. The Developmental Origins of Health and Disease (DOHaD). Am J Lifestyle Med. 2020;14(1):47-50.

[73] Baserga M, Kaur R, Hale MA, Bares A, Yu X, Callaway CW, et al. Fetal growth restriction alters transcription factor binding and epigenetic mechanisms of renal 11beta-hydroxysteroid dehydrogenase type 2 in a sex-specific manner. Am J Physiol Regul Integr Comp Physiol. 2010;299(1):R334-R342.

[74] Zhang D, Yu ZY, Cruz P, Kong Q, Li S, Kone BC. Epigenetics and the control of epithelial sodium channel expression in collecting duct. Kidney Int. 2009;75(3):260-267.

[75] Morinaga Y, Tsuchihashi T, Ohta Y, Matsumura K. Salt intake in 3-year-old Japanese children. Hypertens Res. 2011;34(7):836-839.

[76] Intersalt: an international study of electrolyte excretion and blood pressure. Results for 24 hour urinary sodium and potassium excretion. Intersalt Cooperative Research Group. BMJ. 1988;297(6644):319-28.

[77] Fujita T, Ando K. Hemodynamic and endocrine changes associated with potassium supplementation in sodium-loaded hypertensives. Hypertension. 1984;6(2 Pt 1):184-192.

[78] Eaton SB, Eaton SB, 3rd, Konner MJ, Shostak M. An evolutionary perspective enhances understanding of human nutritional requirements. J Nutr. 1996;126(6):1732-1740.

[79] Whelton PK, He J, Cutler JA, Brancati FL, Appel LJ, Follmann D, et al. Effects of oral potassium on blood pressure. Meta-analysis of randomized controlled clinical trials. JAMA. 1997;277(20):1624-1632.

[80] Akita S, Sacks FM, Svetkey LP, Conlin PR, Kimura G. Effects of the Dietary Approaches to Stop Hypertension (DASH) diet on the pressure-natriuresis relationship. Hypertension. 2003;42(1):8-13.

[81] Appel LJ, Moore TJ, Obarzanek E, Vollmer WM, Svetkey LP, Sacks FM, et al. A clinical trial of the effects of dietary patterns on blood pressure. DASH Collaborative Research Group. N Engl J Med. 1997;336(16):1117-1124.

[82] 82. Umemura S, Arima H, Arima S, Asayama K, Dohi Y, Hirooka Y, et al. The Japanese Society of Hypertension Guidelines for the Management of

Hypertension (JSH 2019). Hypertens Res. 2019;42(9):1235-1481.

[83] Kanno Y, Kanda E, Kato A. Methods and Nutritional Interventions to Improve the Nutritional Status of Dialysis Patients in JAPAN-A Narrative Review. Nutrients. 2021;13(5).

Chapter 11

# Effect of Lifestyle Modification on Glycemic Control of Type 2 Diabetic Patients at Suez Canal University Hospitals

*Fatma Ibrahim Abdel-Latif Megahed,*
*Salwa Abbas Ali Hassan, Hassan Ali Abdelwahid*
*and Hanaa Kassem Farg*

## Abstract

Type 2 Diabetes mellitus, as one of the major universal public health disorders wide spread, requires patients' lifestyle modulation which would be conducive in dominating blood glucose. The aim of the study was to evaluate the effect of lifestyle modification on glycemic control of type 2 diabetic patients at Suez Canal University Hospitals at Ismailia city. A quasi-experimental design made up of a control group and a study group with pre- and post-test administration was applied. This study was carried out at the Family Medicine Outpatient Clinic and the Diabetic Outpatient Clinic of Suez Canal University Hospitals at Ismailia city in Egypt. 92 type 2 diabetic patients were included in this study. The Diabetes Knowledge Questionnaire; Health promoting lifestyle profile II Scale; and Physical assessment sheet were used for data collection in the two groups. After implementing of the program, those patients who received lifestyle modification intervention achieved better total score of knowledge & knowledge related practice about DM, health promoting lifestyle domains values and glycated hemoglobin, compared with the control group. Factors related to lower glycated hemoglobin in the present study were lower fasting blood sugar level and increasing physical activity. Overall, lifestyle modification program has a positive influence on blood glucose control of patients with type 2 diabetes mellitus. Therefore, it is recommended to that lifestyle modification interventions should be integral part of the curative management of type 2 diabetic patients, and further study in other places to investigate the effect of lifestyle modification on glycemic control of those patients.

**Keywords:** "lifestyle modification", "type 2 diabetes mellitus", and "glycemic control"

## 1. Introduction

Diabetes Mellitus (DM) is one of the widespread and universal health problems that affect many people worldwide. It is defined as a metabolic disorder caused by different factors, which is characterized by hyperglycemia (elevated blood glucose level) and is usually associated with carbohydrate, fat and protein metabolism abnormalities [1]. There are two main types of DM: Type 1diabetes mellitus (T1DM) and Type 2 diabetes mellitus (T2DM). T2DM is the commonest form of diabetes, constituting nearly 90% of the diabetic patients in any country [2].

Type 2 diabetes mellitus is a heterogeneous and progressive illness, with an underlying mechanism ranging from predominantly insulin resistance with relative insulin deficiency, to predominantly an insulin secretory defect with lesser degrees of insulin resistance. The spread of T2DM is increasing all over the world, probably due to the expectations of population's long life, a sedentary lifestyle and above all, the increasing rates of obesity. There are two sub-divisions of T2DM. The "Not Insulin Requiring" diabetes, managed by lifestyle measures alone and sometimes oral drugs, and the "Insulin requiring for diabetes control", where insulin is required to control, rather than survival [3].

A recent study proved that the uncontrolled diabetes, particularly elevated blood sugar over a prolonged period of time could lead to a number of short and long-term health complications. Such complications were divided traditionally into two main subtypes: the diabetes specific micro-vascular complications of retinopathy, nephropathy, and neuropathy which were caused by injuries to the small blood vessels; and the thrombotic macro-vascular complications of myocardial infraction, hypertension, and peripheral arterial disease which were presented due to arterial damage [4].

Many chronic diseases, as proved by recent studies, are associated with poor lifestyle and unwise human conduct. Lifestyle is an individual's typical way of life which includes activities and attitudes that influence man's health, whether healthy or unhealthy. A healthy lifestyle often results in better health and happiness. In contrast, an unhealthy lifestyle may cause illness and morbidity. Lifestyle related risk factors are associated with the development and progression of T2DM. These risk factors such as sedentary lifestyle, smoking, alcohol consumption, dietary choices and overweight are modifiable. The cornerstone of DM management includes appropriate lifestyle choices supported by regular medication and blood glucose self-monitoring, where necessary [5, 6].

The core of Type 2 diabetes mellitus treatment depends mainly on physical activity and nutrition therapy. The recent studies have proved the benefits of physical activity on individuals who maintain a physically active lifestyle and therefore, they are less likely to develop insulin resistance, impaired glucose tolerance, or T2DM. The effects of exercise training on glycemic control and related physiological parameters have also been extensively studied in type 2 diabetic patients. On the same line, healthy nutrition is the basis for the treatment of T2DM. It positively maintains blood glucose to be within normal limits and effectively minimizes the complications of the T2DM and weight loss is also an important goal because it improves glycemic control [7, 8].

The community health nurse had an effective role in patient education about all newly lifestyle modification for T2DM. No matter that encouraging and supporting lifestyle modifications could help in enabling type 2 diabetic patients to feel more satisfied in controlling of their disease. Pender's health promotion model (HPM) is one of the widely used models to plan for changing unhealthy behaviors and promote general hygiene. Pender's model was developed after the health belief model, to assist nurses in understanding the major determinants of health behaviors as a basis for behavioral counseling to promote healthy lifestyles. According to Pender's model, health promotion is a dynamic and positive process that encompasses conducts supporting a healthy lifestyle, including physical activity, dieting, spiritual growth, interpersonal relationships, health responsibility, and stress management. In nutshell, a health-promoting lifestyle is a multi-dimensional pattern of voluntary behaviors needed for promoting one's health conditions, self- growth, and perfection [9].

Moreover, a great importance should be paid for the patients' regular follow-up with the health care provider so as to avert any long-term complications. In diabetes Mellitus care, lifestyle modification can prevent or delay the complications and also decrease the need for medication. Because of the alarming and danger threaten DM statistics, the sacred role of nurses in assisting patients to control associated morbidity and mortality is becoming increasingly significant. Nurses, who are always on the front line, can screen patients for early diabetes identification, recognize and initiate corrective measures for inadequate treatment regimens, help patients set and achieve therapeutic goals and assess diabetes-related complications as soon as they arise [10]. DM, as a chronic disease, often has a relapsing and remitting course with substantial impact on function and quality of life (QOL). For chronic illnesses where there is no cure, it is important to establish that therapy which really makes people feel better.

## 1.1 Diabetes mellitus

### *1.1.1 Definition*

Diabetes Mellitus (DM) is a complex, chronic disease that caused by inherited and/or acquired deficiency in production of insulin by the pancreas or by the ineffectiveness of the insulin produced; both require continuous medical care with multifactor risk-reduction strategies beyond glycemic control. It is defined as a metabolic disorder caused by different factors and is characterized by hyperglycemia (elevated level of blood glucose) with disturbances in carbohydrate, fat and protein metabolism. The chronic hyperglycemia is associated with long-term damage, dysfunction and degeneration/deterioration of various organs, particularly eyes, kidney, nerves, heart and blood vessels [8, 11].

### *1.1.2 Etiologic classification of DM*

This classification includes four types:(1) Type 1 diabetes mellitus (T1DM), (2) Type 2 diabetes mellitus (T2DM), (3) Other specific forms of diabetes: Genetic defects of beta cell function; Genetic defects of insulin function; exocrine pancreatic diseases; Endocrinopathies; drugs and chemicals; infections; rare immunologic forms of diabetes; other genetic syndromes associated with diabetes; Latent autoimmune diabetes in adults (LADA); Maturity-onset diabetes of the young (MODY) and (4) Gestational diabetes mellitus (GDM) [8].

The majority of cases of diabetes can be broadly classified into 2categories: T1DM– autoimmune which is primarily a result of pancreatic beta cell destruction with consequent insulin deficiency, which is prone to ketoacidos is. This form includes cases due to an autoimmune process and those for which the etiology of beta cell destruction is unknown; T2DM – may range from predominant insulin resistance with relative insulin deficiency to a predominant secretory defect with insulin resistance. Ketosis is not as common. GDM refers to glucose intolerance with onset or first recognition during pregnancy. Other specific types include a wide variety of relatively uncommon conditions, primarily specific genetically defined forms of diabetes or diabetes associated with other diseases or drug use [12].

### *1.1.3 Latent autoimmune diabetes in adults*

Latent autoimmune diabetes in adults (LADA) is a late manifesting autoimmune form of diabetes in adults, most commonly diagnosed in patients above35years of age, characterized by clinical insulin independence in the first months after the diagnosis, with the presence of serum antibodies against glutamic acid decarboxylase (anti-GAD65) and/or other anti-islet antibodies and a low serum peptide C level. LADA is a form of T1DM with slowly progressive autoimmune-mediated destruction of beta cells. This diabetes subtype is present in 5–10% of subjects with diabetes diagnosed after 35 years of age and categorized asT2DM. Clinical manifestations of LADA do not always allow a definite diagnosis, presenting diagnostic challenges when differentiating with T2DM. A definite diagnosis of LADA requires identification of auto-antibodies typical for T1DM, mostly antiGAD65, and/or a low serum peptide C level [13].

#### *1.1.4 Monogenic diabetes*

Monogenic diabetes amounts to 1–2% of all diabetes cases. It is caused by single gene mutations. Most forms are associated with a defect of insulin secretion, and the most common ones are maturity-onset diabetes of the young (MODY), mitochondrial diabetes, and neonatal diabetes. Considering the monogenic forms in the differential diagnosis of diabetes may contribute to treatment optimization and proper evaluation of prognosis in the patient and his family members. A definite diagnosis of monogenic diabetes is a result of genetic testing. The most common form of MODY is associated with HNF1A and glucokinase gene mutations [13].

Typical clinical presentation of MODY due to an HNF1Agene mutation includes: (1) Early onset of diabetes (typically before 25 years of age; (2) No insulin dependence and keto acidosis, low insulin requirement, detectable peptide C levels despite the disease being present for several years or even longer; (3) Diabetic family history over at least 2 generations, with early-onset diabetes in at least two family members. OGTT performed at an early stage of diabetes usually shows high postprandial glucose level elevation with often normal fasting blood glucose; (4) Absence of auto antibodies typical for T1DM; and (5) Glycosuria higher than expected based on blood glucose levels [13].

### 1.2 Type 2 diabetes mellitus

#### *1.2.1 Type 2 diabetes mellitus (T2DM)*

It is universally known that Type 2 diabetes mellitus is considered a modern-day epidemic of epic proportions, affecting all classes of the society. The prevalence is becoming alarmingly high among younger age groups. Global prevalence of diabetes mellitus is about 9%. The prevalence of diabetes is expected to double by 2030 from 8.3 to 17.6% globally, excluding the high numbers of undiagnosed cases estimated as 175 million. Approximately 1.9% of the global disability adjusted life years (DALY) is attributed to diabetes. The International Diabetes Federation (IDF) estimates that 450 million people are living with diabetes, with 5.1million dying from it annually worldwide. T2DM is the greatest contributor to the burden of diabetes globally accounting for up to 90% of people with diabetes worldwide [14].

T2DM is a chronic and progressive medical condition which results from two major metabolic dysfunctions: insulin resistance and a relative insulin deficiency. Insulin resistance in which clinical signs may include: acanthosisnigricans–characterized by hyper pigmentation (darkening of skin pigment) especially in the neck and axillae; skin tags – benign (non-cancerous) skin growths on the body or face; central obesity – defined by a high waist-to-hip ratio, waist-to-thigh ratio and waist circumference; menstrual irregularities; and hirsutism– excess facial and body hair, especially on women. A relative insulin deficiency in which chronic hyperglycemia with multiple disturbances in carbohydrate, protein and fat metabolism develops when a person's beta cell function is no longer sufficient to meet his/her insulin requirement [15].

### 1.3 Risk factors of T2DM

Several factors contribute to the high incidence of DM, such as population growth rate, ageing population, age structures, urbanization, unhealthy diet habits, obesity, sedentary lifestyles, lack of physical activities, failure to access to healthcare facilities both in rural and urban areas in addition to the economic and health transition of the country. Moreover, the increased case of DM is also triggered by the positive family history of the disease [16]. The literature reveals three interrelated spheres of risk factors that contribute to the development of T2DM: (1) genetics, (2) environment or lifestyle, and (3) metabolic abnormalities. It is imperative to implement appropriate interventions for the prevention and treatment of T2DM among adult patients, where there is an understanding of the risk factors predisposing adults to this disease [17].

#### *1.3.1 Genetic factors*

Although research has not clarified a single gene that is alone responsible for the development of T2DM, there are many findings in literature that support the genetic hypothesis. Higher concordance rates are found among identical (96%) than dizygotic twins in some but not all twin studies which have been a compelling evidence of a significant genetic component in T2DM. Moreover, 40% of first-degree relatives of T2DM patients may develop diabetes, whereas the incident rate is only 6% in the general population [5].

- Environmental or lifestyle factors:

  There are a wide range of lifestyle factors which are of great importance to the development of T2DM disease, such as smoking, alcohol consumption, physical inactivity, obesity, obstructive sleep apnea, unhealthy diet (dietary fiber (a low-fiber diet with a high glycemic index), dietary fat (total and saturated fat intake) and frequent consumption of processed meat [5].

- Metabolic abnormalities or changes:

  A recent study proved that resistance to insulin was the underlying abnormality in most people who develop T2DM. Such resistance resulted from an interaction between both genetic and environmental factors. Those factors were associated with the development of insulin resistance. The initial reaction of the beta cells was to increase output of insulin in order to overcome the insulin resistance and to maintain normal blood glucose levels. Unless insulin resistance was reversed, hyper secretion of insulin was insufficient to maintain normoglycemia indefinitely and progression to the states of impaired glucose metabolism (impaired fasting glucose (IFG), impaired glucose tolerance (IGT) and eventually T2DM) [18].

### 1.4 Pathophysiology of T2DM

The main pathophysiological cause of T2DM is the failure of pancreatic beta cells which leads to inadequate secretion of insulin and increased insulin resistance which refers to decreased tissue (especially the liver, adipose tissues and muscle) sensitivity to insulin. Normally, insulin binds to special receptors on cell surfaces and initiates a series of reactions involved in glucose metabolism. In T2DM; intracellular reactions are diminished, making insulin less effective at stimulating glucose uptake by the liver. Physical inactivity and obesity lead to insulin resistance, increased production of glucose by the liver and decreased glucose uptake in skeletal muscles. In order to compensate beta cells, increase insulin secretion, but the progressive failure of beta cells leads to hyperglycemia and finally T2DM [19, 20].

The inappropriately increased alpha-cell function and consequent hyperglucagonemia, in addition to insulin resistance and beta cell dysfunction, they all have long contributed to hyperglycemia in diabetic patients, by stimulating hepatic glucose production. In fasting state, hyperglycemia is directly related to increase hepatic glucose production while in postprandial state, hyperglycemia results from the combination of insufficient suppression to glucose output and defective insulin stimulation of glucose disposal in target tissues, mainly skeletal muscles. Anti-hyperglycemic agents are directed to one or more of the pathophysiological defects of T2DM; they modify physiological processes related to appetite, nutrient absorption or excretion [21, 22].

### 1.5 Clinical manifestation of T2DM

It is almost traditionally known that classic symptoms of diabetes are polyuria (the need to urinate frequently), polydipsia (increased thirst & fluid intake), polyphagia (increased appetite) and weight loss and the symptoms that may provide cause for testing T2DM include increased thirst or urination, numbing of extremities, impotence, blurred vision and fatigue [23]. Other symptoms that are commonly present at diagnosis include; a history of blurred vision, itchiness, peripheral neuropathy, recurrent vaginal infections, poor healing skin wounds and fatigue. Patients with T2DM may rarely present with non-ketonic hyperosmolar coma, a condition of very high blood sugar associated with a decreased level of consciousness and low blood pressure. Many people however have no symptoms during the first few years which are diagnosed on routine testing [24].

### 1.6 Diagnosis of T2DM

The diagnostic criteria for diabetes mellitus are at least one of the following: [1] Glycated hemoglobin test (HbA1c) $\geq$ 6.5%. That test should be performed in a laboratory using the National Glycohemoglobin Standardization Program (NGSP) method which was certified by the NGSP standardized to the Diabetes Control and Complications Trial (DCCT) assay; [2] The Fasting Plasma Glucose Test (FPG) $\geq$ 126 mg/dl. Fasting is defined as no caloric intake for at least 8h; [3] 2-hour plasma glucose $\geq$ 200 mg/dl during an Oral Glucose Tolerance Test (OGTT). This test should be performed as described by the WHO, using a glucose load containing the equivalent of 75 g, anhydrous glucose dissolved in water; or [4]. In a patient with classic symptoms of hyperglycemia (polyuria, polydipsia, weight loss) or hyperglycemic crisis (Diabetic ketoacidosis (DKA), Hyperglycemic Hyperosmolar State (HHS)), a random plasma glucose $\geq$200mg/dL (11.1mmol/L). In the absence of unequivocal hyperglycemia, results should be confirmed by repeat testing [25].

### 1.7 Complications of T2DM

T2DM is considered as one of the most leading causes of premature morbidity and mortality worldwide as a result of the long-term micro vascular and macro vascular complications associated with this disease. For instance, diabetic retinopathy is the most leading cause of blindness among adults aged 20-74 years; diabetic nephropathy, which affects approximately 40% of type 2 diabetic patients, is the leading cause of chronic kidney disease in patients starting replacement therapy; and diabetic neuropathy, which affects up to 50% of individuals with diabetes, increases the risk of foot ulcers and limb amputation [26].

In fact, more than 80% of non-traumatic limb amputations follow a foot ulcer or injury, and the risk of amputation in individuals with diabetes is up to 25 times greater compared with patients without diabetes. Although micro vascular complications increase morbidity and lead to premature mortality, the major cause of death in individuals with diabetes is cardiovascular disease (CVD), which in turn accounts for approximately 65% of all diabetes-related deaths. For example, transient ischemic attacks are 2-6 times more common in patients with T2DM, while the risk of developing heart failure is a startling 2- to 8-fold higher [26].

The sudden development of short-term complications, such as hyperglycemic crisis (DKA, HHS and severe hypoglycemia) that can lead to coma and, if untreated, death, are a daily threat to the many people worldwide with diabetes who have major difficulty in accessing essential treatment supplies (including insulin) [27].

Recent studies have shed the light on "hypoglycemia" (blood glucose < 3.9 mmol/L or 70 mg/dL) as a common unwanted effect in people treated with insulin and occurs when there is an imbalance in insulin dose, food consumed and activity. Usually the condition is manageable, but occasionally, it can be severe or even life threatening, particularly if the patient fails to recognize the symptoms, especially while continuing to take insulin or other hypoglycemic drugs. The signs of hypoglycemia can vary from person to person and may occur suddenly such as: hunger, perspiration, rapid heartbeat, weakness, feeling sleepy, feeling drunk, difficulty speaking, trembling, dizziness, confusion, and anxiety [28, 29].

DKA results from absolute insulin insufficiency, leading to metabolic acidosis (pH <7.3), hyperglycemia (blood glucose >11 mmol/L). DKA may also be present in up to 25% of young people presenting with T2DM. DKA should be treated as a medical emergency by an experienced medical team [30]. Hyperglycemic Hyperosmolar Non ketonic Syndrome (HHNS) usually occurs with T2DM and can occur with T1DM. It is often triggered by a serious infection, another severe illness, or by medications that lower glucose tolerance or increase fluid loss (especially in people who are not drinking enough fluids). Symptoms of HHNS include; high blood sugar levels, dry mouth, extreme thirst, dry skin and high fever. HHNS leads to loss of consciousness, seizures, coma and death [31].

No doubt, early detection and good glycemic control can slow the progression of the acute and chronic complications of DM, which cause significant mortality and morbidity in both developing and developed countries. Such chronic complications of DM if once developed are irreversible except by early detection and management [4].

### 1.8 Management of T2DM

Both patients and health care professionals are partners in managing T2DM, in which the health professionals support the patients in self-managing their disease. Management of every patient should start with a detailed evaluation of the initial diagnosis including diabetes complications and its risk factors. This, of course, provides basis for continuing treatment plan, treatment administration, monitoring, and review [32]. The main goals of treatment of DM are to reduce complications through control of glycaemia, blood pressure, macro vascular (i.e., coronary,

| S.no | Category | Examples |
|---|---|---|
| 1 | Sulfonylureas First generation | Acetohexamide,Chlorpropamide, Tolbutamide, Tolzamide |
| | Second generation | Glyburide,Glimepiride Glipizide. |
| 2 | Biguanides | Metformin |
| 3 | Meglitinides | Repaglinide,Nataglinide |
| 4 | Thiazolidinediones | Pioglitazone,Rosiglitazone |
| 5 | Alpha-glucosidase Inhibitors | Acorbose, Miglitol |
| 6 | Glucagon like peptide-1-agonist | Exenatide, Liraglutide |
| 7 | Amylinomimetics | Pramlintide acetate |

**Table 1.**
*Oral antihyperglycemic agents for T2DM [35].*

cerebrovascular, peripheral vascular), control of lipids, hypertension and smoking cessation. Metabolic and neurological complications can be reduced through control of glycaemia [33].

The treatment of hyperglycemia should start with the establishment of a target HbA1c that, in most cases, will be ≤ 7.0%, as this has been shown to reduce long-term microvascular complications in newly diagnosed patients with T2DM. HbA1c targets may be higher (up to 8.5%) if the benefits of intensive glycemic control are unlikely to outweigh the risks and burden, such as in individuals with limited life expectancy, high risk of hypoglycemia, multimorbidity, or based on the values and preferences of the person with diabetes. It should be emphasized to people with T2DM that reductions in HbA1c levels are associated with better outcomes even if recommended glycemic targets cannot be reached, and inability to achieve HbA1c target should not be considered a treatment failure [34].

If the level of HbA1c at diagnosis is less than 1.5% above target and the person with T2DM, lacks metabolic decompensate and/or symptoms of hyperglycemia, the first step of treatment should be healthy lifestyle conduct. If healthy behavior interventions are insufficient to achieve target HbA1c levels within 3 months, they should be combined with oral antihyperglycemic medications (**Table 1**) [35].

In the face of significant hyperglycemia (i.e., HbA1c >1.5% above target), pharmacotherapy is usually required at diagnosis concurrent with healthy behavior interventions. People who have evidence of metabolic decompensation (e.g., marked hyperglycemia, ketosis or unintentional weight loss) and/or symptomatic hyperglycemia should be started immediately on insulin, regardless of HbA1c level. Insulin may later be tapered or discontinued once stability is achieved [34].

## 2. Glycemic control

Glycemic control is extremely fundamental to the management of T2DM. Diabetes management aims to delay the onset of disease complications, and to hinder its progression, mostly by improving glycemic control and controlling the risk of cardiovascular disease. Previous studies have provided evidence of the power of good glycemic control to restrict the micro-vascular and macro-vascular complications of diabetes [36].

### 2.1 Assessment of glycemic control

Glycemic control is a very important instrument that prevents or delays the complications associated with DM, such as peripheral vascular disease, vision loss, and renal failure. There are two primary techniques available for both health providers and patients to assess effectiveness of management plan on glycemic control: patient self-monitoring of blood glucose (SMBG) and HbA1c [37].

### *2.1.1 Self-monitoring of blood glucose (SMBG)*

The first primary technique to assess the effectiveness of glycemic control plan for diabetic patients is the self-monitoring of blood glucose since most people with diabetes get benefit from monitoring of blood glucose for a various reasons. SMBG is the optimal way to confirm and appropriately treat hypoglycemia. It can provide feedback on the results of healthy behavior interventions and antihyperglycemic pharmacological treatments. It can increase patient's empowerment and adherence to treatment. It can also provide information to both the diabetic patient and the diabetes health-care team to facilitate longer-term treatment modifications and titrations as well as shorter-term treatment decisions, such as insulin dosing for people with T1DM or T2DM. Finally, in situations where HbA1c does not accurately reflect glycaemia, monitoring of blood glucose is necessary to monitor glycaemia adequately [38].

For people with T2DM treated with healthy behavior interventions, with or without non-insulin antihyperglycemic agents, the effectiveness and frequency of monitoring of blood glucose in improving glycemic control is less clear. The evidence is less certain in people with T2DM treated with insulin, although the above principle likely applies. In a large, non-randomized study of individuals with stable T2DM using insulin, testing at least 3 times a day was associated with improved glycemic control [38].

### *2.1.2 Glycated hemoglobin (HbA1c)*

Glycated hemoglobin (HbA1c) can be used as a diagnostic test for diabetes providing that strict quality assurance tests. An HbA1c of 6.5% is recommended as the cut point for diagnosing diabetes. A value of less than 6.5% does not exclude diabetes diagnosed using glucose tests. HbA1c is a reliable estimate of mean plasma glucose levels over the previous 8 to 12 weeks. The mean blood glucose level in the 30 days immediately preceding the blood sampling (days 0 to 30) contributes 50% of the result and the prior 90 to 120 days contributes 10%. HbA1c is a valuable indicator of treatment effectiveness and should be measured at least every 3 months when glycemic targets are not being met and when diabetes therapy is being adjusted or changed. It is a measure of long-term blood glucose concentration and is not affected by acute changes in glucose levels due to stress or illness. Testing at 6-month intervals may be considered in situations where glycemic targets are consistently achieved. In some circumstances, such as when significant changes are made to therapy, or during pregnancy, it is appropriate to check HbA1c more frequently [38].

An appropriate level of HbA1c is difficult to define exactly; therefore Target HbA1c should be defined based on personal assessment of risks and benefits of treatment. The factors limiting the benefit of tight control are co-morbidities (e.g., end-stage cancer, severe heart failure), advanced diabetes complications (e.g., proliferative retinopathy, renal failure), inability to safely carry out treatment regimen, and limited life expectancy; or factors that heighten the risk of tight control: history of severe hypoglycemia (inability to treat without assistance), hypoglycemia unawareness and advanced cardiovascular or cerebrovascular disease, in addition to autonomic neuropathy (especially cardiac), comorbidities that impair the detection of hypoglycemia (e.g., alteration in mental status, alcoholism, etc...), and/or poor social support [39].

Patients who do not have any of these factors possibly would generally have a target HbA1c of ≤ 7%. Patients who do have one or more of these factors should have a goal of minimizing symptoms of hyperglycemia and to control glucose as well as possible without incurring side effects or excessive treatment burden; while an appropriate HbA1c is difficult to define exactly, treatment should be aimed to keep the HbA1c under 9% [39].

### 2.2 Type 2 diabetes mellitus lifestyle modification

Lifestyle modification or modification of unhealthy lifestyle choices such as: physical inactivity, unhealthy diet, harmful use of tobacco and/or alcohols can reduce the risk of complications and premature death of T2DM, by contributing to a better glycemic control. At diagnosis, highly motivated patients with HbA1c levels (<7.5%) could be given opportunity to engage in lifestyle modification for 3-6 months before staring pharmacotherapy. Encouraging and supporting people to make the best choices about their health can lead to a real difference to people's quality of life. Some studies have conclusively shown that reducing hyperglycemia decreases the onset and progression of microvascular complications and individualized dietary plan, regular physical activity and weight loss, when required, have been recognized as key components of diabetes management [22, 40].

The required lifestyle changes in managing DM are influenced by patient's knowledge, attitudes, practices, culture and values. Lack of knowledge about diabetes has been identified as one of the barriers to self-management of diabetes. Lack of understanding of how to manage diabetes also has a significant impact on limited diabetes knowledge in this population. Lifestyle modification counseling or education is the key component to achieve good glycemic control, to reduce the risk of diabetes complications, improve self-management and enhance the quality of life of type 2 diabetic patients including medical nutrition therapy, regular physical activity, weight reduction, and diabetes self-management education and support. Lifestyle interventions with oral hypoglycemic agents are often effective [8, 41].

### 2.3 Components of the lifestyle modification program

#### *2.3.1 Medical nutrition therapy (MNT) for T2DM*

Type 2 diabetic patients should consult a registered dietician (RD) to know about nutrition therapy for managing DM. MNT for type 2 diabetic patients encourages meal choices based on the patient's own needs and preferences, while awareness of the importance of dietary control promotes planning of meals and adherence to dietary regimen. There are some of the general dietary guidelines to follow to help manage diabetes are not to skip meals, to evenly distribute the meals throughout the day in small portions and to have a diet low in saturated fat [42, 43].

The goals of MNT include improving control of blood glucose levels, lipid profiles, and blood pressure to reduce the risk of cardiovascular disease in patients with T2DM through implementing lifestyle changes which reduce intakes of energy, saturated and trans fatty acids, cholesterol, and sodium and increase physical activity. Achieving these goals requires the dietitian and other professionals to teach and otherwise assist type 2 diabetic patients to modify or manage their nutritional intake in the light of a variety of individual factors such as: medication, exercise. Plasma glucose monitoring can be used to determine whether adjustments to foods and meals will be sufficient to achieve glycemic control or if medication(s) needs to be combined with MNT. MNT has been shown to reduce glycosylated hemoglobin (HbA1c) by 1% to 2% in patients with T2DM [44].

## 2.4 Diet composition

### *2.4.1 Carbohydrates (CHO) in T2DM management*

Type 2 diabetic patients are persuaded to keep track of the amount of CHO they eat. The amount and the type of CHO ingested usually affects postprandial response. The recommended daily allowance (RDA) for CHO (130 g/day) is an average minimum requirement but less than 130 g/day of CHO is not recommended because the brain and central nervous system have an absolute requirement for glucose as an energy source. About 45-60 grams of carbohydrate can be consumed at a meal. Perhaps more or less CHO needed at meal depending on how diabetes is being managed [37].

Carbohydrate intake should be from sources like: fruits, vegetables, whole grains, lentils and legumes, and low-fat dairyproducts. However, carbohydrates should not be avoided completely as carbohydrate containing food is also a good source of fiber, vitamins and minerals which are extremely essential for the proper functioning of the body [45].

### *2.4.2 Glycemic index(GI)*

Glycemic Index concept has best described the type of CHO. Researchers developed the GI of food to compare the physiologic or postprandial effects of carbohydrates (usually 50 g carbohydrate portion) on glucose. Glucose is given a value of 100; other CHOs are given a number relative to glucose. A ranking system indicates how quickly CHO food raises blood glucose15level. The higher the blood glucose responses, the higher the GI ranks carbohydrate foods according to their effect on blood glucose levels. GI ranges, in general: low GI foods < 55, intermediate GI foods 55 – 70, and high GI foods > 70. Foods with low glycemic indexes such as: oats, barely, lentils, beans, fiber... etc., Substituting high GI foods with lower GI foods at mealtime reduces postprandial blood glucose [46]. Detailed lists can be found in the International Tables of Glycemic Index and Glycemic Load Values [47].

### *2.4.3 Dietary fiber*

It is scientifically well known that fibers are non-digestible carbohydrates. Soluble fibers help to slow down the digestion of starches and absorption of glucose. Example: fruit pectin (guava, apples, and plums), oats fiber, and legume fiber (beans & lentils). Some studies proved that consuming a high-fiber diet (50 g fiber/day) improves the postprandial glycemic response, reduces hyperinsulinemia, and lipemia in type 2 diabetic patients. Dietary Reference Intakes (DRI) recommended consumption of 14 g dietary fiber per 1000 kcal (or 25 g for adult women and 38 g for adult men) based on epidemiologic studies but usual fiber intake (up to 24 g daily) not shown to have beneficial effects on glycaemia. Good sources of fibers are: whole grain cereals, fruits, vegetables, beans and peas. Whole grains (contains the entire grain seed, bran, germ & endosperm) are not associated with improved glycemic control but may reduce systemic inflammation. The diabetic patient should consume at least half of all grains as whole grains [48, 49].

### *2.4.4 Nutritive and non-nutritive (calorie-free) sweeteners*

Nutritive sweeteners contain sucrose and fructose. Sucrose (table sugar), a disaccharide-containing glucose and sucrose-containing foods have proven not to have a significant effect on glycemic levels of diabetic patients and therefore, do not need to be restricted but fat ingested with sucrose (ice cream) will increase calories. Fructose produces a lower postprandial glucose response when it replaces sucrose or starch in the diet; however, fructose may adversely affect plasma lipids. Therefore, the use of added fructose as a sweetener in the diabetic diet is not recommended. It is founded in fruits, honey and vegetables. The US Food and Drug Administration (FDA) approved non-nutritive sweeteners such as: aspartame and saccharin are safe for diabetic patients when consumed within the acceptable daily intake levels established by the FDA. Diabetic patients should limit/avoid intake of sugar sweetened beverages to reduce risk for weight gain and worsening of cardio metabolic risk profile [37].

### *2.4.5 Protein in T2DM management*

No ideal amount of protein recommended for patients without evidence of diabetic kidney disease except (protein intake typically 1-1.5 g/kg body weight) so as to optimize glycemic control or to improve one or more CVD risk measures. In T2DM: ingested protein increases insulin response without increasing plasma glucose concentrations. Therefore: CHO sources high in protein should not be used to treat or prevent hypoglycemia. For those with albuminuria and reduced glomerular filtration rate, dietary protein should be maintained at 0.8g/kg body weight/day. Reducing the amount of dietary protein below the recommended daily allowance is not advocated because it does not alter glycemic measures, cardiovascular risk measures or the rate at which glomerular filtration rate declines. Meals with > 75 g protein can raise post prandial glucose at 3-5 hours following consumption. The effect of protein & fat is additive (high fat increases insulin resistance). Protein from fish and chicken may also be included in the diet, however consumption of red and processed meat should be avoided [50, 51].

### *2.4.6 Dietary fat and cholesterol in T2DM management*

It is recommended for type 2 diabetic patients to follow the guidelines for the recommended intakes of saturated fat dietary cholesterol and trans-fat since the type of fatty acids consumed is more important than total amount offal when looking at metabolic goals and CVD risk. Monounsaturated fats may improve glucose metabolism and lower CVD risk and can be an effective alternative to a diet low in total fat but relatively high in CHO. Eating foods rich in Omega-3 fatty acids (fatty fish, nuts and seeds) is recommended to prevent or treat CVD (not supplements though). Monounsaturated and polyunsaturated fats are recommended over saturated fat. In general, trans-fat should be avoided. In animal & observational studies, higher intakes of total dietary fat produce greater insulin resistance. In clinical trials saturated & trans-fats have been shown to cause insulin resistance whereas mono- & polyunsaturated and omega-3 fatty acids do not have an adverse effect. Polyunsaturated fats are as beneficial as monounsaturated fats. Individuals with diabetes and Dyslipidemia may be able to modestly reduce total and low-density lipoprotein (LDL) cholesterol by consuming 1.6-3 g/day of plant stanols or sterols typically found in enriched foods such as: corn and soy <300 mg dietary cholesterol/day is recommended [50, 51].

### *2.4.7 Sodium*

Generally, diabetic patients are advised to limit their sodium consumption to < 2.300 mg/day. Lowering sodium intake (i.e., 1.500 mg/day) could improve blood pressure in certain circumstances. However, other studies suggested caution for universal sodium restriction to 1.500 mg in diabetic patients [8].

#### *2.4.8 Micronutrients and herbal supplements in T2DM management*

There is no clear evidence that supplementation in diabetic patients without deficiencies with vitamins, minerals, herbs or spices can improve diabetes. There is insufficient evidence to support the routine use of chromium, magnesium and vitamin D to improve glycemic control in people with diabetes. There is insufficient evidence to support the use of cinnamon for diabetes treatment. May be safety concerns regarding long-term use of antioxidant supplements such as: vitamin E, vitamin C and carotene [51].

#### *2.4.9 Meal planning*

There is no ideal meal plan that works for everyone with diabetes. Regardless of which meal planning method is used, it should be individualized and modified to put into practice with less difficulty. Meals and snacks should be distributed that is consistent with each individual's way of life, activity patterns and diabetes medication at regular meal times. Spacing of meals: MNT as monotherapy: 3 moderate meals or 4 smaller meals, snacks based on pt's schedule and preferences; MNT with oral anti-diabetes agents: moderate to small in size, snacks not needed unless risk of low BG, and maintain the consistent timing of meals and carbohydrates; and MNT with insulin: keep meals moderate to small in size. Avoid skipping meals. Varieties of eating patterns (combinations of different foods or food groups) are acceptable. Meal planning method ranges from simple guidelines to more complex counting methods. A simple diabetes meal planning approach such as: portion control or healthful food choices may be better suited to individuals with T2DM identified with health and numeric literacy concerns [45, 52].

It is widely acceptable that the healthy nutrition is a basis for T2DM treatment. It contributes positively to the maintenance of blood glucose within normal range and minimizes the disease complications. A balanced diet consisting of 45–60% energy from carbohydrate, 15–20% energy from protein and 20–35% energy from fats is encouraged. There is no ideal eating pattern that is expected to benefit all diabetic patients, but the total energy intake (and thus portion size) is an important factor no matter which eating pattern is chosen [8].

### 2.5 Physical activity for T2DM

Physical activity and exercise are just as important as nutrition for type 2 diabetic patients. Physical activity includes any movement that increases energy use; whereas exercise is considered a more specific form of physical activity designed to improve physical fitness. Exercise has been shown to have several benefits including: improved blood glucose control, reduced cardiovascular risk, increased energy as well as burning extra calories and fat to help manage weight and improve wellbeing. Exercise interventions of at least8 weeks also have shown to lower HbA1c in those with T2DM [42].

### 2.6 The basic principles of an effective exercise program

The basic principles of an effective exercise program are its intensity, its duration, and its exercise frequency. The intensity of exercise should be sufficient to cause changes in the cardiorespiratory system and is determined either by the physical condition of each patient or by the heart rate. In non-fit patients, the intensity can be set to 50-60% of maximum heart rate or to the intensity that increases the resting heart rate by 20 pulses per minute. The duration of the exercise should be 30 minutes in the beginning, starting with 5-10 minutes of warm-up and finish always with recovery exercises. The lower frequency recommended is 3 times/week. Usually, low intensity and long-duration exercise programs are considered the most appropriate and safe for diabetic patients. Finally, the subjective perception of fatigue should be continuously assessed throughout the whole exercise session [53].

There are other important parameters that need to be estimated during exercise sessions are the levels of blood glucose before and during the exercise, the type of food and the time prior to exercise that it was consumed, the time and point of administration of medication. An appropriate environment during exercise is also required. Excessive heat leads to intense sweating and dehydration. Another factor that should not be underestimated during exercise is the use of proper footwear and maintenance of foot cleanness so as to prevent infection [53].

### 2.7 Weight reduction for T2DM

There is solid proof to help lifestyle alterations for those patients with DM who are overweight or obese to enhance glycemic control and lessen the requirement for medications with T2DM. A few examinations have demonstrated a decrease in HbA1c esteems and in addition fasting glucose with low-calorie eats fewer carbohydrates in stout patients with T2DM. Overweight and obese people with DM who are prepared to accomplish weight reduction ought to have an objective of somewhere around 5%weight misfortune through way of life changes [42].

Weight loss is also an important goal because it improves insulin resistance, glycemic control, blood pressure, and lipid profiles. Modest weight loss is defined as a sustained reduction of 5% of initial body weight and has been shown to improve glycemic control & reduce the need for glucose-lowering medications. 5% loss shows benefits but sustained loss of > 7% is optimal. A structured lifestyle plan that combines dietary modification, activity, and behavioral modification, along with ongoing support, is necessary for weight reduction. Lifestyle programs: reduce calories by 500-750/day or provide: For women 1.200-1.500 calories/day, adjusted for baseline weight. For men 1,500-1.800 calories/day adjusted for baseline weight. A reduction in the total calorie intake should allow gradual but systematic body weight reduction (by about 0.5–1 kg/week). The diet choice should be based on health status & preferences [8].

### 2.8 Diabetes self-management education and support for T2DM

Self-management is defined as a set of skilled behaviors engaged in to manage one's own illness. This emphasizes the responsibility and role of the diabetic patients in managing the disease. Self-management of DM can be achieved by self-management education. As part of this education, people with diabetes should receive instruction on how and when to perform self-monitoring; how to record the results in an organized fashion; the meaning of various blood glucose (BG) levels and how behavior and actions affect BG results [38].

Self-management education (SME) is the process of providing the person with diabetes the knowledge and skills needed to perform self-care, manage crisis and make lifestyle changes required to manage the disease. The goal of the process is to enable the patient to become the most knowledgeable and hopefully the most active participant in his or her diabetes care. It provides the information regarding various treatment options and the benefits and costs of each of these strategies, how to make changes in their behaviors and to solve problems [54]. Several meta-analyses have demonstrated that SME is associated with clinically important benefits in people with diabetes, such as reductions in glycated hemoglobin and improvements in cardiovascular risk factors and reductions in foot ulcerations, infections, and amputations [55].

People with diabetes should know how to prevent potential foot problems, recognize early presentation without losing time before referral to doctors. Some tips for preventing problems such as inspecting feet daily and washing for changes in color, texture, odor and firm or hardened areas which may indicate infection and potential ulcers. When washing the feet, the water should be warm (not hot), feet and areas between toes should be thoroughly dried afterward, applying moisturizers, but not between the toes, trimming toenails short and file the edges to avoid cutting adjacent toes and Well-fitting footwear is very important. Be sure the shoe is wide enough [56].

Self-management support (SMS) includes activities that support the implementation and maintenance of behaviors for ongoing diabetes self-management, including education, behavior modification, and psychosocial and/or clinical support. The objective of SME and SMS is to cultivate open doors for individuals with diabetes to end up educated and inspired to take part in viable diabetes self-administration practices and practices ceaselessly. To date, a developing assemblage of research proof shows that the blend of both SME and SMS is most profitable for enhancing glycemic control, self-viability, self-care practices (i.e., observing of blood glucose and good dieting) and decreasing diabetes distress and foot complications [55].

## 3. Conceptual framework

Health promotion theories and models can encourage building up, keeping up, and enhancing solid practices by anticipating factors affecting unsafe practices. The theoretical framework for this study is Pender's health Promotion model (HPM). This model is ideally suited to this study since health-promoting behaviors, especially when coordinated into a healthy lifestyle, result improved health, enhanced functional ability, and better quality of life. Healthy lifestyle behaviors are: health responsibility (one's paying attention to and accepting responsibility for one's own health, being educated about health, and seeking professional assistance when necessary), physical activity, nutrition, spiritual growth (one's sense of self-actualization and purpose), interpersonal relations (one's ability to develop intimacy and closeness), and stress management One's ability to identify and mobilize psychological and physical resources to control (including sleep) or reduce anxiety [57].

Pender et al. [58] believed that, health behavior might be persuaded by a desire to protect one's health by avoiding illness or a desire to increase one's level of health in either the presence or absence of illness. Understanding the mechanisms or the mediators for behavior change and sustainability of these changes is necessary to develop effective health promotion and prevention interventions. Health promotion is the art and science of enabling people to move toward a state of optimal health through lifestyle change and is considered a combination of educational and ecological supports for actions and conditions of living conducive to health. A combination of health promotion strategies is needed to address the multiple determinants of health. Ecological strategies address the social, economic, and physical environments that influence health.

Health promotion has moved from being viewed as an objective or wanted end-point to a process or tool to facilitate movement toward accomplishment of goals. It balances individual health behavior choices with creating environments where healthier choices become easier choices. The nurse's role is to advance a positive atmosphere for change, fill in as an impetus for change, assist with various steps of the change process, and increase the individual's capacity to maintain change [59].

### 3.1 Pender's health promotion model (HPM)

Pender et al. [60] proposed a framework for coordinating nursing and behavioral science points of view with elements affecting health behaviors. This model offered a guide to investigate the complex biopsychosocial processes that motivate individuals to take part in practices coordinated toward improving health. This model aimed to help nursing professionals comprehend the major determinants of health behaviors as a reason for behavioral counseling to advance sound ways of life. The HPM integrated constructs from expectancy-value theory and social cognitive theory, within a nursing perspective of holistic human functioning. The expectancy-value theory is based on the idea that the course of action will likely lead to the desired outcome, and that this outcome will be of positive personal value. The social cognitive theory describes the concept of perceived self-efficacy which is a judgment of one's ability to carry out a particular course of action. The domains of this model include (a) individual characteristics and experiences (previous behaviors and personal factors); (b) behavior specific cognitions and affects (perception of benefits, barriers, self-efficacy, activity related affect, interpersonal influences, and situational influences); and (c) behavioral outcomes (commitment to the plan of action, and demands and preferences).

The first zone, as found in (**Figure 1**) is individual characteristics and experiences, which consists of two aspects that affect the willingness to take health actions. The first aspect is prior related behavior that is related to the health practices and behaviors in the past that influence the existing behavior. The second aspect: personal factors that are related to the biological, psychological, and sociocultural of the individual. These factors affect the individual's behavior. Examples such as age, gender, body mass index comprises biological factors. Psychological factor variables such as; self- esteem, motivation, personal competence, and perceived health status are also represented along with race, ethnicity, education and socioeconomic status [61].

The second zone, behavior-specific cognitions and affect consist of six other aspects: perceived benefits of action, perceived barriers to action, perceived

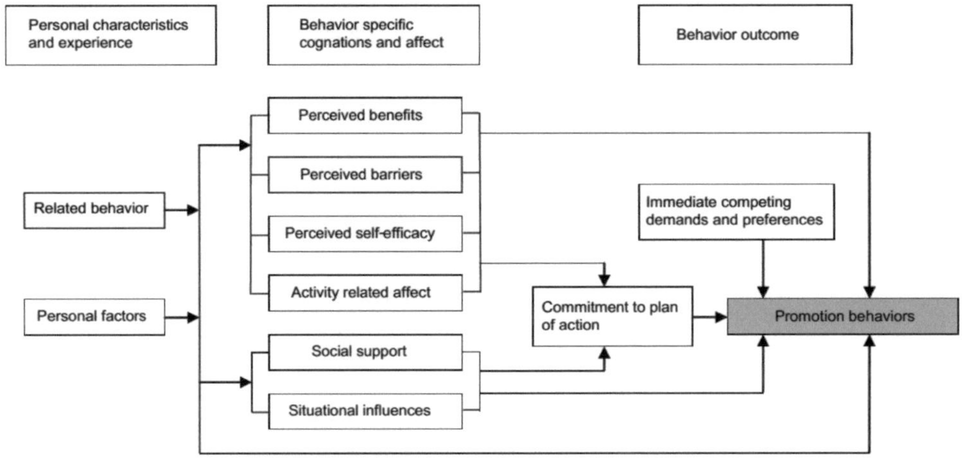


**Figure 1.**
*Diagram of Pender's health promotion model. Source: [61].*

self-efficacy, activity-related affect, interpersonal influences, and situational influences. Perceived benefits are perceptions of the positive or reinforcing benefits of practicing healthy behaviors. Perceived barriers to action suggest that hindrances or obstacles may occur on the process of undertaking healthy behavior. Perceived self-efficacy is the personal capability and self-confidence of performing the health behavior successfully and believing that change is possible. Being self-efficient decreases the perception of barriers to achieving a positive outcome [61].

Activity- related affect is defined as the person's subjective feeling states or emotions before, during and after associated to a specific behavior. A person with positive subjective feeling tends to be self-efficient leading to a positive effect. Interpersonal influences are behaviors, beliefs and attitudes of family, peers, and relevant others in relation to norms, social support and modeling greatly influence undertaking such health behaviors. Lastly, situational influences include options available, demand characteristics and aesthetic features of the behavior environment that influence the action [61].

The third zone, behavioral outcome, has three aspects: immediate competing demands and preferences, commitment to a plan of action and health promoting behavior. The first aspect, immediate competing demands and preferences are behaviors that an individual has low or high control of. Individuals have low control with regards to competing demands such as work and family responsibilities and high control on the competing preferences such as selection of food or diet. These factors infringe the course of action prior to the planned healthy behavior. Second, commitment to a plan of action is the intention to implement health behavior including recognition of strategies to achieve a positive outcome. Lastly, health-promoting behavior is the final, desired, and positive outcome [61].

The HPM recommended that people have one of a kind individual quality and encounters that influence resulting subsequent behavior. The set of variables related to behavior specific cognitions and affect are highly motivational to the individual. Health promoting behavior is the desired outcome although it can be hindered by immediate competing demands and preferences [58]. Individual characteristics are generally viewed as indirect influencers of health promoting behaviors while behavior-specific cognitions and affect are viewed as direct influencers of behavior. Personal factors can be altered by intervention; however, they are generally viewed as fixed factors of HPBs. Behavior-specific cognition variables of the HPM, such as perceived benefits and barriers, are considered to have major motivational significance because they can be altered by nurse intervention [62].

This study concentrated on individual characteristics which are subdivided into prior related behavior and personal factors– demographic, socio-economic, clinical variables and type 2 diabetic patients' knowledge regarding diabetes are considered to be a personal factor; Regarding to the behavior specific cognitions of perceived benefits, the awareness of the lifestyle modification and its positive effect on glycemic control are believed to influence the need to undertake a health behavior, Perceived self-efficacy, social support, and situational influences.; and the behavioral outcomes of health responsibility, physical activity, nutrition, spiritual growth, interpersonal relations, and stress management.

### 3.2 The role of family and community health nursing

The community health nurses play a pivotal role in the detection, monitoring, treatment and prevention of diseases and in health promotion in the whole community. They help patients to learn or relearn lifestyle practices, as concentrating on the patient's reaction to health and illnesses rather than on the disease itself [63, 64]. The focus of community health nursing includes not only the individual, but also the family and the community, meeting these multiple needs requires multiple roles. The seven major roles of a community health nurse are: Care provider, educator, advocate, manager, collaborator, leader and researcher.

The community health nurse as a care provider assists the patient in implementing nursing care plan for disease management. The patient should take an active role in disease management, it is the responsibility of the community health nurse to promote this self-management and to instill the confidence in the patient that they can manage their disease process to remain healthy and decrease the risk of potentially deadly complications [17].

During the treatment process, they follow the progress of the patient and act accordingly with the patient's best interests in mind and therefore leading to improve diabetes coping skills of those patients. They help their patients adjust treatment regimens to ease the burden of diabetes management and to maintain good glycemic control and good health. They are responsible for the holistic care of patients, which includes a wide range of approaches, including medication, education, communication, self-help, and complementary treatment. Holistic care increases self-awareness and self-confidence in patients and causes nurses to better understand the effects of an illness on a person's entire life and his/her true needs. It also improves harmony between mind, body, emotions and spirit in an ever-changing environment [65, 66].

The community health nurse ought to guarantee that the patient is on a strict dietary regimen and that they are checking blood glucose levels regularly. The nurse should also ensure that the patient is complying with medication regimen, checking their feet and getting standard eye examinations, not smoking, and practicing routinely. The community health nurse should monitor the patient's health status and motivate them to be compliant with the prescribed treatment regimen. The nurse should encourage and motivate the patient to take active role in avoiding further complications and to remain compliant with the prescribed treatment regimen and follow up arrangements [17].

The community health nurse as an educator provides health teaching and education through health promotion programs and services. Diabetic health teaching in regard to health promotion and prevention is an ideal role of them because of the overwhelming rate of diabetes and knowledge deficit of the individuals. Concerning diabetes, an individual must be committed to self-health promoting behaviors and to adopting a lifestyle change or else non-compliance will result and complications of the disease process could follow [17].

The community health nurse educates about health and wellness activities such as healthy diet, regular exercise, smoking cessation. The patient should be encouraged and expected to take active role in creating and maintain healthy behaviors. Concerning individualized characteristics and experiences, the patient must examine his or her own behaviors including diet, and level of physical activity, body fat and weight, and settle on a decision to change unhealthy behaviors to health promoting behaviors. The patient will be instructed to be proactive in their own health. The patient will be made to understand that maintain a healthy lifestyle will decrease the chances of getting diabetes. Personal responsibility is the key to diabetes prevention and treatment [17].

The community health nurse assists the patient in early recognition of the signs and symptoms of diabetes and to take control of the disease before potential complications emerge. For those who are prediabetic, it is imperative for community health nurse to clarify the signs and symptoms of hyperglycemia besides what to report to the physician. It is critical to screen those at risk for diabetes. The early diagnosis is similarly as vital. If diabetes is caught prior to the point where complications arise then it will be easier for the patient to be proactive in health promotion. Besides, as blood glucose levels are controlled, the risk of complications diminishes. During educational treatment they are responsible for ensuring that patients are able to understand their health, illnesses, medications, and treatments to the best of their ability. It is fundamental to assess whether the individual with diabetes or a close relative has comprehended the messages and has adequate self-care abilities or skills [17].

The community health nurse as advocator advocates for the patients' rights and maintains the patient's dignity. Every patient has the right to receive, just, equal, and human treatment. This is particularly important for patients who are the poor, the disadvantaged, those without health insurance because they become frustrated, confused, degraded, and unable to cope with the system on their own. The community health nurse often acts as an advocate for patients, pleading their cause or acting on their behalf, Clients may need some one: To explain which services to expect, which services they ought to receive; to make referrals as needed; to write letters to agencies or health care providers for them; and to assure the satisfaction of their needs. The advocate role incorporates four characteristics actions: Being assertive; taking risks; communicating & negating well; and identifying recourses and obtaining results. The community health nurse support the patient and represent the patients best interests at all times, especially when treatment decisions are being made [67].

The community health nurse as a manger exercises administrative direction toward the accomplishment of specified goals by: Assessing patients' needs; planning and organizing to meet those needs; controlling; and evaluating the progress to ensure that goals are met. These activities are sequential and yet also occur simultaneously for managing service objectives. As other health professionals are usually responsible for making the final treatment decisions, nurses should be able to communicate information regarding patient health effectively. In this, the community health nurse facilitates collaboration, coordination, and cooperation among caregivers for continuity of care for the patient and promoting the best patient health outcomes [67].

The community health nurse as a collaborator enables and promotes the interprofessional teamwork and comprehensive care provided by healthcare professionals, paraprofessionals, and volunteers. The collaborator role also may involve functioning as a consultant with other healthcare colleagues to inform decision-making and planning to meet healthcare consumer needs therefore, provide proper care and improve patient outcomes. This role requires communication skills, skill in interpreting the nurse's unique contribution to the team and acting assertively as an equal partner [67, 68].

The community health nurse as a leader focuses on affecting change, thus the nurse becomes an agent of change. The community health nurse seeks to initiate changers that positively affect people's health. They also seek to influence people to think and behave differently about their health and the factors contributing to it. The care for diabetic patients includes adopting a healthy lifestyle where the diet plan represents an important support of care so they can meet their goals. At the community level, the leadership role may involve working with a team of professionals to direct and coordinate such as a campaign to eliminate smoking in public areas [67, 69].

The community health nurse as a researcher engages in systematic investigation, collection, and analysis of data for solving problems and enhancing community health practice. The community health nurse often participates in agency and organizational studies to determine such matters as risks associated with home visiting. The researcher role helps to determine needs, evaluate effectiveness of care, and develop theoretic bases for community health nursing practice. Nurses must become responsible users of research, keeping up-to-date of new knowledge and applying it in practice. Nurses must learn to evaluate nursing research articles critically, assessing their validity and applicability to their own practice. A commitment to use and conduct of research will move the nursing profession forward and enhance its influence on the health of at-risk populations [67].

The main results of the present study could be outlined in the following points:

Results revealed that 68.5% of the studied sample groups were females and 64.1% of them aged from 45-64 years with mean 49.76 ± 9.19 years.

Regarding educational level, 42.4% of the studied sample groups were illiterate. Whereas, 63.0% were unemployed, 68.5% of them came from urban areas, and 76.2% of them had low social class level.

Regarding diabetes history, 43.5% of the studied sample had rare attacks, 96.7% of them have taken oral hypoglycemic agents, 94.6% of them were not following planned diet regimen and 76.1% of them did not do physical activities.

Independent t-test demonstrated high significant difference (P-value < 0.005) between pre-test study and control groups' total score of knowledge & knowledge related practice about DM. Though, this result was of unnecessary inconsistency between the two groups, both levels of their pre-test knowledge and practices about diabetes mellitus were still inadequate. Independent t-test demonstrated also that there was only statistical significant difference (P-value < 0.023) between the two groups regarding pre-test health responsibility domain. It can be concluded from outputs that the mean scores between control and study were successful in achieving homogeneity of most sub-class groups.

However, differences regarding clinical data between pre-test study and control groups were statistically insignificant. Generally, the mean scores of groups between control and study were homogeneous for all sub-class groups.

Results of Paired t-test between total score of knowledge & knowledge related practice about DM, health promoting lifestyle domains values and clinical data, before and after the program intervention in the study group revealed high significant differences represented in (P-value < 0.009 or P-value < 0.001 or P-value < 0.0001). Patients who received lifestyle modification intervention program achieved better total score of knowledge & knowledge related practice about DM, health promoting lifestyle domains values and clinical data.

Statistical results of Paired t-test that was computed between total score of knowledge & knowledge related practice about DM pre- and post-tests in the control group, have illustrated high significant differences (P-value < 0.0001). Those patients were still having inadequate and insufficient total score of knowledge & knowledge related practice about DM.

Statistical results of Paired t-test that were computed between health promoting lifestyle domains pre- and post-tests pre- and post-tests in the control group, have illustrated statistical significant differences of all domains except that for the physical activity and interpersonal relations domains. Patients though didn't receive a lifestyle modification intervention, have had slight increases (with no trend change) in their total scores of overall health promoting lifestyle score, health responsibility, nutrition, spiritual growth, stress management domains.

Statistical results of Paired t-test that were computed between clinical data pre- and post-tests in the control group have not revealed any statistical significance regarding clinical data.

Glycated Hemoglobin multiple linear regressions demonstrated a statistical significant positive independent predictor (fasting plasma glucose; P-value < 0.0001), whereas the Physical Activity Domain was the only statistical significant negative independent predictor (P-value < 0.015) after employing the program in the study group.

## 4. Conclusions

Based on the findings of the current study, it could be concluded that: Type 2 diabetic patients who have received lifestyle modification program (dietary modification, physical activity, self-blood glucose monitoring and diabetes self-care education) and attended to the Family Medicine Outpatient Clinic & the Diabetic Outpatient Clinic of Suez Canal University Hospitals at Ismailia city in Egypt has a positive effect on glycemic control (HbA1c) among patients with type 2 diabetes mellitus and also improved their knowledge and practices about DM post lifestyle modification program.

## Acknowledgements

First and foremost, praise be to Almighty Allah for the countless gifts I have been offered and for helping me and giving me the power to pass safely through all difficulties and overcome them. I would like to express my deepest gratitude to Prof. Salwa Abbas Ali Hassan, Professor of Community Health Nursing, Faculty of Nursing, Zagazig University for her instructive supervision, guidance and continuous encouragement to produce this work. I am indebted to her valuable consultation and direction. My deepest gratitude and sincerest appreciation are also extended to Prof. Dr. Hassan Ali Abdelwahid, Professor of Family Medicine, Faculty of Medicine, Suez Canal University for his instructive supervision, guidance and continuous encouragement to produce this work. I am indebted to his valuable guidance and advice. My deepest gratitude and thanks are also extended to Dr. Hanaa Kassem Farg, lecture of Family and Community Health Nursing, Faculty of Nursing, Suez Canal University for her instructive supervision, guidance and continuous encouragement to produce this work. I am indebted to her valuable consultation and direction. Special thanks to every diabetic patient who participated in the conduction of this study. Finally, I would also like to extend my deepest gratitude to all the team members of Family Medicine Outpatient Clinic and Endocrine Outpatient Clinic at Suez Canal university Hospitals and to all those who helped me to fulfill this study.

## Acronyms and abbreviations

| | |
|---|---|
| ADA | American Diabetes Association |
| BG | Blood Glucose |
| BMI | Body Mass Index |
| CHO | Carbohydrates |
| CVD | Cardiovascular Disease |
| DALY | Disability Adjusted Life Years |
| DCCT | Diabetes Control And Complications Trial |
| DKA | Diabetic Ketoacidosis |
| DKQ | Diabetes Knowledge Questionnaire |
| DM | Diabetes Mellitus |
| DRI | Dietary Reference Intakes |
| FDA | Food and Drug Administration |
| FPG | Fasting Plasma Glucose |
| GDM | Gestational Diabetes Mellitus |
| GI | Glycemic Index |
| HbA1c | Glycated Hemoglobin |

| | |
|---|---|
| HHNS | Hyperglycemic Hyperosmolar Non KetonicSyndrome |
| HHS | Hyperglycemic Hyperosmolar State |
| HPLP II | Health Promoting Lifestyle Profile II |
| HPM | Pender's Health Promotion Model |
| IDF | International Diabetes Federation |
| IFG | Impaired Fasting Glucose |
| IGT | Impaired Glucose Tolerance |
| LADA | Latent Autoimmune Diabetes In Adults |
| LDL | Low-Density Lipoprotein |
| MNT | Medical Nutrition Therapy |
| MODY | Maturity-Onset Diabetes of The Young |
| NCDs | Non-Communicable Diseases |
| NGSP | National Glycohemoglobin Standardization Program |
| OGTT | Oral Glucose Tolerance Test |
| QOL | Quality of Life |
| RDA | Recommended Daily Allowance |

## Author details

Fatma Ibrahim Abdel-Latif Megahed[1*], Salwa Abbas Ali Hassan[2], Hassan Ali Abdelwahid[3] and Hanaa Kassem Farg[1]

1 Faculty of Nursing, Family and Community Health Nursing, Suez Canal University, Egypt

2 Faculty of Nursing, Community Health Nursing, Zagazig University, Egypt

3 Faculty of Medicine, Family Medicine, Suez Canal University, Egypt

*Address all correspondence to: dr.fm_2013@yahoo.com

## References

[1] Sami, W., Ansari, T., Butt, N. & Ab Hamid, M. (2017). Effect of Diet on Type 2 Diabetes Mellitus. International Journal of Health Sciences, 11(2), 1-7.

[2] IDF. (2017). IDF Diabetes Atlas, International Diabetes Federation (8th ed.). Brussels.

[3] Pisimisis, T. (2013). Quality of Life of People with Diabetes Mellitus in Greece. Published Doctorate thesis, Faculty of Population Health Sciences, University College London.

[4] Ahmed, M., Yirdachew, E. and Tefera, G. (2018). Diabetic Complications among Follow-up Patients: A cross-sectional Study at Jimma University Specialized Hospital Diabetic Clinic. Journal of Clinical and Molecular Endocrinology, 3(1), 45.

[5] Wu, Y., Ding, Y., Tanaka, Y. and Zhang, W. (2014). Risk Factors Contributing to Type 2 Diabetes and Recent Advances in the Treatment and Prevention. International Journal of Medical Sciences, 11(11), 1185-1200.

[6] Gheibizadeh, M., Bazpour, M., Saki Malehi, A. and Keikhaei, B. (2017). Health-Promoting lifestyle of Adolescents with β-Thalassemia Based on Precede Model in Ahvaz, Iran, 2016. Jundishapur J Chronic Dis Care, 6(1), e39238.

[7] Mohamed, S. (2014). Effect of Lifestyle Intervention on Health Behaviors Weight and Blood Glucose Level among Patients with Diabetes Mellitus. Journal of Nursing Education and Practice, 4(12), 75-87.

[8] ADA. (2018). Standards of Medical Care in Diabetes—2018. Diabetes Care, 41(suppl. 1), S1- S156.

[9] Chenary, R., Noroozi, A., Tavafian, S. and Firoozabadi, M. (2015). Effective Factors on Health-Promoting Lifestyle among Iranian Chemical Veterans in 2014 Based on Health Promotion Model. Iranian Red Crescent Medical, 18(8), e33467.

[10] Davies, A. and Buxton, C. (2015). Professional Nurses' Knowledge level on Type II Diabetes Mellitus at Selected teaching and Training Hospitals in the Central Region of Ghana. Journal of Nursing & Care, 4(1), 229.

[11] Meng, D., Chunyan, W., Xiaosheng, D. and Xiangren, Y. (2018). The Effects of Qigong on Type 2 Diabetes Mellitus: A Systematic Review and Meta-Analysis. Evidence-Based Complementary and Alternative Medicine, 2018, 1-8.

[12] Punthakee, Z., Goldenberg, R., Katz, P. and Committee DCCPGE. (2018). Definition, Classification and Diagnosis of Diabetes, Prediabetes and Metabolic Syndrome. Canadian journal of diabetes, 42, S10–SS5.

[13] Danilova, L. (2018). 2018 Guidelines on the management of diabetic patients. A position of Diabetes Poland. Clinical Diabetology, 7(1), 1-90.

[14] Gopalakrishnan, S. and Muthulakshmi, M. (2018). Type 2 diabetes mellitus and its determinants among adults in an urban area of Kancheepuram district, Tamil Nadu. International Journal of Community Medicine and Public Health, 5(5), 1956-1962.

[15] The Royal Australian College of General Practitioners and Diabetes Australia. (2014). General practice management of type 2 diabetes – 2014-15. Melbourne. ISBN 978-0-86906-375-0 (web).

[16] Qamar, M., Lau, W., A., Ahmed, F., Khan, J. and Mahmud, A. (2015). Knowledge of Diabetes Mellitus,

Risk Factors and Complications among The General Public in Kuala Lumpur. World Journal of Pharmaceutical Research, 4(12), 154-170.

[17] Shamia, I. (2011). Effectiveness of Educational Intervention Program on Knowledge, Practice, and Blood Glucose Level of Adult Patients with Type 2 Diabetes in Gaza Strip. Un published Master Thesis, Faculty of Nursing, Cairo University.

[18] Abozaid, L. (2006). Impact of Lifestyle Counseling on Knowledge, Practice, and Glycemic Control among Patients with Type 2 Diabetes Mellitus in Port-Said City. Un published Doctorate Thesis, Faculty of Medicine, Suez Canal University.

[19] Inzucchi, S., Bergenstal, R., Buse, J., Diamant, M., Ferrannini, E., Nauck, M., Peters, A., Tsapas, A., Wender, R. and Matthews, D. (2012). Management of hyperglycemia in type 2 diabetes: a patient-centered approach: Position Statement of the American Diabetes Association and the European Association for the Study of Diabetes. Diabetologia, 55(6), 1577-1596.

[20] Thomas, G. (2015). Disease progression in newly diagnosed Type 2 Diabetes Mellitus patients: a statistical analysis using Clinical Practice Research Datalink (CPRD). Published doctorate Thesis, School of Public Health, The University of Queensland.

[21] Godoy-Matos, A. (2014). The role of glucagon on type 2 diabetes at a glance. Diabetology and Metabolic Syndrome, 6(1), 91.

[22] Inzucchi, S., Bergenstal, R., Buse, J., Diamant, M., Ferrannini, E., Nauck, M., Peters, A., Tsapas, A., Wender, R. and Matthews, D. (2015). Management of hyperglycemia in type 2 diabetes, 2015: a patient-centered approach: update to a position statement of the American Diabetes Association and the European Association for the Study of Diabetes. Diabetes care, 38(1), 140-149.

[23] Vijan, S. (2010). Type 2 diabetes. Annals of internal medicine, 152 (5), 15.

[24] Gardner, D. and Shoback, D. (2011). Greenspan's Basic and Clinical Endocrinology (9th ed.). New York: McGraw-Hill Medical: Pp. 599. Chapter 17. ISBN-13: 978-0071622431.

[25] Mandal, B., Shukla, R., Basu, A., Sinha, A., Maiti, A. and Bhattacharjee, K. (2018). Association of ABO blood groups with type-2 diabetes mellitus and its complications. Journal of Diabetes, Metabolic Disorders & Control, 5(1), 1-7.

[26] Pratley, R. (2013). The Early Treatment of Type 2 Diabetes. The American Journal of Medicine, 126, S2-S9.

[27] Lefebvre, P. and Silink, M. (2006). Diabetes fights for recognition. International Diabetes Federation, Belgium. The lancet, 368(9548), 1625-1626.

[28] Davies, M., Heller S., Skinner T., Campbell, M., Carey, M., Cradock, S., Dallosso, H., Daly, H., Doherty, Y., Eaton, S., Fox, C., Oliver, L., Rantell, K., Rayman, G. and Khunti, K. (2008). Effectiveness of the diabetes education and self-management for ongoing and newly diagnosed (DESMOND) program for people with newly diagnosed type 2 diabetes: Cluster randomized controlled trial. British Medical Journal, 336(7642), 491-495.

[29] Fowler, M. (2011). The Diabetes Treatment Trap: Hypoglycemia. Clinical Diabetes, 29(1), 36-39.

[30] Siddiqui, A., Siddiqui, S., Ahmad, S., Siddiqui, S., Ahsan, I. and Sahu, K. (2013). Diabetes: Mechanism, Pathophysiology and Management-A Review. International Journal of Drug Development & Research, 5(2), 1-23.

[31] International Diabetes Federation (IDF). (2010). IDF Diabetes Atlas: morbidity and mortality. Available at: http://www.diabetesatlas.org/content/diabetes-mortality.

[32] Hughes, J., Wibowo, Y., Sunderland, B. and Hoti, K. (2017). The role of the pharmacist in the management of type 2 diabetes: current insights and future directions. Integrated Pharmacy Research and Practice, 6, 15-27.

[33] Inzucchi, S. and Sherwin, R. (2011). T2DM. In: Goldman L, Schafer AI, eds. Goldman's Cecil Medicine (24th ed.). Philadelphia, PA: Elsevier Saunders: chap 237.

[34] Lipscombe, L., Booth, G., Butalia, S., Dasgupta, K., Eurich, D., Goldenberg, R., Khan, N., MacCallum, L., Shah, B. and Simpson, S. (2018). Pharmacologic glycemic management of type 2 diabetes in adults. Canadian journal of diabetes, 42, S88–S103.

[35] Kumar, A., Reddy, V., Parveen, S., Padmakar, S., Lakshmi, V. and Shahzadi, Y. (2018). Evaluation of Medication Adherence in Type-2 DM Patients in a Tertiary Care Teaching Hospital. IOSR Journal of Pharmacy and Biological Sciences, 13(2), 57-67.

[36] Alzaheb, R. and Altemani, A. (2018). The prevalence and determinants of poor glycemic control among adults with type 2 diabetes mellitus in Saudi Arabia. Diabetes, Metabolic Syndrome and Obesity: Targets and Therapy, 11, 15-21.

[37] Mostafa, O. (2013). Effect of Lifestyle Modification on Control of Type 2 Diabetes Mellitus; A Prototype for Primary Health Care Settings. Un-Published Master Thesis, Faculty of Medicine, Cairo University.

[38] Berard, L., Siemens, R. and Woo, V. (2018). 2018 Clinical Practice Guidelines: Monitoring Glycemic Control. Canadian Journal of Diabetes, 42, S47–S53.

[39] University of Michigan Health System (UMHS). (2017). Management of Type 2 Diabetes Mellitus. Available at: http://diabetesresearch.med.umich.edu/

[40] Evert, A. (2013). Nutrition therapy recommendations for the management of adults with diabetes. Diabetes care, 36(11), 3821-3842.

[41] Ntaate, C. (2015). Dietary knowledge, attitude and practices of diabetic patients at Nsambya Hospital Kampala, Uganda. Published Master Thesis, Faculty of Medicine, Stellenbosch University.

[42] ADA. (2017). Standards of medical care in diabetes - 2017. Diabetes Care, 40 (Supplement 1), S1–S135.

[43] Ghosh, S. (2017). Implementation of Proper Nutrition in Managing Diabetes-A Review Article. Journal of Food Science Research, 2(1), 103.

[44] El-Said, A. (2014). Quality of Life among Type 2 Diabetic Patients. Un- published Master Thesis, Faculty of Nursing, Menoufiya University.

[45] Hodorowicz, M. (2015). Nutrition recommendations for adults with type 1 and type 2 diabetes. Available at: http://www.maryannhodorowicz.com.

[46] Ministry of Health Malaysia. (2015). Clinical Practice Guidelines on Management of Type 2 Diabetes Mellitus (5th ed.). Available at: http://www.diabetes.org.my.

[47] Atkinson, F., Foster-Powell, K. and Brand-Miller, J. (2008). International tables of glycemic index and glycemic load values: 2008. Diabetes Care, 31, 2281-2283.

[48] Carvalho, F., Pimazoni-Netto, A., Zach, P., Sachs, A. and Zanella, M.

(2012). Importance of Nutritional Counseling and Dietary Fiber Content on Glycemic Control in Type 2 Diabetic Patients under Intensive Educational Intervention. Arquivos Brasileiros de Endocrinologia & Metabologia, 56(2), 110-119.

[49] Keshani, P. and Farvid, M. (2014). Relationship of Glycemic Control and Stages of Change for Fiber Intake in Type 2 Diabetic Patients: A Cross-sectional Study. Nutrition and Food Sciences Research, 1(2), 11-18.

[50] Evert, A., Boucher, J., Cypress, M., Dunbar, S., Franz, M., Mayer-Davis, E., Neumiller, J., Nwankwo, R., Verdi, C. and Urbanski, P. (2014). Nutrition therapy recommendations for the management of adults with diabetes. Diabetes Care, 37 (Supplement 1), S120-SS43.

[51] ADA. (2016). Standards of Medical Care in Diabetes. Diabetes Care, 39(Supplement 1).

[52] Pastors, J., Waslaski, J. and Gunderson, H. (2005). Nutritional Considerations in Type 2 Diabetes Mellitus.

[53] Polikandrioti, M. and Dokoutsidou, H. (2009). The role of exercise and nutrition in type II diabetes mellitus management. Health Science Journal, 3(4), 216-221.

[54] Kisokanth, G., Prathapan, S., Indrakumar, J. and Joseph, J. (2013). Factors influencing self- management of Diabetes Mellitus; a review article. Journal of Diabetology, 3(1), 1-7.

[55] Sherifali, D., Berard, L., Gucciardi, E., MacDonald, B. and MacNeill, g. (2018). 2018 Clinical Practice Guidelines: Self-Management Education and Support. Canadian Journal of Diabetes, 42, S36–S41.

[56] Agency for Health Care Research and Quality (AHRQ) (2014). TOPIC? Available at: http://www.effectivehealthcare.ahrq.gov.

[57] Roebuck, D. (2017). Health Promotion Lifestyle Profile of Low-Income African American Women During Interconception. Published Doctorate thesis, Faculty of Nursing, Drexel University.

[58] Pender, N., Murdaugh, C. & Parsons, M. (2015). Health Promotion in Nursing Practice (7th ed.). Upper Saddle River, NJ: Prentice Hall.

[59] Dehdari, T., Rahimi, T., Aryaeian, N., and Gohari, M. (2014). Effect of nutrition education intervention based on Pender's Health Promotion Model in improving the frequency and nutrient intake of breakfast consumption among female Iranian students. Public Health Nutrition, 17(3), 657-666.

[60] Pender, N., Murdaugh, C. & Parsons, M. (2002). Health Promotion in Nursing Practice (4th ed.). Upper Saddle River, NJ: Pearson Education, Inc.

[61] Pender, N., Murdaugh, C. & Parsons, M. (2011). Health Promotion in Nursing Practice (6th ed.). Boston, MA: Pearson.

[62] Baldwin, S. (2014). Coronary Heart Disease Knowledge, Health Promoting Behaviors and Perceived Benefits and Barriers to Exercise and Healthy Eating in Montana Females. Published Master thesis, Faculty of Nursing, Montana State University.

[63] Rabelo E.R., Aliti, G.B., Domingues, F.B., Ruschel, K.B., and De Oliveira Brun, A. (2007). What to teach to patients with heart failure and why: the role of nurses in heart failure clinics. Revista Latino-Americana de Enfermagem., 15(1), 165-170.

[64] Guedes, N., Moreira, R., Cavalcante,T., de Araujo, T., Lopes, M.,

Ximenes, L. and Vieira, N. (2012). Nursing interventions related to health promotion in hypertensive patients. Acta Paul Enferm., 25(1), 151-156.

[65] Zamanzadeh, V., Jasemi, M., Valizadeh, L., Keogh, B. and Taleghani, F. (2015). Effective factors in providing holistic care: a qualitative study. Indian journal of palliative care, 21(2), 214-224.

[66] Smith, Y. (2019). Roles of a Nurse. Available at: https://www.news-medical.net/health/Roles-of-a-Nurse.aspx

[67] Allender, J., Rector, C. and Warner, K. (2014). Community & Public Health Nursing: Promoting the Public's Health (8th ed.). Lippincott Williams & Wilkins: p.56-64.

[68] ADA. (2015). Standards of medical care in diabetes. Summary of revisions. Diabetes care, 38(suppl. 1), S4.

[69] Buowari O. (2013). Diabetes Mellitus in Developing Countries and Case Series, Diabetes Mellitus - Insights and Perspectives, Oguntibeju, O. (Ed.), ISBN: 978-953-51-0939-6, In Tech.

Chapter 12

# Psychotherapeutic Interventions for Type 2 Diabetes Mellitus

*Keisha C. Gobin, Jennifer S. Mills and Joel D. Katz*

## Abstract

This chapter explores the efficacy of psychotherapeutic interventions for patients with type 2 diabetes mellitus (T2DM). This condition can lead to serious adverse health outcomes (e.g., cardiovascular disease, blindness, loss of limbs, etc.). Medical interventions alone are often not sufficient to manage the disease. Psychotherapy can promote behavioral change that improves medication adherence, dietary choices, exercise, stress, and other variables that affect blood sugar levels. The current chapter summarizes the trends in recent research for psychotherapeutic interventions for the management of T2DM. The results from 16 randomized controlled trials on cognitive-behavioral therapy, motivational interviewing, counseling, and mindfulness-based therapies are discussed. These interventions varied in length (3 to 18 months) and were conducted in many geographic regions (e.g., Australia, Netherlands, Saudi Arabia, Thailand, and more). Changes in biological health outcomes (i.e., HbA1c levels) were the primary focus of this chapter, but diabetes-related behavioral changes (e.g., diet and exercise) and psychological variables (e.g., stress, depression, and well-being) are also discussed. This chapter highlights that recent research has provided the most support for mindfulness-based therapies for improving blood sugar levels in patients with T2DM.

**Keywords:** Type 2 diabetes mellitus, psychotherapy, intervention, diet, exercise

## 1. Introduction

Diabetes mellitus is a condition marked by an inability to produce or properly use insulin, a hormone that allows cells to use glucose for energy [1]. Approximately 3 million Canadians, or 8% of the general population, are living with diabetes, with the prevalence increasing with age [1]. The condition usually develops in middle aged or older adults, and men are slightly more likely to be diagnosed with this condition (8.7%) than are women (7.6%) [1]. There are two types of diabetes mellitus: type 1, where the body cannot produce a sufficient amount of insulin, and type 2, where the body cannot use the insulin it produces effectively, resulting in high blood sugar levels [1]. Accordingly, blood glucose levels are the most reliable physiological marker by which to diagnose diabetes mellitus [2] and are also used to monitor patients' management of their condition. The main criterion for a diagnosis of diabetes mellitus is a hemoglobin A1c [HbA1c] level above 6.4%, indicating above-average blood sugar levels, for the past 2–3 months. Interventions that produce lower HbA1c levels indicate efficacy at improving patient self-management of their diabetes mellitus. If left untreated or if poorly managed, diabetes mellitus can lead to serious health conditions such as heart disease and stroke, blindness, nerve damage, and loss of limbs [1].

About 90% of people with diabetes mellitus have type 2 (T2DM). This is a chronic disease, which must be carefully managed on an ongoing basis by the patient and/or their caregivers. The biopsychosocial approach combines the use of medication and insulin with self-management behaviors for the purpose of regulating blood glucose levels. Lifestyle changes that are generally recommended for people at higher risk of diabetes and those who are newly diagnosed include sufficient moderate to high intensity exercise, and dietary considerations such as increased intake of fiber and reduced intake of fats (especially saturated fat). As well, overweight individuals are advised to lose weight gradually to achieve a body mass index in the healthy range. Health care professionals working with patients with T2DM aim to teach and encourage appropriate eating habits and physical activity to help patients achieve better glycemic control. However, implementing and adhering to these lifestyle changes is often difficult. Many individuals with T2DM do not adhere to the recommended nutrition and physical activity guidelines. Specifically, many patients exceed the recommended fat and sodium intake, and do not consume enough grains, dairy, fruits and vegetables [3]. Stress is also recognized as a variable that can exacerbate T2DM. Stress triggers the release of hormones that produce a surge in blood glucose levels. For this reason, stress management is considered to be part of a biopsychosocial approach to the management of T2DM. Due to the prevalence and manageability of this type of diabetes mellitus through lifestyle modifications alone, this chapter will focus solely on T2DM.

In addition to pharmacological interventions, various psychotherapeutic interventions are used and have been studied to help people with T2DM achieve better glycemic control. In theory, psychotherapy can promote behavioral changes that would improve medication adherence, dietary choices, exercise, stress levels, and other variables that affect blood sugar levels. Within this chapter, we review various psychotherapeutic interventions that are commonly used for the management of T2DM, including cognitive-behavioral therapy, motivational interviewing, counseling, and mindfulness-based therapies. This chapter explores the trends in recent research to understand the evidence base for various psychotherapeutic interventions in the management of T2DM. Change in HbA1c level is the primary focus of this chapter, since HbA1c is commonly measured and is the most objective and standardized outcome measure across studies. However, trends in diabetes-related behavioral changes (e.g., diet and exercise) and psychological variables (e.g., coping, stress, depression, and well-being) are also discussed.

## 2. Psychotherapeutic interventions for type 2 diabetes mellitus

Previous review papers have demonstrated that psychotherapeutic interventions in general are effective at improving health outcomes for individuals with T2DM. A 2004 meta-analysis of 12 randomized control trials (RCT) of psychological interventions (i.e., cognitive behavior therapy, counseling, or psychodynamic therapy) found lower HbA1c levels and psychological distress compared to different control groups (i.e., treatment as usual, an education group, attentional control, or waitlist control) [4]. There was no difference between treatment groups on weight gain and blood glucose concentration, suggesting that there was no clearly superior psychological intervention for the management of T2DM. A 2013 systematic review similarly concluded that psychotherapy is effective in supporting healthy coping among individuals with diabetes mellitus [5]. More recently, a 2020 meta-analysis of 70

RCTs found that psychological interventions, such as cognitive behavioral therapy, self-help materials, and counseling, were generally effective in reducing HbA1c levels over and above usual care [6].

These research findings cited above support the general use of psychotherapeutic interventions in the management of diabetes mellitus. However, it would be helpful to know whether and how specific interventions can enhance care for patients with T2DM so as to assist with treatment planning. In this chapter we analyze the recent literature on the efficacy of psychotherapeutic interventions for the care of T2DM. There have been 16 relevant RCTs published within the past 8 years (see Appendix A for details of the search strategy), which represent the most up-to-date published scientific findings on the topic. These studies and time period were deemed to give a valid snapshot of the recent literature. The results of specific studies are discussed, and we summarize the most noteworthy findings within each type of psychotherapeutic intervention. The effects of specific interventions on various outcomes relevant to patients with T2DM are discussed in detail. See **Table 1** for a summary of the reviewed studies.

### 2.1 Cognitive-behavioral therapy

Cognitive-behavioral therapy (CBT) is an umbrella term that encompasses various cognitive and behavioral techniques to identify and transform negative thinking patterns. CBT has been used to promote behavioral change in patients with diabetes mellitus [7]. A goal of CBT is to help individuals understand barriers to their own diabetes mellitus self-management and to provide them with the skills necessary to cope with these barriers. For example, a patient with diabetes mellitus may think, "I have a terrible chronic condition and there is nothing I can do about it." This type of cognition can lead to poor treatment adherence, low confidence, and/or high levels of stress. Within a CBT protocol, the therapist helps the patient to identify thinking errors or "cognitive distortions" (e.g., anticipating the worst outcome, focusing on the negative, and thinking in all-or-nothing terms) and to use strategies to challenge these beliefs (e.g., "what evidence is there for and against this thought?"). In addition to developing more balanced or rational thoughts, the therapist and the patient can also work on behavioral changes. They may engage in gradual exposure to challenging activities (e.g., walking for 5 minutes a day, then 10 minutes, then 20 minutes, until they can walk for one hour) or behavioral experiments (e.g., writing down how they feel before and after taking medication in order to help identify that anticipatory anxiety is often worse than any discomfort they feel during or after the avoided task). In CBT, patients receive emotional and psychological support while learning strategies to overcome avoidance and to adhere to their medication, dietary intake, and physical activity goals. CBT for the management of T2DM can be done in weekly individual or group sessions, and is traditionally done in-person with a therapist and over the span of several weeks to months.

For many years, CBT was the most commonly investigated form of psychotherapy for T2DM (for example, see [4–6]) and results confirmed its efficacy in increasing positive outcomes. In recent years, the literature has shifted away from investigating CBT in its traditional application. Instead, new research has begun to examine CBT in alternative delivery formats in an effort to boost accessibility. For instance, a 6-month web-based CBT intervention was found to be more effective than a control group in lowering HbA1c levels ($p$ = .002) among T2DM patients in Saudi Arabia [8]. It also resulted in better diabetes mellitus knowledge ($p$ = .004) and self-efficacy ($p$ < .001) relative to a control group, suggesting that CBT can produce a meaningful change in cognitions that are related to successful self-

| Author (Year) | N | Age | Sex (M, F) | Ethnicity | Country | Intervention | Duration | Outcome | p-value |
|---|---|---|---|---|---|---|---|---|---|
| Abu-Saad, Murad, Barid, Olmer, Ziv, Younis-Zeidan, & Kalter- Leibovici (2019) | 50 | 53 | 21,29 | Arab | Israel | Interactive lifestyle assessment, counseling and education (motivational interviewing) Standard lifestyle advice | 6 months | **Biological** | |
| | | | | | | | | HbA1c | .400 |
| | | | | | | | | **Diabetes-related** | |
| | | | | | | | | Diabetes Knowledge – 3 months | .023 |
| | | | | | | | | Added sugar[a] | .050 |
| | | | | | | | | Dietary fiber[a] | .578 |
| | | | | | | | | Fruit[a] | .203 |
| | | | | | | | | Vegetables[a] | .172 |
| | | | | | | | | Whole grains[a] | .325 |
| | | | | | | | | Physical Activity | |
| Alanzi, Alanzi, Istepan i-an, & Philip (2018) | 20 | NA | 15,5 | NA | Saudi Arabia | Mobile CBT | 6 months | **Biological** | |
| | | | | | | Conventional diabetes treatment | | HbA1c | .002 |
| | | | | | | | | **Diabetes-related** | |
| | | | | | | | | Diabetes Knowledge Test | .004 |
| | | | | | | | | **Psychological** | |
| | | | | | | | | Self-Efficacy Scale | <.001 |
| Armani, Vahdani, Noorbala, Nejatisafa, Arbabi, Zenoozian & Nakhjavani (2018) | 60 | 56 | 11, 49, | NA | Iran | Mindfulness-based stress reduction | 3 months | **Biological** | |
| | | | | | | | | HbA1c | .01 |
| | | | | | | | | Fasting blood sugar | .001 |
| | | | | | | Usual care | | **Psychological** | |
| | | | | | | | | Overall mental health | .001 |
| | | | | | | | | Depression | .01 |
| | | | | | | | | Anxiety | .01 |

| Author (Year) | N | Age | Sex (M, F) | Ethnicity | Country | Intervention | Duration | Outcome | p-value |
|---|---|---|---|---|---|---|---|---|---|
| Chee, Gilcha-ran Singh, Hamdy, Mechanick, Lee, Barua, Ali & Hussein (2017) | 230 | 55 | 85, 145 | Indian (58%) | Malaysia | Motivational interviewing (Trans-cultural diabetes-specific nutrition algorithm+MI) | 6 months | **Intervention Phase** | |
| | | | | Chinese (28%) | | | 6 month follow-up | **Biological** | |
| | | | | Malaysian (14%) | | | | HbA1c | < .001 |
| | | | | | | | | Weight loss | < .001 |
| | | | | | | | | Body Mass Index | < .001 |
| | | | | | | Conventional counselling (Trans-cultural diabetes-specific nutrition algorithm+CC) | | Waist circumference | < .001 |
| | | | | | | | | Body fat | < .001 |
| | | | | | | | | Fasting plasma glucose | .027 |
| | | | | | | | | Systolic blood pressure | .003 |
| | | | | | | | | Diastolic blood pressure | .013 |
| | | | | | | | | Total | |
| | | | | | | Usual Care | | Cholesterol | .741 |
| | | | | | | | | Low-density lipoproteins | .565 |
| | | | | | | | | High-density lipoproteins | .484 |
| | | | | | | | | Triglyceride high sensitivity | .855 |
| | | | | | | | | C-reactive protein | .092 |
| | | | | | | | | **Follow up** | |
| | | | | | | | | **Biological** | |
| | | | | | | | | HbA1c | .006 |
| | | | | | | | | Weight loss | < .001 |
| | | | | | | | | **Diabetes-** | |

| Author (Year) | N | Age | Sex (M, F) | Ethnicity | Country | Intervention | Duration | Outcome | p-value |
|---|---|---|---|---|---|---|---|---|---|
| | | | | | | | | **related** | |
| | | | | | | | | Energy | < .001 |
| | | | | | | | | Carbohydrate | < .001 |
| | | | | | | | | Protein | < .001 |
| | | | | | | | | Fat | < .001 |
| | | | | | | | | Exercise | < .001 |
| Dobler, Herbeck Belnap, Pollmann, Fairn, Raspe & Mittag (2018) | 199 | 52 | 140, 59 | NA | Germany | Telephone follow-up motivational interviewing | 12 months | **Biological** | |
| | | | | | | | | HbA1c | .006 |
| | | | | | | | | Body mass index | .218 |
| | | | | | | Usual care | | Cardiovascular risk | .011 |
| | | | | | | | | **Diabetes-related** | |
| | | | | | | | | Exercise index | .006 |
| | | | | | | | | Dietary index | .633 |
| | | | | | | | | Medication adherence | .633 |
| | | | | | | | | **Psychological** | |
| | | | | | | | | Illness burden | .069 |
| | | | | | | | | Well-being | .044 |
| | | | | | | | | Depression | .057 |

| Author (Year) | N | Age | Sex (M, F) | Ethnicity | Country | Intervention | Duration | Outcome | p-value |
|---|---|---|---|---|---|---|---|---|---|
| Friis, Johnson, Cutfield, & Consedine (2016) | 63 | 43 | 20, 43 | New Zealand European (73%) | New Zealand | Mindful self-compassion program | 3 months | **Biological** | |
| | | | | | | | | HbA1c | .05 |
| | | | | Maori (2%) | | Usual Care | | **Psychological** | |
| | | | | | | | | Self-Compassion | .05 |
| | | | | | | | | Depression | .001 |
| | | | | Asian (8%) | | | | Diabetes Distress | .05 |
| | | | | Other Pacific (5%) | | | | | |
| | | | | Other European (13%) | | | | | |
| Gainey, Himathongkam, Tanaka & Suksom (2016) | 23 | 60 | 4, 19 | NA | Thailand | Traditional walking | 3 months | **Biological** | |
| | | | | | | Walking meditation | | HbA1c | <.05 |
| | | | | | | | | Fasting blood glucose | >.05 |
| | | | | | | | | Insulin resistance | >.05 |
| | | | | | | | | Total | |
| | | | | | | | | Cholesterol | >.05 |
| | | | | | | | | High-density lipoproteins | >.05 |
| | | | | | | | | Low-density lipoproteins | >.05 |
| | | | | | | | | Triglycerides | >.05 |
| | | | | | | | | Cortisol | <.05 |

| Author (Year) | N | Age | Sex (M, F) | Ethnicity | Country | Intervention | Duration | Outcome | p-value |
|---|---|---|---|---|---|---|---|---|---|
| Holmen, Torbjornsen, Wahl, Jenum, Smastuen, Arsand, & Ribu (2014) | 151 | 57 | 89, 62 | NA | Norway | Few Touch Application (FTA) | 12 months | **Biological** | |
| | | | | | | Few Touch Application—Health Counseling (FTA-HC)→Motivational interviewing Control | | HbA1c (FTA x control) | .42 |
| | | | | | | | | HbA1c (FTA-HC x control) | .97 |
| | | | | | | | | **Diabetes-related** | |
| | | | | | | | | Self-management skill and technique acquisition (FTA x control) | .79 |
| | | | | | | | | Self-management skill and technique acquisition (FTA-HC x control) | .04 |
| | | | | | | | | Health service navigation (FTA x control) | .06 |
| | | | | | | | | Health service navigation (FTA-HC x control) | .97 |
| Jansink, Braspenning, Keizer, van der Weijden, Elwyn & Grol (2013) | 521 | 64 | 285, 236 | NA | Netherlands | Nurse motivational interviewing program | 14 months | **Biological** | |
| | | | | | | | | HbA1c | .221 |
| | | | | | | | | Systolic blood pressure | .279 |
| | | | | | | Usual care | | Diastolic blood pressure | .294 |
| | | | | | | | | Low-density lipoproteins | .081 |
| | | | | | | | | Total | |
| | | | | | | | | Cholesterol | .051 |
| | | | | | | | | Body mass index | .198 |
| | | | | | | | | **Diabetes-related** | |
| | | | | | | | | Alcohol consumption | .647 |

| Author (Year) | N | Age | Sex (M, F) | Ethnicity | Country | Intervention | Duration | Outcome | p-value |
|---|---|---|---|---|---|---|---|---|---|
| | | | | | | | | Fat score | .708 |
| | | | | | | | | Vegetables | .518 |
| | | | | | | | | Fruit | .884 |
| | | | | | | | | Physical activity | .839 |
| | | | | | | | | Low activity | .498 |
| | | | | | | | | Medium activity | .592 |
| | | | | | | | | High activity | .669 |
| | | | | | | | | Diary activity | .066 |
| | | | | | | | | VAS score | .441 |
| Juul, Maindal, Zoffmann, Frydenberg & Sandbaek (2014) | 4034 | 60 | 2279, 1755 | NA | Denmark | Nurse motivational interviewing program | 18 months | **Biological** | |
| | | | | | | | | HbA1c | .67 |
| | | | | | | | | HbA1c ≥8% | .59 |
| | | | | | | Usual care | | Total cholesterol (mmol/l) | .02 |
| | | | | | | | | Total cholesterol ≥5 mmol/l | .07 |
| | | | | | | | | **Diabetes-related** | |
| | | | | | | | | Medication –controlled motivation | 1.00 |
| | | | | | | | | Medication –autonomous motivation | 1.00 |
| | | | | | | | | Diet and physical activity – controlled motivation | 0.70 |
| | | | | | | | | Diet and physical activity – autonomous motivation | 0.98 |
| | | | | | | | | Perceived Competence for Diabetes Scale | 0.97 |

| Author (Year) | N | Age | Sex (M, F) | Ethnicity | Country | Intervention | Duration | Outcome | p-value |
|---|---|---|---|---|---|---|---|---|---|
| Mohamed, Al-Lenjawi, Amuna, Zotor, & Elmahdi (2013) | 430 | 53.5 | NA | Arab | Qatar | Culturally sensitive structured education program | 12 months | **Psychological** | |
| | | | | | | | | Problem Areas in Diabetes | .31 |
| | | | | | | Control | | Mental component of the impact of health on daily living (SF-12) | .15 |
| | | | | | | | | Health Care | .43 |
| | | | | | | | | Climate | |
| | | | | | | | | Questionnaire | |
| | | | | | | | | **Biological** | |
| | | | | | | | | HbA1c | .012 |
| | | | | | | | | Fasting plasma glucose | .022 |
| | | | | | | | | Total cholesterol | .204 |
| | | | | | | | | High-density lipoproteins | <.001 |
| | | | | | | | | Low-density lipoproteins | .203 |
| | | | | | | | | Triglyceride | .200 |
| | | | | | | | | Albumin/creatinine ratio | <.001 |
| | | | | | | | | Systolic blood pressure | .631 |
| | | | | | | | | Diastolic blood pressure | .421 |
| | | | | | | | | Body mass index | .001 |
| | | | | | | | | **Diabetes-related** | |
| | | | | | | | | Knowledge | <.001 |
| | | | | | | | | Attitude | <.001 |
| | | | | | | | | Practice | <.001 |
| | | | | | | | | Overall | <.001 |

| Author (Year) | N | Age | Sex (M, F) | Ethnicity | Country | Intervention | Duration | Outcome | p-value |
|---|---|---|---|---|---|---|---|---|---|
| Pearson, Wills, Woods, & Warnecke (2018) | 67 | 59 | 36, 31 | NA | Australia | Mindfulness practice | 3 months | **Biological** | |
| | | | | | | Usual care | | HbA1c | .02 |
| | | | | | | | | Monitoring Blood Glucose | . 06 |
| | | | | | | | | Systolic blood pressure | .78 |
| | | | | | | | | Diastolic blood pressure | . 28 |
| | | | | | | | | **Diabetes-related** | |
| | | | | | | | | Diet | .31 |
| | | | | | | | | Exercise | .12 |
| | | | | | | | | Foot care | .25 |
| | | | | | | | | **Psychological** | |
| | | | | | | | | Depression | .02 |
| | | | | | | | | Anxiety | .18 |
| | | | | | | | | Stress | .03 |
| | | | | | | | | Problem Areas in Diabetes | .78 |
| Tovote, Fleer, Snippe, Peeters, Emmelkamp, Sanderman ... Schroevers (2014) | 94 | 53 | 48, 46 | NA | Netherland | Mindfulness-based cognitive therapy (MBCT) | 3 months | **Biological** | |
| | | | | | | | | HbA1c (MBCT) | .92 |
| | | | | | | Cognitive behaviour therapy (CBT) | | HbA1c (CBT) | .72 |
| | | | | | | | | **Psychological** | |
| | | | | | | Control | | Depression -BDI-II (MBCT x Control) | .004 |
| | | | | | | | | Depression -BDI-II (CBT x Control) | .001 |
| | | | | | | | | Depression -HAM-D7 (MBCT x Control) | .001 |
| | | | | | | | | Depression -HAM-D7 (CBT x Control) | .001 |

| Author (Year) | N | Age | Sex (M, F) | Ethnicity | Country | Intervention | Duration | Outcome | p-value |
|---|---|---|---|---|---|---|---|---|---|
| | | | | | | | | Well-being -WHO-5 (MBCT x Control) | .001 |
| | | | | | | | | Well-being -WHO-5 (CBT x Control) | .001 |
| | | | | | | | | Anxiety - GAD-7 (MBCT x Control) | .004 |
| | | | | | | | | Anxiety - GAD-7 (CBT x Control) | .01 |
| | | | | | | | | Diabetes Distress (MBCT x Control) | .02 |
| | | | | | | | | Diabetes Distress (CBT x Control) | .04 |
| van Son, Nyklicek, Pop, Blonk, Erdtsieck, Spooren, ... Pouwer (2013) | 139 | 56.5 | 70, 69 | NA | Netherland | Mindfulness-based cognitive therapy | 3 months | **Biological** | |
| | | | | | | | | HbA1c | .35 |
| | | | | | | Usual care | | **Diabetes-related** | |
| | | | | | | | | Physical Health Status | .03 |
| | | | | | | | | **Psychological** | |
| | | | | | | | | Perceived Stress Scale | .001 |
| | | | | | | | | Anxiety (HADS) | .02 |
| | | | | | | | | Anxiety (POMS) | .001 |
| | | | | | | | | Depression (HADS) | .01 |
| | | | | | | | | Depression (POMS) | .001 |
| | | | | | | | | Diabetes distress | .49 |
| | | | | | | | | Fatigue (POMS) | .01 |
| | | | | | | | | Mental Health Status | .01 |

DOI: http://dx.doi.org/10.5772/intechopen.97653

| Author (Year) | N | Age | Sex (M, F) | Ethnicity | Country | Intervention | Duration | Outcome | p-value |
|---|---|---|---|---|---|---|---|---|---|
| van Son, Nyklicek, Pop, Blonk, Erdtsieck, & Pouwer (2014) | 139 | 56.5 | 70, 69 | NA | Netherland | Mindfulness-based cognitive therapy | 6 months | **Biological** | |
| | | | | | | Usual care | | HbA1c | .816 |
| | | | | | | | | **Diabetes-related** | |
| | | | | | | | | Physical Health Status | .034 |
| | | | | | | | | Diabetes acceptance | .105 |
| | | | | | | | | **Psychological** | |
| | | | | | | | | Perceived Stress | .001 |
| | | | | | | | | Anxiety (HADS) | .001 |
| | | | | | | | | Anxiety (POMS) | .001 |
| | | | | | | | | Depression (HADS) | .004 |
| | | | | | | | | Depression (POMS) | .16 |
| | | | | | | | | Diabetes distress | .034 |
| | | | | | | | | Mental Health Status | .001 |
| | | | | | | | | Mindfulness | .001 |
| | | | | | | | | Self-Esteem | .597 |
| Varming, Rasmussen, Husted, Olesen, Grønnegaard, & Willaing, (2019) | 97 | 64.3 | 64, 33 | Danish | Denmark | Empowerment, motivation, and medical adherence (EMMA) | 3.5 months | **Intervention phase** | |
| | | | | | | | 6-month follow up | **Biological** | |
| | | | | | | Usual care | | HbA1c | >.05 |
| | | | | | | | | Blood sugar | >.05 |
| | | | | | | | | Body mass index | >.05 |
| | | | | | | | | Systolic blood pressure | >.05 |

| Author (Year) | N | Age | Sex (M, F) | Ethnicity | Country | Intervention | Duration | Outcome | p-value |
|---|---|---|---|---|---|---|---|---|---|
| | | | | | | | | Diastolic blood pressure | >.05 |
| | | | | | | | | **Diabetes-related** | |
| | | | | | | | | Problem areas in diabetes | >.05 |
| | | | | | | | | Diabetes self-care activities | >.05 |
| | | | | | | | | Healthy diet | <.05 |
| | | | | | | | | Physical activity | >.05 |
| | | | | | | | | Diabetes medication | >.05 |
| | | | | | | | | Foot care | >.05 |
| | | | | | | | | Diabetes competence | >.05 |
| | | | | | | | | **Psychological** | |
| | | | | | | | | Well-being | >.05 |
| | | | | | | | | Healthcare support | <.05 |
| | | | | | | | | **Follow-up** | |
| | | | | | | | | **Biological** | |
| | | | | | | | | HbA1c | >.05 |
| | | | | | | | | Blood sugar | >.05 |
| | | | | | | | | Body mass index | >.05 |
| | | | | | | | | Systolic blood pressure | >.05 |
| | | | | | | | | Diastolic blood pressure | >.05 |
| | | | | | | | | **Diabetes-related** | |
| | | | | | | | | Problem areas in diabetes | >.05 |

DOI: http://dx.doi.org/10.5772/intechopen.97653

| Author (Year) | N | Age | Sex (M, F) | Ethnicity | Country | Intervention | Duration | Outcome | p-value |
|---|---|---|---|---|---|---|---|---|---|
| | | | | | | | | Diabetes self-care activities | >.05 |
| | | | | | | | | Healthy diet | >.05 |
| | | | | | | | | Physical activity | >.05 |
| | | | | | | | | Diabetes medication | <.01 |
| | | | | | | | | Foot care | <.05 |
| | | | | | | | | Diabetes competence | >.05 |
| | | | | | | | | **Psychological** | |
| | | | | | | | | Well-being | >.05 |
| | | | | | | | | Healthcare support | >.05 |

Note. *NA = Not available within the article.*
*[a]Within group differences*

**Table 1.**
*Summary of reviewed randomized controlled trials.*

management of the condition. Internet-based CBT protocols offer a promising and accessible psychotherapeutic intervention for T2DM patients, but more randomized controlled trials are needed to further elucidate their efficacy. It is also possible that certain patients will do better than others with web-based CBT interventions. Therefore, treatment matching trials are needed to identify the personal characteristics that best predict positive outcomes with non-traditional formats of CBT for T2DM.

### 2.2 Motivational interviewing

Motivational interviewing (MI) is a collaborative and goal-oriented therapy that focuses on resolving ambivalence toward change [9]. Suggestions or instructions for diabetes mellitus self-management may be met with resistance and non-compliance by patients. MI counters these responses by promoting self-efficacy. The therapist helps the patient to determine what is important to their own well-being and how to achieve that goal [10]. For example, a therapist may explore what the patient likes and does not like about their current behaviors to determine the costs and benefits of behavior change. By putting the patient in the 'driver's seat', intrinsic motivation is developed (e.g., "I will change my diet and exercise because I want to live a long and healthy life"). The therapeutic alliance is seen as fundamental to facilitating positive behavior change. From this starting point, the therapist and patient can work together to set an agenda for items they would like to change (e.g., medication, diet, exercise, and regular monitoring of blood sugar levels) and check in frequently about the patient's perceived importance and confidence regarding the target behavior [10].

Although MI has garnered a lot of research interest, the results of recent studies examining its utility in the management of T2DM have been mixed. In support of this intervention in the care of T2DM, Chee and colleagues (2017) found that patients who received MI for 6 months, in addition to diet and exercise planning, reported greater reductions in HbA1c ($p$ = .006) and weight loss ($p$ < .001) than a control group at 6 month follow up [11]. This study took place in Malaysia with a sample of 230 Indian (58%), Chinese (28%), and Malaysian (14%) participants, aged 30–65 years ($M$ = 55, $SD$ = 8). However, a number of recent studies have not found support for MI over treatment as usual. For example, patients treated by nurses trained in MI in the Netherlands and Denmark had similar HbA1c levels, diet, physical activity, and well-being as those treated by nurses trained in standard care. This pattern of results was found in both 14- and 18-month trials [12, 13]. Notably, the competency of the nurses trained in psychological skills for that study was below beginner-level proficiency and was similar to the standard-care nurses. In other words, it may require extensive training among therapists in order to demonstrate the superiority of MI over control groups.

Recent findings for MI in the management of T2DM are also mixed when MI examined in alternative delivery formats. A 12-month telephone-based delivery of MI in Germany was found to reduce patients' HbA1c levels to a greater extent than usual care (i.e., informational pamphlets; $p$ = .006). It also improved to a greater extent patients' physical activity ($p$ = .006), cardiovascular health ($p$ = .011), psychological well-being ($p$ = .044), illness burden ($p$ = .069), and depression ($p$ = .057) [14]. In another study from Norway, telephone-based MI was provided for 4 months in addition to an interactive mobile self-monitoring application that tracks diet, fitness, and diabetes-related goals. There were no differences in patients' HbA1c levels between app users with and without MI, or those who received usual care (i.e., no psychotherapeutic intervention) [15], suggesting that neither the app nor the MI produced a better health outcome than standard, non-psychotherapeutic care. Similarly, a 6-month web-based counseling software delivery of MI was equivalent to standard lifestyle advice in resulting HbA1c levels among Arab participants [16]. The MI-based intervention was, however, superior to the control group at increasing short-term diabetes-related knowledge ($p = .023$) among patients and trended toward within group improvements in dietary habits ($p = .050$). The discrepancy between the findings within that study further highlight that all MI delivery formats are not equal; long-term direct therapist contact may be an essential component of MI in order to elicit sufficient behavior change that manifests in reductions in HbA1c levels. Further research would be necessary to confirm this hypothesis.

### 2.3 Counseling

Another category of psychological interventions for T2DM involves counseling interventions which tend to provide non-specific support for diabetes mellitus management. Counseling typically promotes self-awareness and self-determination which, in the context of diabetes mellitus, can aid in improving self-management behaviors [17]. Counseling can also provide emotional and psychological support to individuals who are dealing with the stress of living with a chronic disease. In other words, although behavior change is not the focus of counseling interventions, they may, in theory, be helpful for reducing stress and increasing adherence among patients.

RCTs of counseling interventions for T2DM are scarce [4–6], but there have been two recent studies on this modality. One study examined a culturally sensitive 12-month counseling program for T2DM patients in Qatar (i.e., using Arabic language and referencing culturally specific food habits and health beliefs). Within this program, patients were provided with information about diabetes and related complications, how to incorporate a healthy lifestyle and eating habits, the benefits of exercise, and how to use counseling techniques at home. The researchers found that this program led to significant reductions in patients' HbA1c levels ($p = .012$) and BMI ($p < .001$), as well as improved diabetes-related knowledge ($p < .001$), attitudes ($p < .001$), and practices ($p < .001$) over the standard practice of distributing informational booklets [18]. However, in another study of counseling, patients in Denmark who were offered short-term empowerment, motivation and medical adherence (EMMA) therapy, which focuses on goal setting and autonomy support, did not report improvements in HbA1c levels over and above treatment as usual. Individuals who received counseling did, however, demonstrated increases in frequency of healthy eating ($p < .05$) [19].

Based on these findings, counseling may have benefits for improving HbA1c levels in specific cultural contexts, but these therapies may have to be long-term (one year or longer) and follow a structured format to be beneficial for glycemic control.

### 2.4 Mindfulness-based therapies

Mindfulness-based therapies teach meditative practices and promote a non-judgmental awareness of the present moment, including noticing thoughts, emotions, and bodily sensations. In the context of T2DM, noticing negative diabetes-related thoughts can help promote passive observation of the experience and allow the individual to be present in their everyday life without an unhelpful behavioral reaction. For example, noticing internal hunger or satiety cues can influence dietary choices and help patients regulate blood sugar levels. Mindfulness can, in theory, help patients become better attuned to their physiological state, including blood sugar levels. Or a patient who experiences anxiety about increasing their physical activity may learn to nonjudgmentally notice their anxious thoughts and urges to avoid exercise, but intentionally choose to exercise nonetheless. Regular mindfulness practice trains the mind to be less reactive and more intentional in one's choices and experiences.

Mindfulness interventions have increased in popularity in the past decade and there have been a number of recent RCTs that indicate the applicability of mindfulness-based therapies for the treatment of diabetes mellitus. The outcomes are mixed in regard to changes in HbA1c levels. In support of the efficacy of mindfulness programs, an 8-week mindfulness-based stress reduction program in Iran was found to improve HbA1c levels ($p$ = .010), fasting blood sugar ($p$ < .001), depression ($p$ = .010), anxiety ($p$ = .010), and overall mental health ($p$ = .001) compared to a control group [20]. In another study from New Zealand, an 8-week program based in mindful self-compassion led to greater decreases in HbA1c ($p$ = .050) than a waitlist control, as well as reductions in depression ($p$ = .001) and diabetes-related distress ($p$ = .050) [21]. Even when the 8-week program was self-directed, mindfulness practice has been found to improve HbA1c levels ($p$ = .020), stress ($p$ = .030), and depression symptoms ($p$ = .020) compared to a control condition in Australia [22]. Specific techniques within a mindfulness-based practice have been found to be effective. For instance, Thai patients with T2DM who engaged in mindful walking for 3 months demonstrated greater decreases in HbA1c ($p$ < .050) relative to walking alone [23].

A relatively recent variation of mindfulness therapy, mindfulness-based cognitive therapy, involves training patients in both meditation and cognitive therapy (i.e., identifying and challenging cognitive distortions). A series of studies in the Netherlands were recently conducted to investigate the effects of this intervention on the care of patients with T2DM, but none showed any benefit for HbA1c levels. For instance, although van Son and colleagues [24, 25] found improvements in self-reported stress ($p$ = .001), anxiety ($p$ = .020), depression ($p$ = .010), and improved quality of life ($p$ = .010) following mindfulness-based cognitive therapy and that were maintained at 6-month follow-up, they did not find a difference on HbA1c levels when compared to usual care. Another study also did not find differences in glycemic control between mindfulness-based cognitive therapy and a control group, but did report changes in diabetes-related distress ($p$ = .020) and well-being ($p$ = .001) [26]. Within these studies, poor glycemic control was not an inclusion criterion, which may have resulted in a floor effect due to generally low levels among patients regardless of treatment condition. It may be that mindfulness-based cognitive therapy, which was originally developed to treat depression, is less effective at reducing HbA1c levels than traditional mindfulness training practices that do not incorporate cognitive therapy but focus instead on meditation. In other words, the cognitive therapy addition may dilute the efficacy of mindfulness training, which, at this point in time, has more support for it in the care of T2DM. Research designs that compare mindfulness-based cognitive therapy to other mindfulness interventions in patients with poor glycemic control would be necessary to confirm this hypothesis.

## 3. Summary

T2DM is a serious disease with significant morbidity which, if poorly managed, can lead to short- and long-term complications including cardiovascular disease, blindness, nerve damage, and loss of limbs [1]. There has been interest among researchers to examine whether psychotherapeutic interventions aimed at changing thoughts, feelings, and/or behaviors among patients with T2DM have any significant benefit. Recent randomized controlled trials suggest that psychotherapy for T2DM may be an effective treatment option for certain outcomes, but that not all therapies have an evidence base for use with patients with T2DM.

Research from the past 8 years has provided the most support for mindfulness-based therapies at improving health outcomes for patients with T2DM. Numerous studies with different samples have demonstrated statistically significant reductions in HbA1c levels and fasting blood sugar, as well as improvements in psychological variables such as depression, anxiety, stress, diabetes-related distress, and overall mental health. These findings were demonstrated in various geographical regions (including Iran, New Zealand, and Australia) among middle-aged (average age ranged from 23 to 59 years old) men ($n$ = 67) and women ($n$ = 123). Notably, however, mindfulness-based cognitive therapy was only superior to a control group for psychological outcomes, not HbA1c levels. In other words, mindfulness-based therapies that emphasize meditative practices, but not mindfulness-based cognitive therapy, have evidence to support their use in the management of T2DM. Of note, the existing studies on mindfulness-based cognitive therapy that did not show its benefit for glycemic control were conducted with middle-aged (53 to 56.5 years old) men ($n$ = 118) and women ($n$ = 115) from the Netherlands. As such, this form of therapy may not be effective within this relatively young sample. More research is needed to understand whether mindfulness-based cognitive therapy is as good or better than mindfulness therapy.

While research interest in traditional-delivery CBT has declined in recent years, one recent study expanded upon existing literature to demonstrate the effectiveness of CBT in a web-based format in diabetic patients from Saudi Arabia. This program improved HbA1c levels, as well as diabetes mellitus knowledge and self-efficacy, to a greater extent than the control group. The research results are more divided for MI and counseling interventions. In regard to the former, MI was typically found to be as effective as standard care on HbA1c levels and diabetes-related behaviors such as diet and physical activity in patients from Malaysia and parts of Europe (average ages 55 to 64 years old). However, when delivered in a telephone- or web-based format, MI had the added benefits of improving diabetes-related behaviors, such as dietary changes and physical activity, as well as psychological variables, including lowering depression and increasing well-being and diabetes-related knowledge. Notably, this was true in both men and women from diverse backgrounds (i.e., Arab and German). Recent findings for counseling intervention have been mixed whereby culture-specific counseling appears to be more effective at reducing HbA1c levels than informational booklets for middle-aged ($M$ = 53.5 years old) Arab patients. But counseling was no more effective than usual care for diabetes mellitus self-management in older ($M$ = 64.5 years old) Danish patients on improving HbA1c levels.

Commonly used psychotherapeutic interventions, such as mindfulness-based therapies and CBT, have empirical support in recent studies for use in the management of T2DM. This provides an evidence base for the widespread implementation of these treatments by healthcare professionals in their care of patients with T2DM. Training in both of these psychotherapy approaches for health professionals is widely available through professional development workshops or training manuals, and many workshops have been offered remotely during the COVID-19 pandemic. In addition, the recent promising findings from a study of self-directed mindfulness therapy suggests that healthcare professionals can recommend these programs to patients to pursue as a self-help resource, which reduces the potential obstacles of cost and geographic accessibility. Additional research is necessary to understand the efficacy of counseling and alternative-format CBT before practitioners should recommend these interventions in the management of T2DM.

This chapter reveals that psychotherapeutic interventions are an appropriate treatment modality for patients with T2DM and some have support from recent studies in improving health outcomes. These interventions extend beyond treating the physiological concerns of this disorder and can address other psychosocial variables, such as thoughts, feelings, and behaviors related to diabetes mellitus care. As such, not only did HbA1c levels improve in a number of treatments, research has supported changes in diet, physical activity, diabetes-related knowledge, and, in some cases, mood. There are no known negative effects of psychotherapeutic interventions on the health or well-being of patients with T2DM. The evidence for these interventions should be considered in regard to the sample population and size, comparison group, length of intervention, and geographic region.

There are still many gaps in the literature regarding which groups of individuals benefit the most from psychotherapy for T2DM and from which approach. Future research should continue to explore psychotherapeutic interventions especially in the areas of counseling and new delivery formats of CBT to expand treatment options. Of note, a recent RCT of Acceptance and Commitment Therapy for patients with T2DM has demonstrated preliminary success in improving HbA1c levels compared to education alone [27], but more research is needed on this intervention strategy before drawing generalized conclusions. In addition, more attention in future research studies needs to be paid to how different types of patients respond to psychotherapy and whether variables such as age, sex, and ethnicity interact with intervention type to produce different outcomes. Across all psychotherapeutic treatment modalities under investigation for use in the management of T2DM, treatment matching research is warranted to determine which patients may be able to benefit from modified, more accessible and cost-effective (self-help, web-based) formats. With that more targeted research in future research, healthcare professionals can feel even more confident implementing some therapies, such as mindfulness-based therapies, CBT, and some formats of MI, to promote better glycemic control and psychological well-being in their patients with T2DM.

## 4. Conclusions

Psychological interventions can lower HbA1c levels, improve psychological distress, and support healthy coping among patients with T2DM. There is recent and reliable research support for mindfulness-based therapies at improving HbA1c levels, blood sugar, and psychosocial variables. Results are promising, but more research is needed on the efficacy of longer-term culture-sensitive counseling as well as alternative delivery formats of cognitive-behavioral therapy on health outcomes among patients with T2DM.

## Acknowledgements

Dr. Joel Katz is supported by a Canadian Institutes of Health Research Canada Research Chair in Health Psychology. Thank you to Susan Zahir for help with tables and revisions.

## Conflict of interest

The authors have no conflicts of interest to declare.

## Appendix: Search Strategy

To identify relevant studies, the authors used the same search terms as two previously published systematic reviews of psychotherapy for T2DM [4, 5]. The search was conducted by pairing relevant search terms, including "psychotherapy", "cognitive-behavioral therapy", "motivational interviewing", "counseling", "supportive therapy", and "mindfulness-based therapy", with "type 2 diabetes" and "randomized controlled trial" on PsycINFO, PubMed, and Medline using a Boolean "AND". The search was limited to articles published after December 2012 since this was the end of the period reviewed since the last review paper [5]. The original search was conducted on January 24th, 2019, then repeated at each revision, on March 24th, 2019, October 28th, 2019, and November 12th, 2020, to be thorough. The initial search identified 268 articles. After duplicates across search engines were removed, articles were screened by the primary author based on titles and abstracts. For the screening process, full articles were retrieved and reviewed to confirm relevance and eligibility. The primary author extracted data on intervention type, methods, and outcomes. To be included in this review, the article must have been an RCT that examined a psychotherapeutic intervention for participants who met criteria for T2DM at the time of recruitment and must have changes in HbA1c levels as a health outcome. Only RCT's were reviewed so as to include only the most scientifically rigorous research on this topic. Studies that used only pharmacological interventions were not included. In addition, interventions that specifically targeted comorbid disorders (e.g., depression in individuals with T2DM) and studies that were not reported in English were also excluded from this review. In the end, 16 articles remained and were reviewed.

## Author details

Keisha C. Gobin*, Jennifer S. Mills and Joel D. Katz
York University, Toronto, Canada

*Address all correspondence to: kgobin@yorku.ca

## References

[1] Public Health Agency of Canada. (2018). Type 2 diabetes. Retrieved from https://www.canada.ca/en/public-health/services/diseases/type-2-diabetes.html

[2] American Diabetes Association. (2015). Classification and diagnosis of diabetes. *Diabetes Care, 38*, 8-16. doi: 10.2337/dc15-S005

[3] Vitolins, M. Z., Anderson, A. M., Delahanty, L, Raynor, H., Miller, G. D., Mobley, C., ... Look AHEAD Research Group. (2009). Action for health in diabetes (look AHEAD) trial: Baseline evaluation of selected nutrients and food group intake. *Journal of the American Dietetic Association, 109*, 1367-1375.

[4] Ismail, K., Winkley, K., & Rabe-Hesketh, S. (2004). Systematic review and meta-analysis of randomised controlled trials of psychological interventions to improve glycaemic control in patients with type 2 diabetes. *The Lancet, 363*, 1589-1597. doi:10.1016/S0140-6736(04)16202-8

[5] Thorpe, C. T., Fahey, L. E., Johnson, H., Deshpande, M., Thorpe, J. M., & Fisher, E. B. (2013). Facilitating healthy coping in patients with diabetes: A systematic review. *The Diabetes Educator*, 39, 33-52. doi:10.1177/0145721712464400

[6] Winkley, K., Upsher, R., Stahl, D., Pollard, D., Brennan, A., Heller, S. R., & Ismail, K. (2020). Psychological interventions to improve glycemic control in adults with type 2 diabetes: A systematic review and meta-analysis. *BMJ Open Diabetes Research & Care*, 8: e001150. doi:10.1136/bmjdrc-2019-001150

[7] Turner, J. (2010). The use of cognitive behavioural therapy in diabetes care: A review and case study. *Journal of Diabetes Nursing, 14*, 86-92.

[8] Alanzi, T., Alanazi, N. R., Istepanian, R., & Philip, N. (2018). Evaluation of the effectiveness of mobile diabetes management system with social networking and cognitive behavioural therapy (CBT) for T2D. *mHealth, 4*, 35. doi:10.21037/mhealth.2018.06.05

[9] Miller, W. & Rollnick, S.(2002) *Motivational interviewing: Preparing people to change addictive behaviour (second edition)*. New York: Guildford Press.

[10] Welch, G., Rose, G., & Ernst, D. (2006). Motivational interviewing and diabetes: What is it, how is it used, and does it work? *Diabetes Spectrum, 19*, 5-11. doi: 10.2337/diaspect.19.1.5

[11] Chee, W. S. S., Gilcharan Singh, H. K., Hamdy, O., Mechanick, J. I., Lee, V. K. M., Barua, A., Ali, S. Z. M., & Hussein, Z. (2017). Structured lifestyle intervention based on a trans-cultural diabetes-specific nutrition algorithm (tDNA) in individuals with type 2 diabetes: A randomized controlled trial. *BMJ Open Diabetes Research and Care, 5*, e000384. doi: 10.1136/bmjdrc-2016-000384

[12] Jansink, R., Braspenning, J., Keizer, E., van der Weijden, T., Elwyn, G., & Grol, R. (2013). No identifiable Hb1Ac or lifestyle change after a comprehensive diabetes programme including motivational interviewing: a cluster randomised trial. *Scandinavian journal of primary health care, 31*, 119–127. doi:10.3109/02813432.2013.797178

[13] Juul, L., Maindal, H. T., Zoffmann, V., Frydenberg, M., & Sandbaek, A. (2014). Effectiveness of a training course for general practice nurses in motivation support in type 2 diabetes care: a cluster-randomised trial. *PloS one, 9*, e96683. doi: 10.1371/journal.pone.0096683

[14] Döbler, A., Herbeck Belnap, B., Pollmann, H., Farin, E., Raspe, H., &

Mittag, O. (2018). Telephone-delivered lifestyle support with action planning and motivational interviewing techniques to improve rehabilitation outcomes. *Rehabilitation Psychology, 63* (2), 170-181. doi:10.1037/rep0000224

[15] Holmen, H., Torbjørnsen, A., Wahl, A.K., Jenum, A.K., Småstuen, M.C., Årsand, E., & Ribu, L. (2014). A mobile health intervention for self-management and lifestyle change for persons with type 2 diabetes, part 2: One-year results from the Norwegian randomized controlled trial RENEWING HEALTH. *JMIR mHealth and uHealth, 2*, e57. doi: 10.2196/mhealth.3882.

[16] Abu-Saad, K., Murad, H., Barid, R., Olmer, L., Ziv, A., Younis-Zeidan, N., Kalter-Leibovici, O. (2019). Development and efficacy of an electronic, culturally adapted lifestyle counseling tool for improving diabetes-related dietary knowledge: Randomized controlled trial among ethnic minority adults with type 2 diabetes mellitus. *Journal of Medical Internet Research, 21*, e13674. doi:10.2196/13674

[17] Rogers, C. (1961) *On becoming a person: A therapist's view of psychotherapy*. London: Constable.

[18] Mohamed, H., Al-Lenjawi, B., Amuna, P., Zotor, F., & Elmahdi, H. (2013). Culturally sensitive patient-centred educational programme for self-management of type 2 diabetes: A randomized controlled trial. *Primary Care Diabetes, 7*(3), 199-206. doi: 10.1016/j.pcd.2013.05.002

[19] Varming, A. R., Rasmussen, L. B., Husted, G. R., Olesen, K., Grønnegaard, C., & Willaing, I. (2019). Improving empowerment, motivation, and medical adherence in patients with poorly controlled type 2 diabetes: A randomized controlled trial of a patient-centered intervention. *Patient Education and Counseling, 102*(12), 2238-2245. doi: 10.1016/j.pec.2019.06.014

[20] Armani, K. A., Vahdani, B., Noorbala, A., Nejatisafa, A., Arbabi, M., Zenoozian, S., & Nakhjavani, M. (2018). The impact of mindfulness-based stress reduction on emotional wellbeing and glycemic control of patients with type 2 diabetes mellitus. *Journal of Diabetes Research*, 1-6. doi: 10.1155/2018/1986820.

[21] Friis, A., Johnson, M., Cutfield, R., & Consedine, N. (2016). Kindness matters: A randomized controlled trial of mindful self compassion improves depression, distress and HbA1c among patients with diabetes. *Diabetes Care, 39*, 1-9. doi: 10.2337/dc16-0416.

[22] Pearson, S., Wills, K., Woods, M., & Warnecke, E. (2018). Effects of mindfulness on psychological distress and HbA1c in people with diabetes. *Mindfulness, 9*, 1615-1626. doi: 10.1007/s12671-018-0908-1

[23] Gainey, A., Himathongkam, T., Tanaka, H., & Suksom, D. (2016). Effects of buddhist walking meditation on glycemic control and vascular function in patients with type 2 diabetes. *Complementary Therapies in Medicine, 26*, 92-97. doi: 10.1016/j.ctim.2016.03.009

[24] van Son, J., Nyklícek, I., Pop, V. J., Blonk, M., C., Erdtsieck, R. J., Spooren, P. F., ... Pouwer, F. (2013). The effects of a mindfulness-based intervention on emotional distress, quality of life, and HbA^sub 1c^ in outpatients with diabetes (DiaMind): A randomized controlled trial. *Diabetes Care, 3*, 823-30. doi: 10.2337/dc12-1477.

[25] van Son, J., Nyklíček, I., Pop, V. J., Blonk, M. C., Erdtsieck, R. J., & Pouwer, F. (2014). Mindfulness-based cognitive therapy for people with diabetes and emotional problems: Long-term follow-up findings from the DiaMind randomized controlled trial. *Journal of Psychosomatic Research, 77*, 81-84. doi: 10.1016/j.jpsychores.2014.03.013

[26] Tovote, K. A., Fleer, J., Snippe, E., Peeters, A. C. T. M., Emmelkamp, P. M. G., Sanderman, R., . . . Schroevers, M. J. (2014). Individual mindfulness-based cognitive therapy and cognitive behavior therapy for treating depressive symptoms in patients with diabetes: Results of a randomized controlled trial. *Diabetes Care, 37*, 2427-34. doi: 10.2337/dc13-2918

[27] Shayeghian, Z., Hassanabadi, H., Aguilar-Vafaie, M., Amiri, P., & Besharat, M. A. (2016). A randomized controlled trial of acceptance and commitment therapy for type 2 diabetes management: The moderating role of coping styles. *PLoS ONE, 11*(11), 14.

Chapter 13

# Diet and Obesity

*Olariike Oyindasola Kayode*

## Abstract

Obesity is a complex disease that involves an excessive amount of body fat. It is a medical problem that increases the risk of other diseases, such as heart disease, diabetes, high blood pressure and certain cancers. Although there are genetic, behavioral, metabolic and hormonal influences on body weight, obesity occurs when you take in more calories than you burn through exercise and daily activities that is when energy intake exceeds energy expenditure. Diet plays an important role in the pathogenesis of obesity; fatty foods are energy dense and gives 9calories per gram compared to carbohydrate and protein that gives 4calories per gram. Also, if physical activity is inadequate, excess consumption of fat can results into weight gain. It does not take as much energy (about 3%), to convert and store dietary fat as it does to convert and store glucose. Fats are easily stored by the body. The aim of this chapter is to provide an understanding of physiological causes and effects of obesity as this will help to promote positive food choices. It is probable that an understanding of dietary patterns and how it relates to obesity will go a long way in the treatment of this complex problem.

**Keywords:** Food, Diet, Dietary Patterns, Obesity and Dietary fat

## 1. Introduction

Excessive body weight is a growing health problem worldwide. It is a well-known risk factor in cardiovascular disease, diabetes, hypertension, and cancers, among other conditions [1]. According to World Health Organization, obesity has been considered as one of the leading threats to future public health.

Obesity is a complex health issue resulting from a combination of causes and individual factors such as behavior and genetics [2]. Behaviors can include physical activity, inactivity, dietary patterns, medication use, and other exposures. Although there are genetic, behavioral, metabolic and hormonal influences on body weight, obesity occurs when you take in more calories than you burn through exercise and normal daily activities that is when energy intake exceeds energy expenditure. Even though the cause of obesity is complicated, dietary habit or lifestyle plays an important role in developing obese conditions [3].

The increasing westernization, urbanization and mechanization occurring in most countries around the world is associated with changes in the diet towards one of high fat, high energy-dense foods and a sedentary lifestyle [4]. Nutrition transition in developing countries leads to dietary intakes of micronutrient – poor, energy – dense foods, which may be important determinants of overweight/obesity [5].

There is also a direct relationship between the amount of dietary fat and the degree of obesity. High-fat diets induce greater food intake and weight gain than high-carbohydrate diets as indicated by animal studies [6]. Contributing factors are caloric density, satiety properties and post-absorptive processing. The satiating effects after meals with a high fat:carbohydrate ratio is less than for meals with a lower ratio.

Mediterranean pattern of nutrition, has been described as containing high proportion of mono-unsaturated fat acids versus saturated fats and contributes in the preservation of body weight, while expands longevity and life expectancy. This pattern of nutrition has been adopted by many countries and it is diversified according to the cultural and socio-economic features of each country. Several research studies have commented on the beneficial effects of the Mediterranean diet in the preservation or decrease of body weight, in the primary or secondary prevention of coronary disease, in the maintenance of high density cholesterol (HDL) and triglycerides within normal rates, as well as in the significant reduction in mortality rates [7–9].

Current recommendations for weight management emphasize the importance of healthy eating patterns that include a variety of nutrient-dense foods, limit portions of energy-dense foods, and reduce overall energy density [10].

A unifying factor for weight loss across dietary patterns is energy density [11]. When a diet's energy density is reduced; it allows individuals to consume satisfying amounts of food for fewer calories. The goal of dietary therapy in the management of obesity is to reduce the total number of calories consumed.

## 2. Physiological causes and effects of obesity

Obesity is a complex disease that involves an excessive amount of body fat. It is a medical problem that increases your risk of other diseases and health problems, such as heart disease, diabetes, high blood pressure and certain cancers. Although there are genetic, behavioral, metabolic and hormonal influences on body weight, obesity occurs when you take in more calories than you burn through exercise and normal daily activities that is when energy intake exceeds energy expenditure.

Even though the cause of obesity is complicated, dietary habit or lifestyle plays an important role in developing obese conditions [3, 12]. Lifestyle changes and nutritional habits, such as irregular meal patterns; mainly skipping breakfast, consumption of foods and beverages of low nutritional value and sub-optimal intake of dairy products, fruits and vegetables, intake of refined carbohydrates such as sugar sweetened soft drinks are all contributing factors to the development of obesity [12–15].

Obesity as a complex disorder has multiple etiological factors. The primary factor which is considered as a driver of obesity is obesogenic environment and unhealthy eating behavior. Secondary factors such as genetic and neuroendocrine factors, and diseases such as hypothyroidism and polycystic ovary syndrome are also related to excessive weight [16].

In a study carried out among undergraduates in Nigeria observed a significant relationship between vegetable consumption and Body Mass Index ($X^2 = 16.031$, p-value = 0.001) and there exist no significant relationship between cereals consumption and body mass index ($X^2 = 8.916$, p-value = 0.710) [17].

Obesity has been shown to be a predisposing factor in the rising prevalence of morbidity and mortality associated with non – communicable diseases like type-2 diabetes mellitus, hypertension, cancer, stroke among adults [18].

Overweight and obesity increases the likelihood of various diseases, particularly heart diseases, type2 diabetes, breathing difficulties during sleep, certain types of cancer and osteoarthritis [19].

## 3. Dietary fat and obesity

Fat are of various types, some are more beneficial to health than others. Those found in foods are known as dietary fats, the body needs fat to function fully as it has a lot of functions in the body and is essential to health. For instance, fat soluble vitamins (Vitamins A, D, E and K) cannot be transported in the absence of fat. However, a diet with too much fat can increase body weight and also increase the risk of cardiovascular disease.

Dietary fats are believed to play an important role in the development of heart disease [20]. The National health institutions has recommended to reduce the intake of dietary fat to prevent CVDs [21].

### 3.1 Healthy versus unhealthy fat

The healthy fat are primarily unsaturated fats:

**Monounsaturated fat**: This type of fat is found in a variety of foods and oils. Eating foods rich in monounsaturated fats improves blood cholesterol levels, which in turn decrease the risk of heart disease and may also help decrease the risk of type 2 diabetes.

**Polyunsaturated Fat:** This fat is found mostly in plant-based foods and oils. Omega-3 fatty acids, which is a polyunsaturated fat has been attributed to low rate of heart disease [22]. Also, it helps to raise HDL cholesterol level [23].

Oils such as canola oil, olive oil, corn oil, sunflower oil and peanut oil are made up of monounsaturated and polyunsaturated fats and are liquid at room temperature. Fish such as tuna, salmon, trout, mackerel, herring and sardines are high in omega-3 fatty acids. Plant sources of omega-3 fatty acids are soybean oil, flaxseed oil, and nuts (walnuts, butternuts).

### 3.2 Unhealthy fats

Saturated fats and trans fat are often termed unhealthy fats, this is due to the fact that both raise LDL cholesterol levels. High level of LDL cholesterol in the blood increases the risk of heart disease and stroke. A larger amount of saturated fats is from animal sources, including meat and dairy products. Foods high in saturated fat include fatty beef, pork, butter, lard and cream, poultry with skin. Plant-based oils, such as coconut oil, palm oil also contain saturated fats, but do not contain cholesterol.

Trans fat is a product of a process that adds hydrogen to liquid vegetable oils to make them more solid and also refer to as partially hydrogenated oils. These partially hydrogenated oils increase LDL cholesterol and lowers HDL cholesterol which in turn increase the risk of cardiovascular disease. Foods high in trans fat include fried foods, such as French fries, stick margarines and shortenings, pastries, packaged foods, baked goods and pizza dough.

Fatty foods are energy dense and give 9calories per gram compared to carbohydrate and protein that gives 4calories per gram. Also, if physical activity is inadequate, excess consumption of fat can results into weight gain. Also, it does not take as much energy (about 3%), to convert and store dietary fat as it does to convert and store glucose or protein. Fats are quickly and easily stored by the body.

Obesity is a multifactorial and complex affectation that is characterized by a long-term excess energy intake(EI) above energy expenditure (EE) and epidemiological evidence have suggested that a high-fat diet promotes the development of obesity [24].

There is also a direct relationship between the amount of dietary fat and the degree of obesity. An overview of animal studies had indicated that high-fat diets induce greater food intake and weight gain than high-carbohydrate diets [25]. Contributing factors are caloric density, satiety properties and post-absorptive processing. The satiating effects after meals with a high fat:carbohydrate ratio is less than for meals with a lower ratio. It has been reported that the most important variable influencing meal size is the nutrient content of the range of foods consumed and not the level of hunger. Thus dietary fat has a weak effect on satiety and periodic exposure to a high-fat meal, particularly when hunger is high, is sufficient enough to lead to overconsumption of energy as fat in obese patients.

### 3.3 Influence of dietary fat on weight gain

An important determinant of body fat is the percentage of dietary energy from fat. Several mechanisms have been proposed to explain why high fat intake might lead to greater body fat [26]. Dietary fat is the most energy dense macronutrient in the diet, providing 9 kcal/g as opposed to 4 kcal/g for carbohydrate or protein; this could lead to overconsumption of energy if food volume is regulated. Fat adds greater flavor and palatability to foods, which could thus increase their consumption.

Fat has a lower thermogenic effect than carbohydrate and protein and this inhibit energy expenditure. A positive energy balance can be the result of overconsumption of energy, perhaps because a high-fat diet has a lower satiating effect per joule than a low-fat diet. A series of studies has produced robust evidence that the fattening effect of dietary fat is linked mainly to the higher energy density of fatty foods compared with carbohydrate and protein rich foods.

In addition, when studied under careful metabolic conditions for short periods, carbohydrate produces a greater thermogenic effect than fat, suggesting that dietary fat may be utilized more efficiently and accumulate as body fat [27]. Carbohydrate intake, but not fat intake, is regulated; thus, individuals on a high-fat diet would tend to consume more total energy to gain the required amount of carbohydrate than would someone on a low-fat diet [28]. Although these mechanisms may seem compelling at face value, foods are not eaten in isolation, and the energy for weight of foods is more determined by the water and fiber content.

Different types of fat contain the same amount of energy, although there are differences in their respective influence on energy balance, energy expenditure and satiety. Low-fat diets and in weight-maintenance diets, have been shown to be affected by the quality of dietary fat. Animal studies have shown that rats fed a diet rich in safflower oil polyunsaturated fats accumulate less body fat than rats fed a diet rich in beef tallow which is a saturated fat [29].

Monounsaturated was found to induce a lower level of postingestive satiety and a larger subsequent energy intake than polyunsaturated and saturated fat in a study on the effect in lean subjects of high-fat meals, differing in fatty acid composition [30].

## 4. Dietary patterns and obesity

Dietary patterns that have inverse relationship with obesity include vegan diet, Mediterranean diet and prudent diet. Western diet is directly associated with obesity.

### 4.1 The vegan diet

This is a form of vegetarian diet that eliminates meat and animal product, this diet is beneficial to health because it reduces the intake of cholesterol and saturated fat that is predominant in animal product. It has been proven that those who practice a vegan diet minimize their overall risk of coronary heart disease, obesity and high blood pressure.

### 4.2 The Mediterranean diet

This diet recommends the use of plant based oil as alternative to butter, it emphasizes adding vegetables to each meal. Avoidance of meat is recommended, though not eliminated. This diet has been proven to help with depression, in addition to controlling blood sugar levels and helping with weight loss. Whole grains, nuts and herbs are also used in larger amounts.

### 4.3 Prudent diet

This diet protects against heart disease, stroke, and other common diseases. It consists of fruits, vegetables, whole grains, legumes, nuts, fish, and low-fat dairy products rather than refined or processed foods, red meats, high concentrated sweets, eggs, and butter.

### 4.4 Western diet

This diet is characterized by high intake of processed food, red meat, high-sugar foods and pre-packaged foods, that increase the risk of chronic illness. Eating junk foods, which are part of the western diet, could impair the part of the brain tied to self-control, in turn result to overeating and weight gain.

## 5. Dietay management of obesity

Recommendations for weight management emphasize the importance of healthy eating patterns which include consumption of nutrient-dense foods, limiting portion size of energy-dense foods, and reduce overall energy density. A unifying factor for weight loss across dietary patterns is energy density, when a diet's energy density is reduced; individuals consume satisfying amounts of food for fewer calories. The goal of dietary therapy is to reduce the total number of calories consumed.

The optimal diet for prevention of weight gain, obesity, metabolic syndrome, and type 2 diabetes is fat-reduced, fiber-rich and high in low-energy density carbohydrates (fruit, vegetables, and whole grain products). The Mediterranean eating pattern that emphasizes intake of low-energy dense fruits, vegetables, legumes, seafood, and dairy foods has proved effective in the management of obesity. However, higher amounts of fat (30–40% of total energy), especially from olive oil, are recommended with the Mediterranean diet. Even with this level of healthy fats, the Mediterranean diet recommends high proportion of fruit and vegetable which can help to keep the overall diet relatively low in energy density.

It has been established that different types of carbohydrate have varying effects on metabolism and health. Some carbohydrates are healthier than others; those with lower glycemic indexes (or GI) have a slower and flatter blood glucose response. They take longer to digest and can help us feel full thus preventing overeating and weight gain. Lower GI foods are less refined (or processed) such as whole grains, legumes, fruit, and vegetable. High GI foods are refined carbohydrate and contribute to weight gain.

Many high-carbohydrate foods common to Western diets produce a high glycemic response, promoting postprandial carbohydrate oxidation at the expense of fat oxidation, thus altering fuel partitioning in a way that may be conducive to body fat gain [31].

### 5.1 Daily intake patterns that can help to lower dietary energy density

**Breakfast**: The pattern of food consumption over a day as either meals or snacks could affect weight management. Epidemiological studies have also found breakfast consumption to be associated with lower body weights and lower daily energy density. If individuals consume breakfast daily, including higher amounts of protein and fiber during breakfast may help increase satiety, decrease energy intake, and lower dietary energy density.

**Snacking**: Snacks are often refers to processed, high-calorie items like chips and cookies. Snacking refers to the consumption of foods and beverages between regular meals, regardless of whether the food is healthy [32]. Many a times people consume snacks when appetizing food is available; even though they are not hungry. Snacking in the absence of hunger leads to the consumption of fat, sugar, and sodium-rich foods [33]. Unnecessary snacking promotes "weight gain and poor nutrition" [33].

If snacks should be consumed, it should be chosen wisely; high energy-dense snacks, nutrient-poor snacks (such as chips, cookies, confectionary) may be associated with high BMI should be limited [32]. However, lower – energy dense snacks (such as fruit and vegetable) which enhance satiety and improves diet quality should be consumed in large amount.

### 5.2 Manage fat to lower energy density and moderate energy intake

Evidence from multiple clinical trials shows that both low- and moderate-fat diets combined with an energy restriction can be used to achieve weight loss. High-fat foods are energy dense, low-fat diet is therefore recommended for weight loss. Also, there is need for moderation of portion size to stay within recommended energy intakes. Methods for moderating fat intake include switching to lower-fat alternatives such as grilled chicken instead of fried chicken or low-fat Greek yogurt instead of sour cream. Also, the amount of solid fats, which contain saturated and trans fat should decrease, and to substitute with oils containing polyunsaturated and monounsaturated fats to improve diet quality and overall health.

### 5.3 Add more protein and fiber to meals

Protein and fiber have been suggested to promote satiety or feelings of fullness. The most satiating macronutrient is protein, incorporating more protein in the diet may increase satiety and decrease daily energy intake. Patients should be encouraged to incorporate recommended amounts of lean protein sources such as grilled chicken breast, legumes, or low-fat dairy to create satisfying low-energy-dense meals. Dietary fiber is thought to promote feelings of fullness by increasing chewing time, promoting stomach expansion, and decreasing absorption efficiency. Studies show that increasing fiber at meals can lead to decreased energy intake and increased ratings of fullness. Also, diets containing higher amounts of fiber are associated with lower body weights and reduced disease risks.

## 6. Conclusion

Dietary fat induces overconsumption and weight gain through its low satiety properties and high caloric density. Obese and post-obese subjects do not appear to adapt to dietary fat, and therefore fat storage is increased. Both total fat and individual fatty acids have to be considered when reaching conclusions about dietary fat and obesity. The optimal diet for prevention of weight gain, obesity, metabolic syndrome, and type 2 diabetes is fat-reduced, fiber-rich and high in low-energy density carbohydrates (fruit, vegetables, and whole grain products).

## Conflict of interest

The authors declare no conflict of interest.

## Author details

Olariike Oyindasola Kayode
Adeleke University, Ede, Nigeria

*Address all correspondence to: okeyoyinolariike@yahoo.com;
okeyoyin.olariike@adelekeuniversity.edu.ng

## References

[1] Kopelman, P. (2007). Health risks associated with overweight and obesity. Obesity Reviews 8, 13 –17.

[2] Centre for Disease Control and Prevention (2020). COVID - 19: Obesity and Excess Weight Increase Severe Illness Risk; Racial and Ethnic Disparities Persist

[3] Danielsen K.K., Svendsen M., Mæhlum S., Sundgot-Borgen J. (2013). Changes in body composition, cardiovascular disease risk factors, and eating behavior after an intensive lifestyle intervention with high volume of physical activity in severely obese subjects: A prospective clinical controlled trial. J Obes. 325464. PUBMED | CROSSREF

[4] Popkin B.M. (2001). The nutrition transition and obesity in the developing world. Journal of Nutrition; 131(3): 871S–873S.

[5] Troesch B., Biesalski H.K., Bos R., Buskens E., Calder P.C., Saris W.H., et al. (2015). Increased intake of foods with high nutrient density can help to break the intergenerational cycle of malnutrition and obesity. Nutrients. 7(7):6016

[6] Rolls BJ, Hammer VA. Fat, carbo-hydrate, and the regulation of energy intake. Am J Clin Nutr 1995;62(5 suppl):1086S– 1095S

[7] Sanders T.A. (2001). Olive oil and the Mediterranean diet. Int J Vitam Nutr Res. 71(3):179-184.

[8] Flynn G., Colquhoun D. (2004). Mediterranean diet improves lipid profiles over three months. Asia Pac J Clin.Nutr. 13(Suppl):S 138.

[9] Katsilambros N. (2004). Clinical Nutrition. Beta Publishers. Athens.

[10] U.S. Department of Health and Human Services and U.S. Department of Agriculture. 2015-2020 Dietary guidelines for Americans. 8thAvailable at http://health.gov/dietaryguidelines/2015/guidelines/. Published December 2015. Accessed February 11, 2017

[11] Smethers AD and Rolls BJ (2018). Dietary Management of Obesity: Cornerstones of healthy eating patterns med. Clin north Am.102(1):107-124 DOI: 10.1016/j.mcna.2017.08.009

[12] Chin J.H., Chang K.J. (2005). College student's attitude toward body weight control, health-related lifestyle and dietary behavior by self-perception on body image and obesity index. J Korean Soc food Sci Nutr;34:1559-65. CROSSREF

[13] Otemuyiwa I.O., Adewusi S.R. (2012). Food choice and meal consumption pattern among undergraduate students in two universities in southwestern Nigeria. Nutr Health. 21(4):233-245. https://doi.org/10.1177/0260106013510994

[14] Alfaris N.A., Al-Tamimi J.Z., Al-Jobair M.O., Al-Shwaiyat N.M., (2015). Trends of fast food consumption among adolescent and young adult Saudi girls living in Riyadh. Food Nutr Res. 59:26488. http://dx.doi.org/10.3402/fnr.v59.26488 PMID:25792229

[15] Binish K., Sukhsohale, N. D., Khamgaonkar, M.B. (2015). Nutritional status and dietary pattern of under-graduate medical students of Central India Sch. J. App. Med. Sci., 3(1A): 49-52.

[16] Kadouh H.C., Acosta A. (2017). Current paradigms in the etiology of obesity. Techniq Gastrointestinal Endoscopy 19:2 11.

[17] Kayode, O.O., Quadri K. Alabi (2020). Food consumption patterns, physical activity and overweight and

obesity among undergraduates of a private university in Nigeria. Clinical nutrition experimental. https://doi.org/10.1016/j.yclnex.2020.01.001

[18] Chopra S.M., Misra, A., Gulati S., Gupta R. (2013) Overweight, obesity and related non-communicable diseases in Asian Indian girls and women. European journal of clinical nutrition volume 67, pages688-696

[19] Leinum C.J., Dopp J.M., Morgan B.J., (2009). Sleep-disordered breathing and obesity: Pathophysiology, complications, and treatment. Nutr Clin Pract.24(6): 675-687

[20] Hooper L., Martin N., Abdelhamid A., Davey Smith G. (2015). Reduction in saturated fat intake for cardiovascular disease. Cochrane database Syst rev. 10:Cd011737.

[21] FAO/WHO (2010). Summary of Conclusions and Dietary Recommendations on Total Fat and Fatty Acids in Fats and Fatty Acids in Human Nutrition—Report of an Expert Consultation. Geneva: FAO/WHO.

[22] Alexander Leaf (2008). Historical overview of n-3 fatty acids and coronary heart disease Am J Clin Nutri. 87(6): 1978S-1980S. doi: 10.1093/ajcn/87.6.1978S

[23] Bernstein A. M., Ding, E.L., Willett, W.C., Rimm, E.B (2012). A meta-analysis shows that docosahexaenoic acid from algal oil reduces serum triglycerides and increases HDL-cholesterol and LDL-cholesterol in persons without coronary heart disease.

[24] Doucet E. and Tremblay A. (1997). Food intake, energy balance and body weight control Eur J Clin Nutr. 51(12): 846-855. doi: 10.1038/sj.ejcn.1600497

[25] Golay A. and Bobbioni E. (1997) The role of dietary fat in obesity. Int J Obes Relat Metab Disord. Jun; 21 Suppl 3: S2 – 11.

[26] Gershoff S.N. (1995). Nutrition evaluation of dietary fat substitutes. Nutr Rev;53: 305 – 313.

[27] Astrup A. (1993). Dietary composition, substrate balances and body fat in subjects with a predisposition to obesity. Int J Obes 1993; 17(Suppl 3): S32 – S36.

[28] Flatt J.P. (1985). Energetics of intermediary metabolism. In: Garrow JS, Halliday D, eds. Substrate and Energy Metabolism in Man. London: John Libbey; 1985. p. 58 – 69.

[29] Shimomura Y, Tamura T, Suzuki M. (1990). Less body fat accumulation in rats fed a safflower oil diet than in rats fed a beef tallow diet. J Nutr. 120:1291-1296

[30] Lawton C.L., Delargy H.J., Brockman J. (2000). The degree of saturation of fatty acids influences post-ingestive satiety. Br J Nutr 83: 473-482

[31] Brand-Miller, J.C., Holt, S.H., Pawlak, D.B., McMillan J.(2002). Glycemic index and obesity m J Clin Nutr. 76(1):281S-285S. doi: 10.1093/ajcn/76/1.281S.

[32] Hess J.M., Jonnalagadda S.S., Slavin, J.L. (2016). What is a snack, why do we snack, and how can we choose better snacks? A review of the definitions of snacking, motivations to snack, contributions to dietary intake, and recommendations for improvement. Advances in nutrition. 7(3):466-475. doi: 10.3945/an.115.009571.

[33] Bellisle F.(2014). Meals and snacking, diet quality and energy balance. Physiol Behav 134:38-43.

Chapter 14

# The Outcome of Eating Disorders: Relapse, Childbirth, Postnatal Depression, Family Support

*Mariko Makino, Mitsuo Yasushi*
*and Masahiro Hashizume*

## Abstract

This study was aimed to identify eating disorder (ED) relapse, childbirth, postnatal depression,and the family support. Of the ED patients during treatment from 1994 to 2004,55 were pregnant and had ED recovery. Of them, 25 (21 Bulimia Nervosa (BN)and 4 Anorexia Nervosa (AN)) agreed to take part in this study. We interviewed them every 2 wk. both during the pregnancy and after childbirth. We also interviewed family members each month. The Eating Attitudes Test-26 (EAT-26) and Edinburgh Postnatal Depression Scale (EPDS) were helpful for diagnosing the EDs and postnatal depression. As the statistical analysis, We conducted t-test.67%relapsed ED while pregnant and 50%relapsed postnatal. In the non-relapse group, all the subjects had vaginal delivery and their infants were male. 50% of the subjects had postnatal depression. Non-Postnatal depression group had average body- weight infants. With regard to family support, there was no relationship between ED relapse and postnatal depression. We found that the rate of ED relapse and that of suffering from postnatal depression were remarkable in this group, suggesting the necessity for long-term follow-up for the EDs.

**Keywords:** eating disorders, pregnancy, relapse, postpartum depression

## 1. Introduction

Anorexia nervosa (AN) and Bulimia nervosa (BN), are characterized by clinical conditions in body shape and eating attitudes. The core feature of AN is cognitive abd affective disturbance in body image. For example, subjects with AN thought themselves as fat even when they are very thin. They deny the severe thinness to their body weight and have afear of weight gain together with a constant desire for thinness. Thus, they fail to maintain an adequate body weight and shape; girls and women with AN may experience amenorrhea.BN is always concern about their body weight and shape, leading to binging and self-vomiting [1–3]. Claydon et al. [4] concluded that higher risk for relapse of ED was a maternal period and it was a difficult time for EDs with mind and body. In addition, Nakai et al. [5] reported postnatal depression had a close relationship with EDs. One of the recent studies, Watson et al. [6] showed both mothers and their infants complications were detected during pregnancy and afterbirth.Ex-EDwomen may give birth to premature babies; infants born to these women's' infants may not have an appropriate weight. This study was designed to assess ED relapse rate during pregnancy and after childbirth as well as postnatal depression in women experienced complete remission from EDs. Moreover, we investigated the relationship between ED relapse and postnatal depression, and family support.

## 2. Methods

This study was conducted at the Makino Clinic. The ethical committee of the Makino Clinic approved this research (Approved 002). The study purpose and outline were explained to patients, and written informed consent acquired. We treated 1008 EDs at our outpatient clinic between 1994 and 2004. Of these patients, 55 patients experienced ED recovery, pregnancy, and childbirth. Of which, 21 BN and 4 AN agreed to partake in this study; However, we examined 24,because unfortunately, 1 patient experienced a miscarriage. These participants had long-term treatment for EDs. However, they acquired complete remission. We determined remission as 6-months symptoms -free condition. There were some reports for definition of recoveries. Symptoms-free status in the previous 90 d.by Levallious et al. [7] Bardone-Cone et al. [8] reported it as the absence of symptoms in the previous 3 mon, while Zerwas et al. [9] indicating the recovery by 1 y without no symptoms. We chosed a midpoint of these reports. The Diagnostic and Statistical Manual of Mental Disorders (American Psychiatric Association 2013) [2] does not precisely outline the criteria to consider ED in remission. In Japan, there were no particular determined symptoms used to define remission or recovery. Thus, we made to meet the contents for the including and excluding criteria of the patients and for diagnosing ED remission according to the literature [10, 11]. Then, we examined participants experienced the remission for 6 mon. The Japanese version of the Eating Attitudes Test-26 (EAT-26) made by Ujiie and Kono [12] was adopted for diagnosing of EDs. The Japanese version of the Edinburgh Depression Scale (JEPDS), a self-filled questionnaire, developed by Okano [13] was used as a reference to diagnose postnatal depression as well as the interview.

## 3. Contents of the including and excluding criteria and questions in detail

### 3.1 Inclusion and remission criteria

EAT26 $\leq 9$, healthy eating behavior, ability to do ordinary activities without difficulties, working for the members of the society to some extent, having no other psychotic disorders, having not irregular menstruation: For AN patients, normal menstruation,weight increase was not always necessary.

### 3.2 Exclusion criteria

EAT26 $\geq 9$, Complication suffering from other psychotic disorders, such as depression and addiction, serious dependency or obsession with food, preoccupation with thinness, afraid of being fat seriously, having irregular menstruation.

### 3.3 Interview questions during pregnancy and after delivery

We asked the patients if they had panic, depressed about being mother, always preoccupied with food, unsatisfied with their body weight and shape,and if they have an urge to binge or vomit. Using the structured interview according to DSM-4 [14]. Once a month, their husbands were also asked if their spouse had an abnormal eating attitudes or obsessive compulsive thinking for eating etc.

We interviewed the patients every 2 weeks both during gestation period and after birth.

### 3.4 Postnatal depression

We used the JEPDS. In JEPDS, Usually scored >12 were diagnosed as depression, though, we interviewed those who scored>9.because they could have postnatal depression [13].

### 3.5 Relapse group (TRED group)

In hyperemesis symptoms or pregnancy sickness, pregnant women experienced nausea overeating and vomiting. These symptoms were very similar to those of ED symptoms. However, if the patients were motivated to reduce their weight to become thinner these thoughts were dissimilar from those suffered from hyperemesis. Thus, we decided those who had vomit and binge and feelings above mentioned was given name as the relapse group. In our cases, their symptoms disappeared during pregnancy, they were given name as the temporary relapse group during pregnancy. (TRED group).TRED group recovered within 3 mon of pregnancy. Also non-relapse participants during pregnancy was given name as non-relapsing group (NRED group).

### 3.6 Statistical analyses

We conducted t-test to determine the statistical difference between means of two different groups.

We compared the results of the TRED group and NRED group while pregnant and postnatally. Moreover, we examined the results of the postnatal depression and the non-depression group for 3 months following childbirth. A p value of, $\leqq 0.05$ was considered significant, and a p value of $\leq 0.1$ was considered marginally significant.

## 4. Results

### 4.1 Patients characteristics

The characteristics of interviewed women who were recovering from EDs,assessed during their pregnancy and after childbirth are showed in **Table 1**. Sixteen patients (67%)had temporary ED relapse. We made the **Figure 1** to highlight these results clearly after **Table 1**.

We have previously reported that characteristics of women who have recovered from EDs in detail [1].

### 4.2 TRED group and NRED group

Sixteen (67%)showed temporary relapse within 3 mon of pregnancy. All the infants in the NRED group were male. With respect to ED relapse after childbirth,

| | |
|---|---|
| **Age at onset of diagnosis** | 16.6 (SD 3.3) |
| **Disease duration (years)** | 9.5 (SD 5.4) |
| **Age at remission(years)** | 26.1 (SD 5.3) |
| **Maternal age(years)** | 28.1 (SD 5.4) |
| **Temporary ED relapse during pregnancy (%)**<br>**Family support (husband)** | 16 (67%)<br>19(79%) |
| **Gestational age at delivery(week)** | 39 (SD 1.1) |
| **Complications (%)** | 17 (67%) |
| **Complications in the infants (%)** | 3 (13%) |
| **Vaginal delivery (%)** | 19 (79%) |
| **Infant weight(g)**<br>**Male infant(%)** | 2928 (SD 540)<br>67% |
| **ED relapse after delivery(%)** | 12 (50%) |
| **Postnatal depression (%)** | 12 (50%) |

**Table 1.**
*A summary of the characteristics of women who have recovered from EDs and who were interviewed during pregnancy and after childbirth. We made new tables different from previous report [1].*

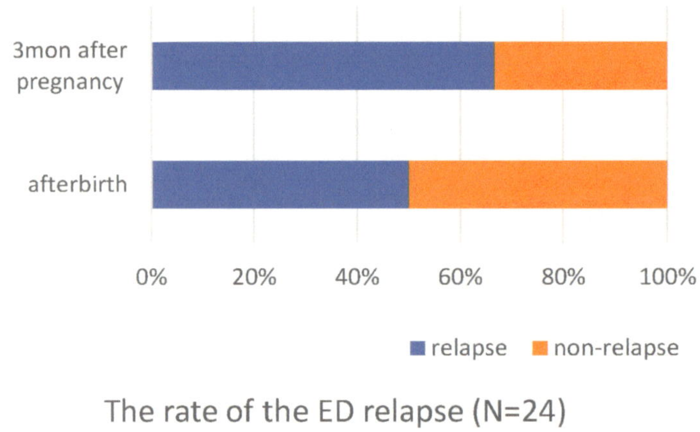


**Figure 1.**
*The rate of the ED relapse: patients with relapse after 3mon of delivery tended to relapse afterbirth.*

there was a significant difference between RED group and NRED group. **Figure 2** shows the comparison of these two groups. **Figure 3** shows the infant sex ratio afterbirth between two groups.

No statistical difference could be seen between RED group and NRED group with regard to family support (**Table 2**).

### 4.3 TRED group and NRED group were compared after childbirth

All NRED group had a vaginal delivery, and most of them gave birth to male infants. However, for the postpnatal depression rate, these two groups were the same. There was a significant difference between age at remission, and age at pregnancy ($P \leq 0.05$); further, difference for ED relapse during pregnancy reached statistical significance ($P \leq 0.05$) between these two groups (**Table 3**).

No significant difference could be seen between RED group and NRED group with respect to postnatal depression and family support.

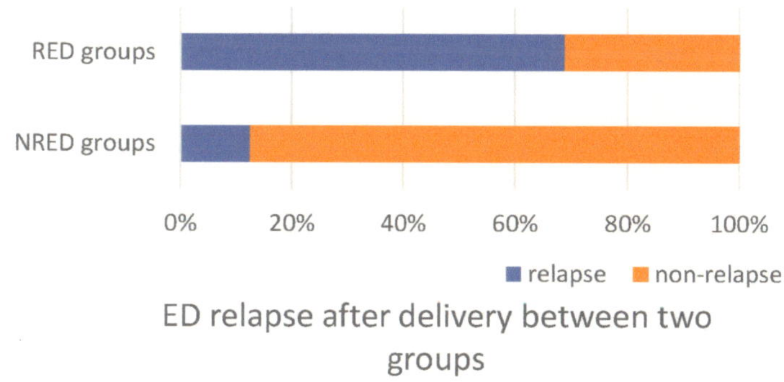


**Figure 2.**
*Showed ED relapse after delivery between two groups. (RED means NRED).*

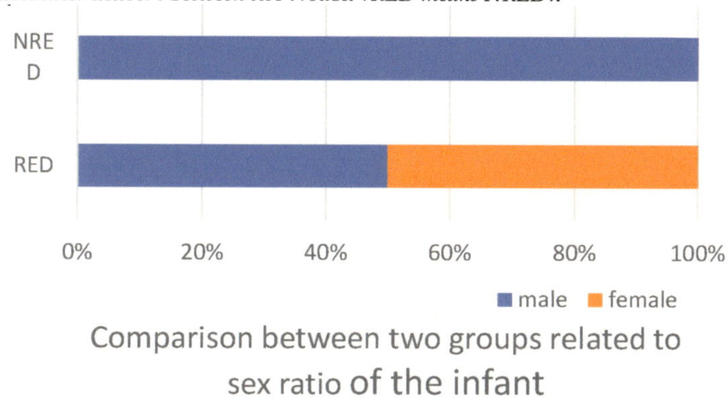


**Figure 3.**
*Showed the infant sex afterbirth between two groups.*

| | RED group (N = 16) | NRED group (N = 8) | |
|---|---|---|---|
| **Age at onset of diagnosis(years)** | 15.9(SD 1.2) | 18.0 (SD 5.4) | NS |
| **Disease duration(years)** | 9.1(SD 4.0) | 10.3(SD7.9) | NS |
| **Age at remission(years)** | 25.1(SD 4.4) | 28.3(SD 6.5) | NS |
| **age at pregnancy (years))** | 27.1(SD 5.0) | 30.1(SD5.8) | NS |
| **Gestational age at delivery(weeks)** | 38.3(SD1.3) | 39 (SD 0.5) | NS |
| **Maternal complications (%)** | 12(75%) | 6 (75%) | NS |
| **Problems in the infants (%)** | 6 (12.5%) | 1 (12.5%) | NS |
| **Vaginal delivery(%)** | 11(68.8%) | 8 (100%) | NS |
| **Infant weight(g)** | 2763 (SD 392) | 3259(SD664) | P < 0.1 |
| **Male infant(%)** | 50% | 100% | P < 0.05 |
| **Family support husband** | 13 (81,3%) | 6 (75%) | NS |
| **Postnatal depression (%)** | 10 (62.5%) | 2 (25%) | NS |
| **ED relapse after delivery (%)** | 11 (68.8%) | 1 (12.5%) | P < 0.05 |

**Table 2.**
*Characteristics of women with RED group and NRED group.*

### 4.4 A comparison between patients with postnatal depression and those who did not develop depression afterbirth

The infant body weight was found to be the only difference (**Table 4**).

| | TRED group (N = 12) | NRED group (N = 12) | |
|---|---|---|---|
| Age at onset of diagnosis (years) | 15.9 (SD 1.4) | 17.3 (SD4.4) | NS |
| Disease duration(years) | 7.5 (SD 3.0) | 11.5 (SD 6.6) | NS |
| Age at remission (Years) | 23.4 (SD 3.9) | 28.8 (SD 5.2) | P < 0.05 |
| Age at pregnancy (years) | 24.8 (SD 1.4) | 31.5 (SD 4.3) | P < 0.05 |
| Gestational age at delivery (weeks) | 38.3 (SD 1.4) | 38.8 (SD 0.7) | NS |
| ED relapse during pregnancy (%) | 11 (91.7%) | 5 (41.7%) | P < 0.05 |
| Family support husband | 11 (91.7%) | 8 (66,7%) | NS |
| Maternal Complications(%) | 9 (75%9 | 9 (75%) | NS |
| Problems in the infant(%) | 2 (12.5%) | 1 (12.5%) | NS |
| Vaginal delivery(%) | 7 (58.3%) | 12 (100%) | P < 0.1 |
| Infant weight(g) | 2813 (SD 446) | 3044 (SD 618) | NS |
| Postnatal depression | 6 (50%) | 6 (50%) | NS |

**Table 3.**
*Comparison between TRED group and NRED group after childbirth.*

| | Depression group(N = 12) | Non-depression group(N = 12) | |
|---|---|---|---|
| Age at onset of diagnosis(years) | 15.8(SD 0.8) | 17.4 (SD 4.5) | NS |
| Disease duration(years) | 10.4(SD 3.3) | 8.6 (SD 7.6) | NS |
| Age at remission(years) | 26.3(SD 3.4) | 26.0 (SD 6.9) | NS |
| Age at pregnancy(years) | 28.3 (SD 3.4) | 27.9 (SD 6.8) | NS |
| Gestational age at delivery (week) | 38.4 (SD 1.3) | 38.8 (SD 0.9) | NS |
| Temporary ED relapse during pregnancy (%) | 10 (83.3%) | 6 (50%) | NS |
| Family support husband | 9 (75%) | 10 (83.3%) | |
| Maternal complications (%) | 7 (58.3%) | 9 (75%) | NS |
| Problems in the infant (%) | 2 (16.7%) | 1 (8.3%) | NS |
| Vaginal delivery(%) | 11 (91.7%) | 8 (66.7%) | NS |
| Infant weight (g) | 2669 (SD 406) | 3188 (SD 544) | P < 0.1 |
| ED relapse after delivery (%) | 6 (50%) | 6 (50%) | NS |

**Table 4.**
*A comparison between postnatal depression and patients who did not develop depression following childbirth.*

## 4.5 Complications among mothers

Our research exhibited a variety of complications such as diabetes mellitus in 5 patients, anemia in 3, threatened miscarriage in 2, kidney stones in 2, nephrosis in 1, eclampsia in1, hypertension in 1, placenta previa in 1, miscarriage in 1, cesarean sections in 5, Although the sample size was small, We detected various complications.

### 4.6 Main summary of the results

#### *4.6.1 The relapse rate of EDs during pregnancy*

67% of the patients relapsed after delivery and of them were belong to RED group.

#### *4.6.2 Relapse of EDs afterbirth*

50% of the participants relapsed.

#### *4.6.3 What kind of the participants experienced relapse of EDs afterbirth*

The group relapsed during pregnancy (TRED group) tended to be relapsed afterbirth.

#### *4.6.4 Infants sex*

50%of the infants in the TRED group had male infants, while 100% of the infants in the NRED group were male.

#### *4.6.5 Postnatal depression*

50% of the participants had postnatal depression.

## 5. Discussions

We hypothesized that Ex-ED patients were vulnerable to relapse ED during body transition period such as pregnancy and giving birth. In addition, after birth, they tended to be anxious and depressed with their body image and weight, leading to have possibility to suffer from postnatal depression. Our results may supported our hypothesis.

Further we anticipated that family support played an important role in preventing relapse and postnatal depression. However, our result was not supported by our anticipation.

As per the literature, partners attitudes to EDs could help prevent ED relapse [15] and postpartum depression [16].

In our samples, all the supporters were partners and not mothers. Ikuno [17] reported there was problematic relationship between mother and daughter; daughter used her thinness as a weapon to draw her mother's attention, and involved her mother in her frustration. This is the problematic relationship of mother and daughter, that had not overcomed for a long time, as a result they hate each other. Owing to this problematic relation, mother might not support her daughter and daughter do not want to be supported by her mother.

We believed that the supporters for patients with EDs are very sensitive and some cases their behavior might worsen the symptoms of ED.

We investigated pregnant women recovered from EDs completely. Keel et al. [18] showed that among the patients who recovered from EDs, relapse rate was 36% in AN patients, and 35% in BN patients. Compared to these results, our rate of TRED group was 67%. Thus, Pregnancy was a crucial event for relapse for patients with ED. Our data showed that the TRED group improved within the first 3mon of pregnancy.

We found the in spite of the relapse, mothers and infants complications were not different compared to NRED group.

Nevertheless, the prevalence of postnatal depression was lower and the infant body weight was greater in the NRED group. Following childbirth, we found that the rate of postnatal depression and complications were similar in the RED and the NRED group. Further, we showed that the infants belonging to the postnatal depression group had a lower body weight than those in the non-depression group.

Angela [19] showed that patients with ex-EDs commonly experienced relapse;in AN 36%, in BN 35%, the figure was similar to that reported by Keel et at al [18]. Hetman et al. [20] showed that ED patients experienced relapse when they go to start to school or to go to college, or to start a new job, to be pregnant, and to have a baby.

Our data (67% of the patients relapsed during pregnancy and 50% of the patients relapsed ED after childbirth.) showed that pregnancy and childbirth represented the transition period for EDs, and postnatal term. Patients had been treated from the time of diagnosis up until the time of giving birth and postnatal period. We treated them twice a month, and we taught them how to coping with their eating attitudes and negative feelings.

A study out of Kelty Mental Health Center in British Columbia, Canada. [21] suggested that ED relapse could be averted by encouraging a support system for EDs, such as teaching them how to eat healthier,and control their unstable feelings. The Authority also taught EDs how to cope with their negative influences; to identify disease triggers, to create personal coping strategies, and to eat meals regularly. Our attitudes to them was that we encouraged them continuously to change their eating attitudes promoting self-control and encouraging the development of healthy relationships with the others, particularly their spouses and close family members. Our strategy may be equivalent to that of Kelty. Therefore, that we should followed -up the ED patients for a long term was the one of the strategies to prevent ED relapse. We think this is also appropriate even for pregnant women with EDs.

Hetman et al. [20] stated that pregnancy was risk factor for ED relapse. Especially AN patients wanted to be thinner seriously, leading to reducing their food, tended have a higher risk of relapse even when they are pregnant, regardless of their desire to be pregnant. They did not want to eat an adequate amount of food. In a similar way, Mancini [22] stated that it was usual that even pregnant healthy women had body image dissatisfaction. Our results suggested that having a prior history of an EDs with body image unsatisfaction was serious risk factors for relapsing for EDs.

Our patients had many complications during gestation. In EKeus et al. [23], it was reported that BN women experienced an increased risk of miscarriage. Similarly, our findings demonstrated that a woman who had a history of BN experienced a miscarriage. In Koubaa et al. [24], they reported that the fetus among AN mothers grew less efficiently in the intrauterine environment, leading to lower body weight infants. The Japanese Nikkei Health [25] describes that an average infants' body weight in Japan, where a male infants' average weight should be 2980 g and a female infants' weight should be 2910 g. Our findings showed an average body weight of 2928 ± 540 g infants, which was comparable to Nikkei Health Report.

However, our RED group regained during the first 3 months of gestation. The mechanism for this change remains unclear. The body weight of infants in the RED group was lower than that infants weight in the NRED group. Nevertheless, the final body weight of infants measured in this study was similar to the average body infant weight in Japan. Thus, the first 3 mon of pregnancy may not be important for the infant growth. Middle ages patients, such as hypertension, the presence of coronary heart disease, and non- insulin-dependent diabetes mellitus can be caused by intrauterine growth restriction, leading to lower birth weight [26]. Thus, low body weight infants should be followed -up for a long duration, which can be important to prove for Barker's hypothesis. Our data showed that all subjects in the NRED group gave birth to male infants. However, the underlying reason remains still unclear.

Franco et al. [27] showed that most women with active EDs had normal progress during gestation period, and the newborn babies were healthy. Our results are in line with those reported by Franco et al.; Further, the patients in our research did not have active EDs; thus their babies were more likely to be normal weight than those from mothers with active EDs.

Bennet et al. [28] demonstrated that in ED patients, half developed postnatal depression and the rate of postnatal depression among healthy women was about 13%. Our results agree with this report. Nasreen et al. also [29] reported that low birth weight infants was strongly related to postnatal depression. Moreover, our results demonstrated that following birth infants in whose mothers' developed depression, had a decreased infant body weight, when compared to those whose mothers did not develop depression. Our results supported Bennet and Narsreen.

Because of the small sample size, we did not reached the result that BN patients had a higher chance for developing postnatal depression. Nevertheless, since about half of BN patients developed postnatal depression, BN has possibility to increase the risk of having postnatal depression. Moreover, within the AN patients group, 75% of the patients developed postnatal depression. However, the underlying reason remains unclear. Mazzeo et al. [30] demonstrated that patients with a history of EDs were at increased risk of relapse during gestation period, which lead to an increased incidence of postnatal depression and anxiety. Chan et al. [31] demonstrated that a higher level of disordered eating during pregnancy was related to an increased incidence of postnatal depression. However, in contrast, our findings did not demonstrate a higher rate of postnatal depression in RED group compared to the NRED group. Therefore, when considering pregnant women who have a history of ED, there may be a higher risk of postnatal depression and long-term follow-up should be considered. In the current study, we demonstrate that approximately half of the patients with pre-existing EDs relapsed within 1 y of delivery. Morgan et al. [32] reported that among mothers with pre-existing EDs 66% of experienced binging and vomiting after childbirth. However, we do not have detect the patients' types precisely about the type of EDs relapse experienced after childbirth. Thus, we are not able to confirm the findings of Morgan. Patients were seen in our outpatient clinic every 2 wk. and we counseled them about the management of their stress coping and anxiety etc., that might helped EDs to prevent relapse.

There are some limitations of this study. Sample size was smaller. An increase in the sample size would have strengthened the statistical power of our study and made us to compare between groups with EDs. Our findings supported our hypothesis that suggested that women with pre-existing EDs were vulnerable to relapse during pregnancy and after childbirth as well as suffering from postnatal depression. Another limitation was that we included only women with AN and BN. Our samples were limited to the following two groups: women with AN and women with BN. As such other subtypes of EDs such as binge eating disorder etc. were not included, and should be examined to verify our results. The most important limitation in our current study was the lack of a control that included healthy women, who did not have any EDs.

In order to anticipate the risk of postnatal depression, we need to consider various questions, including the patients' social support system, and their feeling of becoming a mother and how they perceive their body shape and weight, because Chan et al. [31] demonstrated a relationship between postnatal anxiety, irritability, and depressive symptoms for 6 mon afterbirth had a serious relationship with body dissatisfaction, leading to postnatal depression.

## 6. Conclusions

The findings from our long-term follow-up for EDs as well as our previous research [1] suggest that despite our small sample size, 67% of the patients relapse after childbirth, and they relapsed within the 3mon of the pregnancy. The rate of the postnatal depression was higher compared to healthy women. There was no relation between ED patients and their husband with regard to family support. Thus the long-term follow-up for the patients with EDs were very important.

## Acknowledgements

The authors would like to thank enago (www.enago.jp)for the English language review.

I wish to express my sincere thanks to:

Professor Sueharu Tsutsui for encouraging my study. Supervision of the research and for providing the opportunity to work with Makino Clinic.

Mr. Mitsuo Yasushi of Chu-o University, for providing on statistical analysis.

## Conflict of interest

The authors declare no conflict of interest.

## Ethics approval and consent to participate

Makino Clinic Ethics Committee approved this study (No. 002).

## Consent for publications

The patients provided written informed consent to participate in this study.

## Competing interests

The authors declare that they have no competing interests.

## Availability of data and materials

All data generated or analyzed during this study are included in this published article.

## List of abbreviations

| | |
|---|---|
| AN | Anorexia nervosa |
| BN | Bulimia nervosa |
| DM | Diabetes Mellitus |
| EAT | Eating Attitudes Test |
| ED | Eating disorders |
| EPDS | Edinburgh postnatal Depression Scale |

*DOI: http://dx.doi.org/10.5772/intechopen.95452*

## Author details

Mariko Makino[1*], Mitsuo Yasushi[2] and Masahiro Hashizume[1]

1 Toho-University, School of Psychosomatic Medicine, 1-16-6 Omorinishi, Ota-ku, Tokyo, Japan

2 Faculty of Science and Engineering, Chuo University, Tokyo, Japan

*Address all correspondence to: makimakimakimariko@gmail.com

## References

[1] Mariko M, MitsuoY, Sueharu Tsutsui: The risk of eating disorder relapse during pregnancy and after delivery and postpartum depression among women recovered from eating disorders. BMC Pregnancy and Childbirth 2020;20(323) https://bmcpregnancychildbirth.biomedcentral.com/articles/10.1186/s12884-020-03006-7#main-cntent

[2] American Psychiatric Association. Diagnostic and statistical manual of mental disorders: DSM-5. 5th ed. Arlington, VA: American Psychiatric Association;2013

[3] Strober M: Stressful life events associated with bulimia and anorexia nervosa. International Journal of Eating Disorders.1984;3:1-6.

[4] Claydon EA, Davidov DM, Zullg KJ, et al: Waking up everyday in a body that is not yours: a qualitative research inquiry into the intersection between eating disorders and pregnancy. BMC Pregnancy and Childbirth.2018;18:463.

[5] Nakai Y, Kazuo N, Shuichi N: Outcomes of eating disorders in Japan. Seishin Igaku.2004;46:481-486

[6] Watson HJ, Zerwas S, Torgersen L et al: Maternal eating disorders and perinatal outcomes: A three-generation study in the Norwegian Mother and Child Cohort Study. Journal of Abnormal Psychology.2017;126:552-564

[7] Levallius J, Clinton D, Backstrom M et al:Who do you think you are? Personality in eating disorder patients. Journal of Eating Disorders.2015;3:3

[8] Bardone-Cone AM, Hunt RA, Watson HJ: An overview of conceptualization of eating disorder recovery, recent findings, and future directions. Current Psychiatry Report. 2018;20:79

[9] Zerwas S, Lund BC, Von Holle et al: Factors associated with recovery from anorexia nervosa. Journal of Psychiatric Research. 2013; 47: 972-979

[10] Eddy KT, Tabri N, Thomas JJ et al: Recovery from anorexia nervosa and bulimia nervosa at 22-year follow-up. Journal of Clinical Psychiatry. 2017;78:184-189

[11] Tachikawa H: What is remission in eating disorders?. Seishinka. 2009;15:447-452

[12] Ujiie T, Kono M: Eating attitudes test in Japan. Japanese Journal of Psychiatry and Nuurology. 1994;48:557-565

[13] Okano T: Validation and reliability of a Japanese version of the EPDS. Psychiatric diagnosis and clinical evaluation. 1996;7:525-533

[14] American Psychiatric Association. Diagnostic and Statistical Manual of Mental Disorders:DSM-IVth ed.Arlington,VA:American Psychiatric Association;1994

[15] Koenig.KR: 6ways Eating disorders Can Affect Your(Romantic) Relationships.https://www.recoveryearriors.com/eating-disorders-can-affect-romantic-relationships.2016 August 18

[16] Pregnancy -related depression linked to eating disorders and abuse histories. http://www.med.unc.edu/www/newsarchive/2011/june/pregnancy-related-depression-linked-to-eating-disorders-and-abuse-histories

[17] Ikuno T:Eating disorders and Mother-Daughter relationships. jyoseigaku hyoron koubejyogakuin daigaku 2015;1-22

[18] Keel PK, Dorer DJ, Franco DL et al: Post -remission predictors of

relapse in women with eating disorders. American Journal of Psychiatry. 2005;162(12):2263-2268

[19] Angela D: Eating disorder relapse is common, A therapist's perspective. http://www. Eatingrecoverycenter. com/blog/November-2019/ eating-disorder-relapse.

[20] Hetman I, Klomek AB, Goldzweig G et al: Percentage from target weight predicts re-hospitalization in adolescent anorexia nervosa. Israel Journal of Psychiatry. 2017;54:28-34

[21] Provincial Health Services Authority, Kelty Mental Health(eating disorders)http://www. keltyeatingdisorders.ca/recovery/ relapse-prevention/

[22] Mancini K: Body image, eating attitudes and breastfeeding intention: implications for mental health and maternal child nurses. Issues Mental health Nursing.2017;38:750-7552

[23] EKeus C, Lindberg L, Lindberg F et al: A Birth outcomes and pregnancy complications in women with a history of anorexia nervosa. British Journal of Obstetrics and Gynecology.2006;105:255-260

[24] Koubaa S, Hallstrom T, Lindholm C et al: Pregnancy and neonatal outcomes in women with eating disorders. Obstetrics and Gynecology.2005;105:255-260

[25] Japanese Nikkei Health. http:// www.style.nikkei.com/article/ DGXMZO77271820Z10C14A9000000/ Accessed 12 OCT 2014

[26] Barker DJ: Fetal origins of coronary heart disease. British Medical Journal.1995; 311:171-174

[27] Franco DL, Blais MA, Becker AE et al: Pregnancy complications and neonatal outcomes in women with eating disorders. American Journal of Psychiatry.2001;158:1461-1466

[28] Bennet HA, Einarson A, Taddio A et al: Prevalence of depression during pregnancy : systematic review. Obstetrics and Gynecology.2004;103:698-709

[29] Nasreen HE, Kabir ZN, Forsell Y et al: Low birth weight offspring of women with depressive and anxiety symptoms during pregnancy:results from a population based study in Bangladesh. BMC Public Health. 2010;10:515

[30] Mazzeo SE, Slof'Op't Landt MC, Jones I et al: Associations among postpartum depression, eating disorders, and perfectionism in a population -based sample of adult women. International Journal of Eating Disorders.2006;39:202-211

[31] Chan CY, Lee AM, Koh YW et al: Course, risk factors, and adverse outcomes of disordered eating in pregnancy. International Journal of Eating Disorders. 2019;52:652-658

[32] Morgan JF,Lacey JH,Sedgwick PM: Impact of pregnancy on bulimia nervosa. British Journal of Psychiatry.1999,174.135-140